Psychiatry in Transition

Psychiatry in Transition

SECOND EDITION

Judd Marmor

With a new introduction by the author

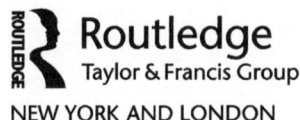

Routledge
Taylor & Francis Group

NEW YORK AND LONDON

Originally published in 1974 by Brunner/Mazel, Inc.

First published 1994 by Transaction Publishers

Published 2021 by Routledge
605 Third Avenue, New York, NY 10017
2 Park Square, Milton Park, Abingdon, Oxon OX14 4RN

Routledge is an imprint of the Taylor & Francis Group, an informa business

Library of Congress Catalog Number: 94-3844

Library of Congress Cataloging-in-Publication Data

Marmor, Judd.
    Psychiatry in transition   /   Judd Marmor, with a new introduction by the
author. — 2nd ed.
        p. cm.
    Includes bibliographical references and index.
    ISBN 1-56000-736-2
    1. Psychiatry. I. Title.
RC458.M26   1994
616.89—dc20   94-3844
                                                                 CIP

ISBN 13: 978-1-56000-736-4 (pbk)

TO **KATHERINE**

CONTENTS

INTRODUCTION TO THE TRANSACTION EDITION   ix

INTRODUCTION by Leon Eisenberg   xiii

PREFACE   xvii

PART I: GENERAL PSYCHIATRY

1. The Role of Instinct in Human Behavior   3
2. Toward an Integrative Conception of Mental Disorder (with E. Pumpian-Mindlin)   17
3. Some Observations on Superstition in Contemporary Life   30
4. The Individual, the Family and the Community   46
5. The Cancer Patient and His Family   61
6. The Crisis of Middle Age   71
7. "Normal" and "Deviant" Sexual Behavior   77

PART II: PSYCHOANALYSIS

8. The Theory and Practice of Psychoanalysis   93
9. Psychoanalysis and Dialectical Materialism   119
10. Some Considerations Concerning Orgasm in the Female   143
11. Orality in the Hysterical Personality   154
12. The Psychodynamics of Realistic Worry   169
13. Some Comments on Ego Psychology   180
14. Psychoanalysis and Psychiatric Practice   186
15. Psychoanalytic Therapy as an Educational Process   195
16. Psychoanalytic Therapy and Theories of Learning   210
17. Psychoanalysis at the Crossroads   226
18. Changing Patterns of Femininity: Psychoanalytic Implications   235
19. New Directions in Psychoanalytic Theory and Therapy   251
20. Limitations of Free Association   265

PART III: PSYCHOTHERAPY

21. The Feeling of Superiority: An Occupational Hazard in
    the Practice of Psychotherapy   279
22. The Doctor-Patient Relationship in Psychotherapy   291
23. The Nature of the Psychotherapeutic Process   296
24. Dynamic Psychotherapy and Behavior Therapy: Are They
    Irreconcilable?   310
25. Sexual Acting-Out in Psychotherapy   327
26. Changing Trends in Psychotherapy   336

PART IV: SOCIAL PSYCHIATRY

27. Psychodynamics of Group Opposition to Health
    Programs (with Bernard & Ottenberg)   355
28. The Psychology of Man in a Warless World   374
29. Nationalism, Internationalism, and Emotional Maturity   388
30. The Psychodynamics of Political Extremism   395
31. Some Psychosocial Aspects of Contemporary Urban
    Violence   406
32. Psychiatry and the Future of Man   416

33. Short-Term Dynamic Psychotherapy   433

ACKNOWLEDGMENTS   449

INDEX OF NAMES   452

INDEX OF SUBJECTS   457

INTRODUCTION TO THE
TRANSACTION EDITION

In the course of the twenty years since this volume was first published, there have been significant developments in psychiatry, but my basic premise, as outlined in my original introduction, namely that systems-theory thinking provides the best and most dependable foundation for understanding and treating disorders of human thought and behavior, still holds true and I am encouraged to believe therefore that the reissuance of these essays will be meaningful and useful to a new generation of readers.

In the area of general psychiatry, the most notable developments have revolved around the great expansion of our knowledge of brain chemistry which in turn has contributed richly to the development of more sophisticated psychopharmacological agents. Indeed some practitioners have been so encouraged by these developments as to envision a time when all clinical disorders will be curable by appropriate medication. Without minimizing the usefulness of pharmacotherapy in many aspects of psychiatric practice, I believe that those who subscribe to the above-mentioned hope are falling victim to a form of biological reductionism in which they are losing sight of the total bio-psycho-social nidus in which all psychopathology develops. Environmental events affect the way people think and feel; the way they think and feel results in complex reverberations within the neuro-humeral and immunological systems; these in turn have consequences for how they think, feel, and interact with other persons and with the adaptive demands of their life situations. An understanding of this constant dynamic back and forth interaction of all of these factors upon one another is essential not only with respect to "psychiatric" disorders, it is equally relevant to the total range of "psychosomatic" disorders as well as to purely "somatic" disorders.

ix

In the area of psychoanalysis, there continues to be a shift from the original focus on instinctual conflict and the Oedipus complex to an emphasis on pre-Oedipal developmental vicissitudes and object relationships. The work of John Bowlby on "Attachment Theory" and Daniel Stern on "The Interpersonal World of the Infant" have both greatly enriched the understanding of this process. Accompanying this shift has been the emergence of Kohutian self-psychology and a new appreciation of object-relations theory although both of these developments owe a greater debt than they acknowledge to the "ego-psychologists" of the fifties and sixties (Horney, Kardiner, Rado) and the interpersonal psychology of Harry Stack Sullivan.

As for the nature of the psychotherapeutic process, I believe the reader of the volume will find that the material in section III is as meaningful and relevant today as it was twenty years ago. All of the significant research on the nature of the psychotherapeutic process over the past score of years has simply served to reaffirm and strengthen the principles set forth in the third part of this volume. It has become increasingly apparent that it is not insight in and of itself, but the nature of the patient-therapist relationship that is critical in effecting psychotherapeutic change. This recognition has found expression in the growing literature on counter-transference, empathy in the psychotherapist, and "inter-subjectivity" between patient and therapist. One important development in the area of psychotherapy that reflects the changing social milieu, has been the growing interest in short-term techniques. Psychoanalysis and long-term psychotherapy are both expensive and time-consuming processes that the vast majority of people who need psychotherapeutic help cannot afford. With expanding sociocultural demands for more equitable health care delivery systems and the growing influence of third party payors, there has been and will undoubtedly continue to be increasing pressure on psychiatrists and psychotherapists to find ways of helping people that involve less time and consequently less cost. Because of the importance of this development, I have included an essay on the historical background and the basic principles involved in brief dynamic psychotherapy in a new article appended at the end of this volume.

Finally, in the area of social psychiatry the unprecedented break up of the Soviet Union and the end of the Cold War have dramatically changed the nature of many of the sociopolitical factors impinging upon the lives of individuals. At this writing, the shadow of nuclear war, hopefully, no longer hangs as heavily over humanity as it did twenty years ago. On the other hand, the rise of ethnic and nationalistic internecine killings all around the globe and the rising rate of urban violence, particularly in the United States but now beginning to show its face in other parts of the world too, make the chapters on nationalism, internationalism, political extremism, and urban violence unhappily more relevant than ever. The final chapter of the original volume, "Psychiatry and the Future of Man," still reflects my basic thinking about many of the problems that mankind faces. If I have changed my views in any respect over the past twenty years, it is that I am no longer as sanguine as I once was about the possibility of totally eliminating the aggression and violence in our society. Even though I still believe that it is *theoretically* possible, I have come to recognize how great the deeply ingrained institutional obstacles are. But I do *not* think that the so-called nature of man is one of those obstacles. On the contrary, it is only the extraordinary adaptive potential of the human brain, with its capacity to anticipate the future and construct models with which to deal with that future, that gives me any reason at all to hope that it is even within the realm of possibility to create a "higher synergy"society, to use Ruth Benedict's felicitous term (see chapter 32), in which the need for aggression and violence will become less relevant. But the history of the twentieth century thus far has demonstrated how difficult it is to overcome the powerful cultural lag that continues to make many people strive to aggrandize themselves at the expense of others, even in so-called socialist countries. Our extraordinary technological advances have made it possible for people to kill one another more efficiently than ever before, but they have not been equally applied to the solution of the problems of hunger, poverty, disease, overpopulation, and environmental spoliation that threaten our long-term existence on this planet.

Perhaps it is our fate ever since the development of civilization began to erode the primitive beauty of life on our rich little planet, to have been doomed, like Sisyphus, to strive eternally for a paradise that we can never fully achieve. But continue to strive we must. Even though aggression and violence can never be totally eliminated, it is

not beyond hope that with continued effort humankind can ultimately succeed in creating social institutions that will put a greater
premium on affiliative behavior than on aggressive behavior and to
which people can adapt themselves more constructively. That in the
words of the great Bard, would be a "consummation devoutly to be
wish'd"!

INTRODUCTION

Those readers familiar with some or most of Judd Marmor's writings will have in this volume a permanent resource for frequent consultation as they confront issues of theory and practice which his papers so admirably serve to clarify. Those who have known few or perhaps even none of them have an intellectual feast in store as they devour these pages, as surely they will, once they are introduced to the lucidity, the brilliance and the unfailing good common sense that characterize his work. He illumines many obscure areas both in the theory of psychiatry and in the clinical dilemmas provided by the very human problems of patients.

My acquaintance with his work began mid-way in my own career. I would have spared myself considerable blundering about had I known it sooner. The occasion of preparing this introduction provided an opportunity for reading his papers through from first to last, some of them old friends I recognized at once, some new friends I was delighted to make, though perturbed that I had failed to meet them when first they made their debut. I suppose few of us manage to keep up with the productivity of even our favorite authors; I excuse my own lack of assiduousness by the busy work that preempts time. Be that as it may, for me and for the rest of us, the appearance of this signal volume now offers in one place an impressive distillate of clinical acumen that cannot fail to make us the wiser for it.

One of the most remarkable qualities of Judd Marmor's writing is the extent to which it has survived the usages of time. All too often, one recalls a paper which had seemed profound when it first appeared because it was responsive to a topical issue, only to find it disappointingly trivial and evanescent when it is re-encountered five or ten years later. A few of the chapters in this book deal with peripheral matters or serve as ceremonial pieces. But the great majority have focused on problems no less central to contemporary psychiatry than they were when the papers first appeared. That I consider a rare tribute to their author. If it is true that the papers occasionally repeat points made in earlier articles (which one of us is not preoccupied with matters which we work over repetitively?), it is almost always with nuances and meanings that the author had not as fully appreciated in his first attempt to grapple with the issue. What *is* striking is the freshness, the breadth and the progression of ideas expressed in a series of papers not initially planned for a single volume and yet together making up an admirable vade mecum of dynamic psychiatry for both resident-in-training and clinician-in-practice.

No critical reader will be in agreement with all that he will find in these pages; even an admiring friend and colleague will acknowledge points of disagreement. It is true that certain of the concepts Freud set forth are now incorporated into the corpus of current psychiatric thought. Indeed, it would be an historical anachronism to judge Freud's social views of the early twentieth century in the light of contemporary sociology, anthropology and political ideology. Freud's position on many issues was well in advance of that of his contemporaries; he is not to be faulted for having failed to anticipate concepts and facts that it took further decades of work to bring into the forefront of our consciousness. However, I would be much less generous in my estimate of the overall impact of what arrogates to itself the term "dynamic psychiatry" on the development of our field. I do not see the wedding of academic psychiatry and psychoanalysis (Chapter 14) that Marmor anticipated (in 1961) as following from the further evolution of each. The rigid impress of orthodoxy (an orthodoxy, to be sure, that he has continually opposed) has nonetheless served to stifle the potential creativity of many of the younger adherents of psychoanalysis. The social impact of psychoanalytic training—its costs and the consequent deferred indebtedness of the student, its ad hominem characteristics which transmute the questioning of theory into matters of "unsuccessfully analyzed" negative transference, its very "completeness" which leads to premature intellectual closure and the stultifying of curiosity—has acted to turn away many of its followers from academic investigation and from the formulation of alternative hypotheses. It must be admitted that analytic training and member-ship in establishment societies have happily failed to act as a brake on the wide ranging application of a free intelligence by the author of this volume. Unhappily, there have been too few like him.

It is difficult to restrain the impulse to comment seriatim on each of his contributions. The reader is not—and should not be—interested in this essayist's opinions but rather will be eager to turn to the book itself. Perhaps I can be forgiven for singling out the several papers on instinct (Chapters 1, 2, 8, 9) as singularly perspicacious treatments of a biological theory no less controversial today than when they were written thirty years ago. Some of the experimental evidence employed to bolster the author's argument no longer holds as firmly as it appeared to then, but even stronger examples could be cited now to support a position that seems to me as valid as when it was first set forth. Indeed, the very same issues continue to occupy center stage. It is difficult to avoid the conclusion that neither evidence nor logic will settle this dispute in the near future; it rests upon value judgments which proponents of the one or the other position on instinct adhere to by force of personal convictions about the nature of the human condition. Here, Judd Marmor is on the side of the angels—in my opinion—and I salute him as one of those happy few willing to battle for the liberation of man's spirit.

In the end, no reader can fail to sense the compassion, the perceptiveness and the heterodoxy of these collected papers. Their author has a point of view, but people come before theories. He is acutely aware of the struggles, the contradictions and the unique-nesses of each of the troubled persons who seek his help. In respond-ing to their needs, he refuses to be bound by what ought to be so and insists upon recognizing what *is* so. To his work, he brings a richness of experience, a treasury of scholarship, a life committed to trying to be of help and humbled by an awareness of the limitations to even the best informed effort to meet that challenge. Add to this his clear and literate style of writing, and we have a volume to be read and reread.

A final personal note may not be inappropriate. Those who know me as a critic (some would say opponent) of psychoanalysis may find my contributing this introduction somewhat anomalous. I would argue that a critic can also be an appreciator and a conservator of what he deems worthwhile in a body of work with which he nonetheless takes issue. Sigmund Freud and that small band of adherents who recognized his genius and furthered the evolution of his doctrines contributed important ideas to the culture of this century. In the beginning, it took courage even to associate oneself with a movement that was broadly condemned and that promised little in the way of income or glory to those who joined it. There was simply no such thing as a tradition of psychiatry outside the asylum and little chance of supporting oneself from the practice of psychotherapy. It is perhaps for this reason that so many of that small and singular group made original contributions to its genesis—and indeed that so many split off with schools and ideas of their own because these were men of integrity and individuality. Once psychoanalysis had become the established doctrine, it attracted to itself the time-servers and the self-servers who, like a medieval guild, took upon themselves the role of official guardians of the revealed truth. In this latter era, the movers and the shakers now became the dissidents and the "splitters," bitterly criticized as heretics, courageous enough to question the received truth in the same spirit as the founding fathers who had in their time dared to challenge conventional wisdom. Judd Marmor is today a kindred spirit to those willing to face excommunication from the establishment in order to pursue truth wherever it might lead.

We are far today from a satisfactory general theory of human behavior. That theory, when it is evolved, will contain some of Freud's insights, others radically revised, and still other ideas yet only barely dreamt of. Among the contributors to its genesis will be Judd Marmor. He does me the honor in inviting me to present this brief prologue, not I him in the writing of it. Enough of introduction, on to the substance! It reads easily, it reads profoundly, and it invites rereading.

Leon Eisenberg, M.D.
Professor of Psychiatry
Harvard Medical School

PREFACE

The essays in this volume cover a span of almost 40 years of psychiatric and psychoanalytic practice; thus they reflect many of the changes that have taken place in my theoretical and clinical perspectives during this period. Nevertheless, I believe the reader will find certain themes weaving persistently through the material.

It has always been my firm conviction that both theory and practice should rest on a sound foundation of scientific thought. Where a theory fails to do so, one must be prepared to alter the theory. Where practice fails to do so and yet is pragmatically effective, one must continue to search for an explanation of the effectiveness that falls within scientifically verifiable boundaries. Psychiatry is a field in which there has always been a profusion of diverse approaches and claims; this has never been more true than it is now. Therapeutic results are promised (and indeed even sometimes achieved!) by methods as widely diverse as hypnosis, electroshock therapy, megavitamins, nude marathons, transcendental meditation, biofeedback, progressive muscular relaxation, tension-maximizing "implosion" techniques, massage therapy, pharmacotherapy, psychosurgery, psychoanalysis, and many others too numerous to list. If we are ever to find our way out of this confusing maze of claims and counterclaims, it will be only by clinging steadfastly to the compass of scientific thought and method. To abandon that is to run the danger of falling into the dark morass of magical and muddled thinking that characterized the Middle Ages.

An important factor in my own efforts at achieving some clarification of the confusion in our field has been my resistance from the beginning to the siren call of simplistic, unitary, or "linear" explanations of complex problems—to what Franz Alexander once characterized as "one of the greatest weaknesses of the human mind . . . the urge to find either/or solutions and to explain everything from one single principle . . .." Rather, I have always tended to think of causation in psychiatry in field-theoretical terms, as a resultant of the interaction of many variables. The contemporary term for this approach is systems theory, and I believe its ultimate implications for the understanding of human behavior are far-reaching. Within this frame of reference, the living human organism is seen as an open-system in which inner, self-activating mechanisms as well as constant feedback processes are involved in a continuous exchange of energy and information with the outer world. Interpersonal relationships, too, are organized in a variety of systems, from the earliest child-mother system, to that of the family, to others ranging in size from small social groups to the largest which we call civilizations. Every person from the beginning of his emergence into the world is enmeshed in a series of dynamic interactions with his environment and with other people all of whose inner processes and perceptions have been shaped and altered by their interactions with a wide variety of systems also. Only an appreciation of all of these interactions can give us a true insight into the complex sources of human thought and behavior. Within this context it should not be surprising to find that individual reactions can be modified by many different approaches—from those that alter our biochemistry, to those that change our intrapsychic perceptions and values, to those dealing with family relationships, to others that focus on community programs, and finally to those whose goal is modification of the large outer system comprising our basic social and cultural institutions.

Another continuing theme in this volume is the search for common denominators underlying the numerous divergent views that characterize our field. In retrospect it may have been my good fortune to have received my psychoanalytic training at the hub of the stormy ideological conflicts that shook the foundations of the American psychoanalytic movement during the nineteen-thirties. As a student at the New York Psychoanalytic Institute during those exciting years, I was exposed to the germinal ideas of people like Karen Horney, Clara Thompson, Abram Kardiner, and Sandor Rado, while also receiving a thorough grounding in classical Freudian theory from outstanding teachers like A. A. Brill, Bertram Lewin, Lawrence Kubie, Herman Nunberg, and Gregory Zilboorg. Thus, early in my professional life I was able to acquire a historical perspective about psychoanalysis as a discipline in the process of development and change, rather than as a fixed and immutable one.

At the same time I could not help noting that, despite the fact that these various leaders held sharply divergent views, each had his or her devoted camp followers and grateful patients. However, a long-standing aversion to idol-worship prevented me from becoming anyone's "disciple"; thus I was preserved from developing the kind of blind emotional commitment to any one particular school of thought that might have compelled me to reject modifications in my theoretical views or therapeutic techniques as my knowledge and experience broadened with time. Indeed, if I can take any credit as a psychiatrist who has lived and worked in the midst of the profound changes that have taken place in our field over the past four decades, it is that I have tried to keep an open mind to new currents of thought and have not been afraid to modify either my theories or my practices in the light of new developments. The history of ideas has shown too well how frequently hallowed hypotheses become transformed into rigid dogmas which with the passage of time are ultimately reduced to myths or at best to only half-truths. One of my favorite James Thurber fables highlights this point. It is about the barnyard rooster who found a gilded goose egg, and insisted, despite the skepticism of the hens, that it would eventually hatch into a golden goose of priceless value. So he stubbornly sat on it, while all of his former friends gradually drifted away. Finally one day the egg broke, and that was the end of his dream. Thurber's moral, which is as applicable to the field of psychiatry as it is to all of science, is that it is wiser to be hendubious than cocksure!

Still another persistent motif has been a search for common denominators underlying the numerous divergent views that characterize psychiatric thought and practice. Some of the differences are essentially semantic in nature, but others seem to be based on a failure to encompass all the variables that play a role in shaping human development. Like the blind men of the fable, some schools of thought are dealing with only a part of the "elephant," and each insists on the validity of its description to the exclusion of the others. Thus the biologically-oriented psychiatrist seeks to explain

human behavior primarily on biological determinants, the psychoanalyst bases his explanations primarily on intrapsychic factors, and
the social psychiatrist rests his on essentially cultural grounds. Clearly,
any comprehensive explanation of human behavior must encompass
all of these vectors, not in sum, but in dynamic interaction with
one another.

Perhaps as pervasive as anything else in these essays is a concern
with betterment of the human predicament. Although this is most
obvious in the social issues section of this volume, it can be found
in almost every essay, beginning with the very first. This preoccupation may, of course, be part of the complex motivational pattern
that so often shapes an interest in psychiatry in the first place,
but in my case it also stems from a background deeply steeped
in a concern for social justice.

The essays in the volume have fallen rather naturally into four
major groupings, with the essays in each section arranged in the
order in which they were written. The first group contains articles
of general psychiatric interest. The second section deals with psychoanalytically oriented subjects and reflects the evolution of my psychoanalytic views over the years. The third section has to do with my
deep and continuing interest in the nature of the psychotherapeutic
process and some of the evolving new techniques of psychotherapy.
The fourth and final section reflects my increasing concern in recent
years with some of the broad social issues confronting our contemporary civilization.

These, then, are some of the major themes with which I have
struggled in the course of a crowded psychiatric career. If the
sampling of the ideas that are encompassed within these pages gives
the reader some awareness of the challenges and gratifications
involved in this struggle, I shall feel amply rewarded.

JUDD MARMOR

February, 1973

ACKNOWLEDGMENT

It would be impossible for me to do justice to all the people—teachers, colleagues, friends and patients—who, in one way or another, have contributed to the shaping of the ideas expressed in these pages. No body of work is ever the production of one man alone. We always build on the foundation provided for us by the influence, not only of those who have gone before us, but also of all those persons with whom we have interacted significantly in the course of our lives.

I want to give special thanks to my friend, Dr. Gene L. Usdin, for certain editorial suggestions and to my Executive Assistant, Mrs. Leona H. Light, for invaluable assistance in preparing the manuscript for publication. I am most appreciative to the various journals and publishing houses which granted permission to reprint many of the essays in this volume. The specific acknowledgments are separately listed on pages 449–451.

Part 1

GENERAL PSYCHIATRY

1

THE ROLE OF INSTINCT IN HUMAN BEHAVIOR

(1942)

The concept of "instinct" has probably been more subject to misuse and confusion than any other in modern psychological thought. This term has been used to cover so many divergent conceptions that discussion seems difficult unless it can first be agreed that the general or popular notion of it—as any seemingly automatic activity or habitual inclination—should be eliminated. Consider the description of a person as being instinctively kind or orderly, having an instinctive liking or distrust for someone, or having instinctive beliefs. It is clear that such employment of this concept does not fulfill the need for scientific precision and accuracy. So widespread has this usage become, however, so deeply is it a part of daily thought and speech that it has had an enormous effect upon the writings and formulations of many introspective psychologists and psychoanalysts. In large measure the confusion has been due to failure to make a clear distinction between a biological *need*—hunger, thirst, sex; its presumed *aim*—reproduction, hunting, self-preservation; its *motor pattern*—walking, running, grasping; and its *emotional concomitants*—fear, anger, sympathy. The result has been a hodge-podge of loose usage in which almost every observable human reaction has at one time or another been characterized as instinctive.

Thus some psychologists of the McDougall school have described instincts of acquisitiveness, possessiveness, hunting, habitation, greed, kindliness, teasing, bullying, cleanliness, adornment, and superstition, to mention but a few. Among psychoanalysts the

3

term has been used with almost equal prodigality. Freud on the whole has been less guilty in this regard than many of his followers. But, apart from his broad dualistic classifications of ego and sex instincts, and life and death instincts, Freud also speaks of instincts of watching, of recovery, of mastery and aggression. Jung enumerates egoistic, altruistic, religious, herd, and animal instincts, and an instinct of intuition; A. A. Brill mentions mating, love, and animal instincts, and a feminine instinct of the desire for children; Wm. Alanson White specifies instincts to be cruel, to fight, hate, kill, love, submit, dominate, to be curious, and those of an acquisitive, gregarious, creative, maternal and paternal pattern; and Adler speaks of congenital, sadistic, murderous, and criminal instincts.

Generally speaking, most scientific definitions of instinct conceive of it as an inherited complex pattern of behavior, entirely automatic and unlearned, and comprising within its inherited scope the *cause* of an activity, its *goal*, the *behavior* necessary to consummate it, and its *emotional concomitant*, if any.*

The most perfect examples of such patterns are observed in insects. Thus a fly, when hatched and dry, makes its first circuit as accurately as though it had practiced it for days; or a solitary mud wasp, even though its mother is dead when it is hatched, and it has no opportunity for learning or imitation, is able to build its nest, hunt spiders of a particular sort, paralyze them by stinging, store them in the nest, lay an egg with them, and seal them in. Similarly the behavior of animals—their modes of hunting prey, of bringing up their young, of courting, mating, running, swimming and flying—has generally been considered phylogenetically predetermined, and not requiring any learning process.

It was by analogy with these observations, and under the influence of the new biological and evolutionary orientation which had just

*Although this was an accurate statement in 1942, the concept of instinct has undergone considerable modification since then. Modern biologists now recognize that, even in lower animals, instinctual patterns of behavior are subject to considerable environmental modification, as exemplified in this paper. There is a growing trend among some biologists to discard the term "instinct" entirely as an archaic and outmoded concept, and to talk instead of inherited biological structures and "behavioral systems," some of which are relatively uninfluenced by environmental variations (i.e., environmentally stable) while others are more influenceable (i.e., environmentally labile). (J. M., 1973)

been initiated by Darwin, that Freud, in common with other psychologists of his time, was led to approach the problem of human behavior from the standpoint of its phylogenetic, biological roots, and to postulate theories of human behavior based on the concept of instinct.

With the development of experimental psychology, however, there has been gradually accumulating a body of facts which has tended to cast serious doubt upon the validity of the entire concept of instinct, and to question its applicability in particular to the behavior of higher mammals and especially to the behavior of man.

But so tenacious and long-standing has been the hold of this concept, that relatively little of this newer knowledge has seeped into general consciousness, although in most academic psychological and sociological circles it has become commonplace. It is particularly striking, when one surveys the literature of psychiatry and psychoanalysis, to note how little awareness there has been of the progress which has been made in a field with so important a bearing upon the understanding of human behavior.

Without completely surveying this work, I would like to indicate briefly a few of the outstanding facts which have been uncovered.

Beginning near the lower end of the evolutionary scale, it is generally agreed that of all phyla and classes of animals, the insects show the highest degree of complex instinctual activity. The social life of ants and bees has long been considered as a prime example of the inheritance of highly complicated integrations, and they have been regarded as impelled entirely by instinct, incapable of intelligent learned responses. Experimental studies (1), however, have demonstrated that insects are superior in learning ability to all other invertebrates, with the possible exception of certain mollusks. Ants, for example, can readily be taught to learn maze habits and to "remember" them for a month or more without retraining (2). This tends to confirm the observation of the naturalist, Romanes, that the ant does not come into the world with a complete equipment of tendencies to perform its many functions, but that it is led about the nest and apparently trained to do its domestic duties and to distinguish between friend and foe. Forel (3) demonstrated this by putting into one glass case the baby ants of three hostile species with the pupae of six other hostile species. The young ants did not fight as their elders would have done, but instead cooperated in the tending of the pupae, and on the hatching of the latter, a peaceful colony was formed.

Ascending the evolutionary ladder to the vertebrates it is seen that more and more of the patterns of behavior which have been assumed to be native or instinctual are in reality learned, adaptive reactions.

The sexual behavior of an organism as far down on the vertebrate scale as the guppy fish is an example. It has been shown by Noble (4) that if guppies are reared from birth in separate containers, males are found to attempt mating as readily with other males as with females. Noble found that the male guppies gradually *learn* to avoid other males, because the males bite at the courter, while females do not. A reaction of avoidance to all guppies with male color patterns is thus gradually established, while those with female color patterns continue to be pursued. Moreover, when female guppies are painted with male colors, even experienced male guppies will tend to avoid them.

The evidence increases in the evolutionary scale to birds. Consider, for example, the findings in connection with the supposedly distinctive songs of various bird species. Scott (5) isolated Baltimore orioles before they had an opportunity to hear the song of their species. Although they eventually became good singers their song did not resemble that of the oriole. When baby orioles were then placed with two of these isolated birds, the former were found to adopt the atypical song of the latter. Scott also found that when birds of different species were reared together within hearing of each other there were interesting modifications of their singing. In one instance, a red-winged blackbird crowed constantly in imitation of a bantam rooster. Conradi (6) secured similar results with sparrows which he reared from incubation in the same room with canaries. None of these sparrows ever developed the call-notes characteristic of wild sparrows, but instead adopted those of the canaries, imitating them perfectly although the quality of their voices was not as good.

Isolation of birds from birth has shown other interesting results. Thus Craig (7) reared three male doves in isolation for periods of one to three years and found that all showed maladaptation to mating behavior when first paired with females. Two of the three isolated doves, moreover, made positive sexual overtures to the hand of the experimenter who fed them. Craig also noted several examples of homosexuality in pigeons. Brückner (8) reared two domestic chicks in isolation—"Kaspar Hauser chicks." When finally released into a group they showed bewilderment and retreated to secluded nesting places as soon as possible. Pattie (9) brought up isolated chicks in the company of white mice and found that they subsequently preferred the company of white mice to other chicks.*

The observation of mammalian life shows further evidence of the diminishing importance of instinct. The maternal responses of lower mammals, for instance, is still often referred to as an outstanding example of a complex behavior pattern dependent upon inherited, physiological changes which take place at certain times in the life of the individual animal. Reasoning by analogy, many psychologists and psychoanalysts have long assumed that maternal behavior in humans is similarly instinctual in origin. Here again, however, recent experimental evidence indicates that even in lower mammals the reaction is far more complex than supposed. Thus, in a scholarly monograph on the maternal responses of the rat, Wiesner and Sheard (10) demonstrate conclusively that these responses "are not fixed patterns, but are largely determined by (and vary with) actual environmental conditions." Their conclusions were subsequently confirmed by Leblond (11) who found that so-called "maternal" behavior could be elicited in almost all adult mice, *whether male or female, parturient or nonparturient.* In males and virgin females, however, it is first necessary to "sensitize" the maternal behavior by leaving newborn young in the cage of the tested animals for one to four days—concaveation. Leblond demonstrates that the more uniform expression of maternal behavior by lactating females may be due in large part to the continuous presence of their young. That hormonal factors play a role is not denied, but that their mediation is not essential is indicated by the fact that both castrated and hypophysectomized animals may show this behavior after concaveation.

The mouse-killing reaction of cats is another behavior pattern which has generally been considered as instinctive. The aggressive rage and attack on the one hand, and the panicky flight on the

---

*Today this reaction would be attributed to imprinting. (J. M., 1973)

other, were believed to be the inborn and inevitable responses of
the one species to the sight or smell of the other. However, in
1930, Kuo (12) performed some simple experiments which effectively
disproved this idea. Kuo reared one group of kittens with mothers
who killed rats in their presence, another group with no contact
with rats until they were several months old, and a third group
with rats as companions from birth. In the first group, 85 per
cent killed rats before they were four months old. In the second
group, only 45 per cent became rat-killers. In the third group *no*
cat killed any of its companion rats, or any strange rats of the
same variety, and only 16 per cent killed rats of other varieties.
As a result of these and similar experiments, Kuo concludes that
"kittens can be made to kill a rat, to love it, to hate it, to fear
it, or to play with it; it depends on the life history of the kitten."
Moreover, it should be noted that, conversely, young mice on their
part showed no initial fear or excitement in the presence of kittens
until the heavy paws and sharp claws and teeth of the latter had
come into play.

Parenthetically, it may be remarked that it is not merely under
the artificial conditions of the laboratory, but even in states of
"nature," that changes have been observed in animal behavior
patterns previously considered instinctual. As far back as 1891 the
noted biologist, C. Lloyd Morgan, wrote (13):

> Mr. G. L. Grant has recently observed that the sparrows near
> Auckland, New Zealand, have taken to burrowing holes in cliffs,
> like the sand-martin. The cliff swallow of the Eastern United
> States has almost ceased to build nests in the cliffs like its
> progenitors and now avails itself of the protection afforded by
> the eaves of homes. The surviving beavers of Europe are said
> to have abandoned the instinct (sic! J. M.) of building huts and
> dams. The race being no longer sufficiently numerous to live
> in communities, the survivors live in deep burrows.. . . . The
> Kea, a brush-tongued parrot of New Zealand, which normally
> feeds on honey, fruit, and berries, has since the introduction
> of sheep taken to a carnivorous diet. It is said to have begun
> by picking at the sheep skins hung out to dry; subsequently
> it began to attack living sheep, and now it has learned to tear
> its way down to the fat which surrounds the kidneys.

According to Linton (14), lions in Kenya Colony, Africa, have taken to hunting in packs rather than alone or in pairs—a new pattern of behavior evidently dependent on a changing environment—diminishing game—rather than on any change in their instinctive endowment.

It is when the level of the infrahuman primates is reached, however, that the widest range of behavior variability next to that of man is observed. Consider, for instance, so fundamental a reaction as the sexual behavior of these primates. Both Bingham (15) and Maslow (16) have observed that in contrast to the smooth, efficient performance of experienced males, young male apes or monkeys, or adults that have had no opportunity for sexual experience or sexual observation, reveal themselves completely ignorant of how to proceed when first mated, and go "through a long series of fumbling approximations and adjustments that look remarkably like trial-and-error learning." Moreover, sexual desire and mating in these primates do not, as a rule, follow any cyclic, hormonally-determined rhythm but may occur at any time and serve a variety of purposes besides sexual ones. Thus Kempf (17) is authority for the statement that monkeys often give sexual favors in exchange for food or protection, which he likens to prostitution. The importance of dominance in the sexual behavior of primates has been emphasized by a number of observers (18), especially by Maslow. It has been noted that the less dominant animal, *whether male or female,* tends to assume the "feminine" copulatory attitude when threatened or attacked, while the more dominant animal, regardless of *its* sex, assumes the "masculine" copulatory position, mounting the former. The significance of these facts in terms of the common conception—inherent also in the Freudian theories about women— that passivity is "normally" or biologically a "female" attribute, while aggressiveness is "normally" or biologically a "male" attribute, is self-evident.

The sexual positions and methods of mutual genital stimulation used by the apes are also variable, and favored positions develop only gradually and are altered with experience and expediency. It should be noted that variations occur not only from animal to animal, within the same species, but even within the same animal at different times. Homosexuality is normally displayed among primates (19) even, it should be noted, where heterosexual opportunities exist. It is more frequent between males than females, and among younger animals than older ones, but it is not restricted to preadolescent males, as has sometimes been supposed. Masturbatory behavior occurs in either sex, especially in the absence of homosexual or heterosexual objects (20). In fact, practically all the so-called "human" sexual perversions have been observed in primates—fellatio, fetishism, exhibitionism, coprophagy, necrophilia, self-mutilation, bestiality—with cats, dogs, for instance—and the use of the very young animal as a sexual object.

Finally, let me speak of man. It is not necessary to rehearse the almost infinite variability of human behavior, nor to repeat the convincing evidence which anthropologists have been accumulating of the profound differences which exist in people under differing social conditions. The fundamental error which the instinct theorists—including Freud—have made in this regard is to assume that the various characteristics which they correctly observed in all human beings *in a particular time and social mileu* were inherent in *all* human beings, in *all* times, and in *all* social milieus—that is to say, were expressions of a universal, biologically determined "human nature." The writings of Benedict (21), Linton (14), Mead (22), Malinowski (23), Sapir (24), and Kardiner (25) are particularly relevant to this problem.

I should like to call attention, however, to another aspect of this problem, namely, the behavior of human beings who have been reared among wild animals—"feral children," or otherwise isolated from human company since birth or early infancy. Gesell (26) has published an account of one of these feral children—Kamala, a girl of India—who was adopted by a wolf-mother at about six months of age, and was not discovered again until she was eight years old. When found she was more beast than human. She ran on all fours, and could not stand erect. She saw better by night than by day. She was terrified of human beings and preferred the company of animals. She rejected all human food, and had a decided preference for raw carrion meat. She tended to sleep by day and prowl around by night, and in the early hours of the morning would lift her head to the moon and howl mournfully, like a wolf. Where was the "human nature" in this child? After six years of patient teaching, she was able to stand erect and walk, but still used all fours when she wished to run. She still retained an unusually acute sense of hearing and smell, and could still see better by night than by day. She had learned to speak but forty words, and only exhibited the intelligence of a three-year-old child. There was no evidence at her death two years later that she would ever have achieved normal human intelligence. This, in the main, is the story of all children isolated in infancy; they are never able to learn to speak normally, they exhibit various sensory and motor abnormalities, and they remain permanently "feebleminded."

Kingsley Davis (27) reported the case of Anna, a child in a small Pennsylvania community, who because she was illegitimate was kept isolated in an attic room from the age of ten months to the age of six years. When discovered, she could not stand or walk, could not speak, and had no sphincter control. One and one-half years later, despite training and constant human companionship, she was still unable to speak, had no sphincter control, and her mental age was still that of a one-year-old idiot. Davis concludes the facts "indicate . . . the stages of socialization are necessarily related to the stages of organic development. If the delicate, complex, and logically prior stages of socialization are not acquired when the organism is plastic, they will never be acquired and the later stages never achieved, except crudely. Anna's history, like others, seems to demonstrate . . . that human nature is determined by the child's communicative social contacts as much as by his organic equipment."

What conclusions can be drawn from this array of evidence? I believe it has been amply demonstrated that the higher the ascent in the evolutionary scale the more variable is the behavior of the individual animal, and the wider its range of adaptability; the less can its adult behavior be explained in terms of phylogenetically predetermined patterns, and the more is it dependent on postnatal environmental influences. The reasons for this are inherent in the neural structure of the organism. The lower the animal form, the more completely developed is its neural structure at birth, and the more totally is it equipped to cope with its environment. This early maturation of the neural structure, however, also means that the capacity for plasticity and variability of behavior is extremely limited.

The higher the animal form, on the other hand, the more helpless is the infant and the less fully developed at birth is its neural structure, until in humans the most prolonged period of infantile helplessness and neural maturation is encountered. This means that the completion of the process of myelinization, and the development of sensory-motor executive functions are effected in relationship to environmental influences. The result is a marked broadening of the plasticity and adaptive possibilities of the organism. That these environmental influences in early infancy are an essential prerequisite to the development of the full functional capacity of the brain is clearly illustrated by the permanent mental retardation which results in isolated children whose brains have completed their myelinization in the absence of social influences.

In other words, the vast range and complexity of modern human behavior are dependent not only on the inheritance of a human brain and body, but equally importantly, upon that vast *social* inheritance called culture. This represents the transmitted learning and experience which one generation of men has handed down to its successors during thousands of years through the medium of language. It is this unique factor which qualitatively distinguishes man from all other animal forms. Without it, as in the instance of isolated children, the son of a civilized man becomes nearer to the beast in his behavior than to his own father.

To speak of "human nature," then, as some form of human behavior, thought, or emotion which is determined by purely biological factors, and which exists even in a state of isolation, is clearly erroneous. There can be no "human" nature apart from some form of human society, and the character of that "nature" will inevitably reflect the character of that society.

This formulation does not in any way deny the existence of basic biological drives or needs which man has in common with all other animals—need for food, water, sexual gratification, and protection from the elements. But the *aims* of these drives in humans, and the *objects* towards which they are expressed, can only be understood in terms of the specific social relationships to which the human being has been exposed.

The failure to make this distinction is one of the fundamental errors involved in the Freudian concept of *Trieb*. There has been a tendency in recent years to defend this concept as being restricted solely to the idea of biological drive, rather than of an instinct in the sense with which the term has been used in this paper. Actually, however, the Freudian concept of *Trieb* is not very far removed from that of instinct, for Freud uses it to denote not merely the biological impulse but also its aim and developmental pattern, both of which he also considers biologically determined. Thus his conception of the biological roots of the Oedipus complex, and his formulation of the libido theory in terms of a phylogenetically predetermined—oral, anal, phallic—pathway of "normal" sexual development clearly illustrates this error. Such concepts as *Lebens-Trieb* and *Todes-Trieb* embrace a wide and complex variety of reactive processes in humans, most of which are learned; their use as explanatory concepts of human motivation can only lead to the kind of unprecise thinking which has made psychoanalytic theory so vulnerable to scientific criticism in the past. It is to the credit of psychoanalysis that it is independently beginning to free itself from these less valuable heritages of its past (28).

Even such popular concepts as the "instinct of self-preservation" and the "instinct of reproduction," or "race-preservation," have no validity in precise scientific thinking about human beings. They too not only embrace a wide variety of behavior patterns, most of which are learned, but also are teleological concepts attributing to inheritance goals which are not innately present. Thus the hunger drive of an infant does not distinguish between what is good for it or bad for it; it will drink poison with as much avidity as it will milk, until it learns better. At birth the child cannot distinguish between edible and non-edible matter, between the breast and a rubber ball. It is only gradually that he learns it is the class of objects known as food that he must look for when he is hungry, or for certain liquids when he is thirsty. Similarly, with regard to the sexual drive the higher one rises in the evolutionary scale, the less bound is the sexual drive to the purpose of reproduction, and the more does it tend to subserve a variety of other functions which have nothing to do with the preservation of the race.

CONCLUSION

The time is now long overdue for psychiatry, and particularly for psychoanalysis, to divest itself of the inaccurate concept of instinct as applied to human behavior. In the past quarter of a century the advances made in the fields of experimental psychology, biology, and anthropology leave little doubt that this concept has diminishing scientific validity at each stage of ascent in the evolutionary scale, and least of all when applied to man.

Similarly, the old conflicts of heredity versus environment or biology versus culture become meaningless when viewed from the organismic approach of modern psychology. Even in the lower forms of animal life, the organism is immersed in an environment from the very beginning of the life cycle. Each stage of development is determined by the cooperation of hereditary and environmental forces. Since the earlier stages influence the character of the development of the later stages, the hereditary and environmental factors become more and more interpenetrated as development proceeds. Nowhere is this more true than in humans, where the cultural factors become indissolubly interrelated with organic processes through the laying down of language patterns in the association centers of the cortex. Thus there develops a new unity which is qualitatively unique in the animal world—a sociobiological unity—called human nature. This interpenetration is so complex and so complete that one cannot separate the hereditary from the environmental factors in man without destroying the specific quality which constitutes the nature of man, just as water cannot be separated into hydrogen and oxygen without destroying that quality which constitutes water.

The emerging fact of major importance is that there is no such entity as a fixed, immutable, universal "human nature." Since the nature of man depends equally upon his biological and social inheritances, significant changes in either sphere may alter it. It was the failure to fully appreciate this fact which made Freud's outlook upon society and upon the results of psychoanalytic therapy inevitably so pessimistic (29). In recognition of this fact, however, rest the conviction and hope that out of the titanic world struggle (World War II) which is now going on there will emerge a better world in which to live, in which the potentialities of man may be raised to ever greater heights of creativeness and self-fulfillment.

REFERENCES

1. WARDEN, C. J., JENKINS, T. N., and WARNER L. H., *Introduction to Comparative Psychology*; New York, Ronald Press, 1934 (581 pp.).

2. SCHNEIRLA, T. C., Learning and Orientation in Ants. *Comp. Psychol. Monograph* (1929) 6; 143 pp.
3. FOREL, AUGUST, *The Social World of the Ants Compared with that of Man;* New York, Boni, 1929 (996 pp.).
4. NOBLE, G. K., Sexual Selection Among Fishes. *Biol. Rev.* (1938) 13:133–158.
5. SCOTT, W. E., Data on Song in Birds. *Science* (1901) 14:522–526, and (1902) 15:179–181.
6. CONRADI, EDWARD, Song and Call-Notes of English Sparrows when Reared by Canaries. *Amer. J. Psychol.* (1905) 16:190-198.
7. CRAIG, WALLACE, Male Doves Reared in Isolation. *J. Animal Behavior* (1914) 4:121–133.
8. BRÜCKNER, G. H., Untersuchungen zur Tiersoziologie, inbezondere zur Auflosung der Familie. *Zeitschr. f. Psychol.* (1933) 128:1–110.
9. PATTIE, F. A., The Gregarious Behavior of Normal Chicks, and Chicks Hatched in Isolation. *J. Comp. Psychol.* (1936) 21:161–178.
10. WIESNER, B. P., and SHEARD, N. M., *Maternal Behavior in the Rat;* Edinburgh, Oliver and Boyd, 1933 (244 pp.).
11. LEBLOND, C. P., Extra-Hormonal Factors in Maternal Behavior. *Proceedings Soc. Exper. Biol. and Med.* (1938) 38:66–70.
12. KUO, Z. Y., Genesis of the Cat's Responses Toward the Rat. *J. Comp. Psychol.* (1930) 11:1-36.
13. MORGAN, C. L., *Animal Life and Intelligence;* London, Arnold, 1891 (519 pp.).
14. LINTON, RALPH, *The Study of Man;* New York, Appleton-Century, 1936 (ix and 503 pp.).
15. BINGHAM, H. C., Sex Development in Apes. *Comp. Psychol. Monograph* (1928) 5; 165 pp.
16. MASLOW, A. H., Rôle of Dominance in the Social and Sexual Behavior of Infra-Human Primates. *J. Genetic Psychol.* (1936) 48:261–277, and 310–338.
17. KEMPF, E. J., The Social and Sexual Behavior of the Infra-Human Primates and Some Comparable Facts in Human Behavior. *Psychoanalytic Rev.* (1917) 4:127–154.
18. HAMILTON, G. V., Sexual Tendencies of Monkeys and Baboons. *J. Animal Behavior* (1914) 4:295–318. See also references 15 and 16.
19. ZUCKERMAN, SOLLY, *The Social Life of Apes and Monkeys;* New York, Harcourt Brace, 1932 (xii and 356 pp.); TINKLEPAUGH, O. L., The Self-Mutilation of a Male Macacus Rhesus Monkey. *J. Mammal.* (1928) 9:293–300. Compare also references 15, 16 and 17.
20. References 15, 16 and 17.
21. BENEDICT, RUTH, *Patterns of Culture;* Boston, Houghton-Mifflin, 1934 (xii and 290 pp.).
22. MEAD, MARGARET, *Sex and Temperament in Three Primitive Societies;* New York, William Morrow, 1935 (xxii and 335 pp.).
23. MALINOWSKI, BRONISLAW, *Crime and Custom in Savage Society;* New York, Harcourt Brace, 1926 (xii and 132 pp.).
24. SAPIR, EDWARD, Cultural Anthropology and Psychiatry. *J. Abnormal and Social Psychol.* (1932) 27:229–242.
25. KARDINER, ABRAM, *The Individual and His Society;* New York, Columbia University Press, 1939 (xxvi and 503 pp.).
26. GESELL, ARNOLD, *Wolf-Child and Human Child;* New York, Harper, 1941 (xvi and 107 pp.).

27. DAVIS, KINGSLEY, Extreme Social Isolation of a Child. *Amer. J. Sociol.* (1940)
    45:554–565.
28. FROMM, ERICH, *Escape from Freedom;* New York, Farrar and Rinehart, 1941
    (ix and 305 pp.); HORNEY, KAREN, *The Neurotic Personality of Our Time;*
    New York, Norton, 1937 (xii and 290 pp.); HORNEY, KAREN, *New Ways
    in Psychoanalysis;* New York, Norton, 1939 (313 pp.); KARDINER, ABRAM,
    The Traumatic Neuroses of War; New York, Hoeber, 1941 (270 pp.). See
    also reference 25; SULLIVAN, HARRY STACK, Conceptions of Modern Psychiatry.
    Psychiatry (1940) 3:1–117.
29. FREUD, SIGMUND, *Civilization and Its Discontents;* London, Hogarth Press, 1930
    (144 pp.); FREUD, SIGMUND, Analysis Terminable and Interminable. *Internat.
    J. Psychoanal.* (1937) 18:373–405.

2

TOWARD AN INTEGRATIVE
CONCEPTION OF MENTAL DISORDER
(1950)

In the past two or three decades there has been a significant, far-reaching change in the fundamental philosophy underlying medical thinking. Virchow's static pathology of individual cells and organs has given way to the study of the pathophysiology of the living organism and the interrelationship of organ systems. The purely mechanistic idea of disease being "caused" solely by a noxious agent has been abandoned. It has been replaced by the more dynamic concept of a functional interrelationship between the individual and a so-called pathogenic agent. Thus an organism which under certain conditions lives in a state of harmless equilibrium with its host may, under changed conditions, become lethal to him. The resistance of the host, the virulence of the organism, the portal of entry and the size of the invasion at any point in time constitute some of the variable factors which may determine whether or not a pathological process will develop. An important consequence of this conception of disease etiology has been a diminution of the tendency to "explain" diseases in terms of inheritance or constitution. The genetic factor is now recognized as but one element in a parallelogram of forces. Thus while we may recognize a constitutional factor in such conditions as diabetes, hypertension, or rheumatoid arthritis, we do not consider it per se as causative.

One of the most lucid presentations of this modern viewpoint on etiology has been that of Halliday (9), who states: "Illness is

_____

Dr. Eugene Pumpian-Mindlin collaborated in the writing of this essay.

17

regarded not as a fault in the parts, but as a *reaction* or mode of behavior, or vital expression of a living unit in response to those forces which he encounters as he moves and grows in time. Cause is therefore *two-fold* and is to be found in the nature of the individual and the nature of his environment at a particular point in time."

IMPLICATIONS FOR PSYCHIATRY

What are the implications of this approach to the nature of illness when applied to the field of psychiatry? The whole conception of personality in a static sense has changed to one of a constant dynamic interplay between the individual and his environment. Events and situations may at certain times be traumatic, at others relatively innocuous. The receptivity of the organism for the stimulus has become as important as the stimulus itself. Stated broadly, this concept implies that all human behavior is the expression, at a psycho-physiological level, of a dynamic interrelationship between the individual and his environment—a relationship which is in a constant state of motion and change. *Mental health, psychopathy, and psychosis can then be understood as expressions of varying quantitative aspects of this interrelationship, which at certain crucial levels result in qualitative changes. Moreover, this concept implies that these changes are potentially reversible.*

This thesis may be broadly schematized in the following diagram (Figure 1), which endeavors to present in highly schematized form the interrelationship between the individual and his environment in the production of mental disease. The vertical line represents the nature of the individual. This is a dynamic complex made up of the dialectical interrelationship of the inherited biological constitution with the individual's life experiences up to that point in time (Table 1). Together they form a unit which constitutes the individual's personality structure at a given point in time. Depending upon the nature of these forces, this structure may have a high resistance to environmental stress (in which event we call it stable), or a low resistance to environmental stress (in which event we call it unstable). The horizontal line, on the other hand, represents the nature of the environment at any particular point in time. This may be broken down into component elements (Table 2), which together form a

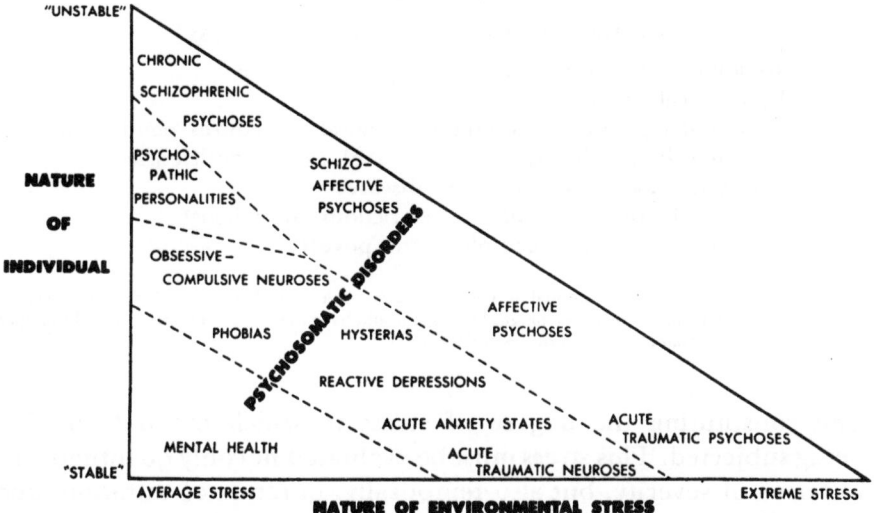

FIGURE 1. NATURE OF THE INDIVIDUAL: NATURE OF ENVIRONMENTAL STRESS.

TABLE 1

NATURE OF THE INDIVIDUAL ("PERSONALITY STRUCTURE")

Biological factors ("constitution")

1. Physical appearance
2. Endocrine balance
3. Intellectual endowment
4. Natural immunity
5. Sex
6. Age

Life experiences

1. Family relationships
2. Interpersonal relationships
3. Education
4. Social status
   a. Religion
   b. Race
   c. Class position
   d. National origin
5. Sexual development
6. Cultural factors

TABLE 2
NATURE OF THE ENVIRONMENTAL STRESS
1. Psychological stress; e.g., bereavement, loss of love
2. Physiological stress:
   a. Physical; e.g., heat, cold, fatigue, surgical procedures, bodily injury*
   b. Chemical; e.g., drugs, poisons, alcohol, dietary deficiencies
   c. Bacteriological; e.g., infectious diseases
3. Sociological stress; e.g., cultural restrictions and taboos*
4. Economic stress; e.g., unemployment, poverty

*Unhappily, the roster of potential physical stresses would now have to include the effects of nuclear radiation, while potential sociological stresses would have to include the effects of technological change, cold war, urbanization and overpopulation.

unit constituting the degree of stress to which the individual is being subjected. This stress must be evaluated not only quantitatively, in terms of severity, but also temporally, in terms of duration, and qualitatively, in terms of its special significance for the particular individual involved. Thus, for a soldier in combat, the quantitative factor is represented by the immediate severity of the battle conditions; the temporal factor, not only by the duration of the immediate combat situation, but also by the duration of previous exposure to combat conditions; and the qualitative factor, by the specific conscious and unconscious significance of the total war situation to the particular soldier.*

Relative Factors

The relative nature of these factors is of the greatest importance. What is considered psychologically healthy in one era or culture may not be considered so in another. For example, the normal sexual behavior of an adolescent girl among the Marquesans or Trobrianders (12) would in our society be set down as constituting nymphomania or "psychopathic personality." Again, while we label homosexuality as pathological in our Western culture, among the Tanalans and Japanese (4, 12) it is accepted as a normal behavior variant and meets with no opprobrium. In our own Western culture,

*Inasmuch as this article was written in the years immediately following World War II, many of the clinical examples cited reflected the recent military experiences of Dr. Pumpian-Mindlin and myself. (J. M., 1973)

within the span of the last five hundred years, individuals who insist that they see visions, hear voices, and communicate directly with God have at varying times been revered as prophets, burned as witches, or hospitalized as psychotic. Moreover, even within the same broad cultural group there may be significant variations in standards of accepted behavior (14).

Again, what is traumatic for a single individual may not be traumatic in a group situation. The experience of the London blitz is a case in point. The number of neurotic casualties was far less than was anticipated owing to the fact that danger was experienced in a group setting. Further, a situation which is traumatic for one individual may be a source of gratification for another. It was not too infrequent for psychiatrists in World War II to see individuals who were previously maladjusted in civilian life make a good adjustment in the Army.

Examining Figure 1, we now see that mental health can be hypothecated as that state in the interrelationship of the individual and his environment in which the personality structure is relatively stable and the environmental stresses are within its absorptive capacity. Ideally, this implies socially adequate behavior in an individual who is consciously and unconsciously well integrated. If the level of the environmental stresses is increased beyond a certain point, however, neurotic symptoms will develop in the most stable individual, and in cases of extreme stress even psychotic symptoms may develop. Thus the first important point which is implicit in this conception is that there is no such thing as *absolute* immunity to mental disease. "Every man has his breaking point." This is borne out clinically in numerous ways. Mild anxiety states, manifesting themselves in insomnia, digestive disturbances, or headaches, are universal under stress. Experiences with normal selected males under conditions of inordinate stress, such as those undergone by American soldiers at Guadalcanal, revealed that entire companies developed transitory acute traumatic syndromes of striking similarity (22). Other psychiatrists have dramatically described the transitory psychotic states which previously well-adjusted soldiers may develop in the face of extreme danger or stress (8).

The one characteristic which all of these mental disorders developing in previously stable personalities have in common is their benignness. Rest, quiet, and relaxation—in other words, removal of the environmental stress—often result in rapid return to normal even in the absence of any direct psychotherapy (22).

Scale of Disorder

When, on the other hand, the individual personality structure is unstable owing to unfavorable hereditary or early environmental influences, the amount of environmental stress necessary to produce abnormal symptoms is correspondingly less. Thus at one end of our scale we have our theoretically perfectly-integrated individual whom only realistic threats of greatest severity and duration can succeed in unsettling; while at the other extreme we have individuals whose personality structure is so poorly equilibrated, so fraught with internal tensions and contradictions, that the simplest routine of everyday living is too much for it, and it gradually disintegrates in the form of an insidious schizophrenia. Between these two extremes there are infinite gradations. At the "stable" end of the scale the clinical picture is more likely to be colored by the "traumatic situation," as in the acute reactive anxiety states, reactive depressions, and the traumatic syndrome. At the "unstable" end of the scale, on the other hand, the traumatic situation itself tends to leave little mark upon the clinical picture, which is dominated by the individual's preexisting conflicts and personality structure. Between these two extremes one finds infinite variations and admixtures.

This conception has considerable usefulness in prognostication. One could anticipate, for example, in a group of soldiers, all manifesting similar neurotic or psychotic symptoms, that those whose past history reveals an unstable personality structure will have the poorest prognosis. Similarly, the more acute the onset of a syndrome and the greater the environmental stress with which it is associated, the better the prognosis is apt to be. These criteria have been found to be equally useful in prognosticating the long-term results of shock therapy in psychotics.

Another implication of this conception, which follows from our diagram (Figure 1), is that an unbroken line of continuity exists from normal behavior through neurotic to psychotic behavior. This corresponds to the general principle in modern scientific thinking that "no boundary in nature is fixed and no category airtight," and that " 'mesoforms' are found at the transition point of one level of organization to the next" (18). In the field of mental disorders such mesoforms are encountered in the frequent borderline cases in which one is hard put to make a definite commitment as to whether an individual is normal, neurotic, or psychotic. This does not mean, however, that there are no qualitative differences between these categories. As in other fields of matter, the quantitative differences at certain levels result in real qualitative changes—just as raising the temperature of water to a certain level results in its qualitative transformation into steam, or lowering its temperature transforms it to ice.

This in turn leads to another significant implication, namely, that it is possible for the same individual, under varying circumstances, to pass from normal to psychotic behavior and back again. Neurosis and psychosis should not be regarded as static and fixed entities. *They are dynamic and changeable states of behavior which are potentially reversible, the borders of which are often indistinct.* One of the residuals of mechanistic thinking in the field of psychiatry is the still commonly held conviction that a neurotic individual can never become psychotic, and vice versa. When the facts tend to disprove this theory, they are sometimes tailored to fit it by post hoc reasoning. For example, if a neurotic individual becomes psychotic, it is stated that he really had been a "latent psychotic" all along. Conversely, the psychotic who ends up with a picture of neurosis is said not to have really had a genuine psychosis, or else is considered as still a "latent psychotic." Used in this post hoc manner, latent psychosis obviously means nothing more than the possibility that an individual may become psychotic under certain conditions. The term thus actually becomes meaningless, for, as we have indicated, given the appropriate environmental conditions, any person may become psychotic. There are numerous examples in the literature of typical neuroses which under observation have changed into psychoses. Myerson (17), Miller (16), Caldwell (5), Zilboorg (25), and Jung (11), among others, have described such cases. In this regard it is also of interest to note that Rorschach records of psychotic patients often show the intermingled presence of neurotic elements (23).

Interaction in Human Behavior

Still another implication of this point of view is that, strictly speaking, there is no such thing as an "endogenous" mental illness. Human behavior, whether normal or abnormal, is always the resultant of an *interaction* between the nature of the individual and the nature of his environment. The fact that not infrequently a neurosis, psychopathy, or psychosis develops insidiously without any apparent outward contributory factor has led to a widespread conception that such conditions are of "endogenous" origin—that is, that they are either inherited or "constitutional," or else the result of certain changes which take place within the individual and which have no relationship whatever to environmental factors. Occasionally one encounters this belief as a result of a faulty understanding of the psychoanalytic formulation that mental illness arises out of conflict between the ego and the id, or between the ego and the superego. This is due to the mistaken conception that these designated aspects of personality are intrinsic within the individual and bear no relationship to the environment. Actually, of course, only the id represents the reservoir of biological impulses, and even the strength of id impulses can be affected by such environmental influences as stimulation, fatigue, malnutrition, disease, and physical castration. But the ego and superego are *always* resultants of interaction with environmental influences. Thus, no conflict which includes one or the other of them (as every conflict must) can be said to be independent of environmental influences. The term "cryptogenic," as used in general medicine, would seem a more appropriate designation than "endogenous" because it implies that external factors, although present, are at the moment unknown.

Every psychiatrist has had the experience of having patients come to him with stories of neurotic or psychotic illnesses "coming on for no reason at all," only to discover on careful study of the patients' past history considerable material pointing to prolonged and severe conflicts with various factors in the environment. Zilboorg (25) and Schilder (21), among others, have described patients with schizophrenias of apparently insidious and nontraumatic origins in whom psychoanalytic study disclosed a wealth of environmental factors. Evidence is accumulating as a result of such studies that schizophrenias of insidious onset are the resultants of the exposure of susceptible individuals to severe and painfully crushing experiences very early in their ego development, probably in the first three or four years of their lives, with consequent serious crippling of their capacity to adapt to other people.* The schizophrenic withdraws from life because he has been deeply hurt—not because he is unable to relate to people but because he is *afraid* to. The therapeutic problem, as Fromm-Reichmann (7) has shown, is that of overcoming an overwhelming and overpowering distrust.

Similarly David Levy (15), Lauretta Bender (3), and others have demonstrated that the study of the early life of the so-called psychopathic personality reveals most often that these patients have suffered a deprivation of warmth and affection from maternal or maternal-surrogate sources in the first two or three years of their lives.† The result has been a distortion of the affective life of these patients.

With our increasing understanding of the dynamics of these conditions, they are gradually becoming accessible to various psychotherapeutic approaches (17, 24). This indicates their essential reversibility and their accessibility to environmental influences.

ROLE OF CONSTITUTIONAL FACTORS

Today it is fairly generally conceded that neurotic disorders arise in connection with various environmental stresses or frustrations in the course of individual development. But psychopathic personality, schizophrenia, and manic-depressive psychosis are still widely regarded as conditions which result primarily from hereditary or constitutional factors. Consequently, they are considered therapeutically more or less hopeless and preventable mainly by eugenic measures. In our opinion this viewpoint is untenable, both on theoretical and clinical grounds. This is not to deny that constitutional (genetic) factors play a role in schizophrenia, manic-depressive

---

*Genetically determined variations in neurochemical responses to stress are probably also involved.

†Another group of psychopathic personalities develops as the result of excessive parental indulgence unaccompanied by any form of discipline (15).

psychosis, and psychopathic personality. Constitutional factors are operative in *all* human behavior, whether normal or abnormal. One has only to go through a ward of newborn infants to see that babies differ from one another biologically. But from the moment of birth on, all human behavior becomes an increasingly complex resultant of the interaction of these genetic factors with environmental forces. Abnormal behavior must always be evaluated in terms of this twofold aspect of causality. Constitutional factors do not operate directly in the production of psychological phenomena, but function as a dynamic substrate, being molded by, and in turn molding, the environmental impact. It is doubtful whether heredity ever contributes more than a greater or lesser propensity to mental disease, a sort of psychological threshold which is analogous to levels of so-called natural immunity in the field of general medicine. But like natural immunity, it is never absolute, and its relative importance depends on the quality, quantity, and timing of the environmental stress.

It will be noted further from Figure 1 that no attempt has been made sharply to "compartmentalize" or segregate the different descriptive types of neurotic and psychotic reactions. The more minutely one examines the mental reactions of neurotics, the more one finds that there are no sharp lines of demarcation between the various types. It is most rare, for example, to find a "pure" hysteria or "pure" obsessional neurosis. Most neurotics when studied intensively are found to be mixed types, with hysterical, obsessional, anxiety, and psychosomatic manifestations. Even the psychopathic personality is not always sharply demarcated from the neurotic. Mixed clinical pictures in which neurotic and psychopathic traits are intermingled are not unusual.

This is not intended to imply that there are no differences between the various types of neuroses and psychopathies. Obviously there are; the quantitative predominance of one or another group of symptoms at certain crucial levels leads to genuine qualitative differences. It is not that there are no differences, but rather that there are no sharp mechanical lines of differentiation between any of these varied mental disorders.

Nowhere are these interwoven dynamics more clearly exemplified than in the whole group of so-called psychosomatic disorders. These represent the exaggerated physiological response of the organism to prolonged psychological stress or tension. As such they may occur in all human beings, normal, neurotic, psychopathic, or psychotic. Most of the classical psychosomatic disorders, such as asthma, migraine, hypertension, ulcer, and colitis, are found on analysis to be accompanied by psychoneuroses and to have similar dynamic background and structure as the psychoneuroses. Why the same amount of anxiety or tension tends to provoke so much greater somatic reaction in some individuals than in others is still one of the important unsolved questions of medicine. It is likely that further elucidation of the physiology of the autonomic nervous system and the individual differences which exist in this regard among human beings may help to clarify this point. There is evidence that in some cases the choice of organ symptomatology may be psychological-ly determined (2).

In the field of the psychoses, also, it may be worth considering whether the sharp differentiation hitherto made between schizo-phrenia and manic-depressive psychosis is warranted. Anyone who has ever worked in a state hospital will recall the countless hours spent in clinical conferences discussing whether a particular case should be placed in one or the other category.* Psychiatric literature is replete with investigations endeavoring to establish the differences between them. For example, Rachlin (19, 20) and Hoch (10), in a series of careful papers, demonstrate conclusively that many cases originally diagnosed as manic-depressive psychosis eventually end up as clear-cut schizophrenia. They do not, however, conclude from this that one condition may merge into the other, or that our descriptive categories are inadequate, but instead assume that wher-ever this has happened, the original diagnosis was incorrect. This kind of post hoc reasoning requires careful reevaluation. Is it not possible that the difficulty in differentiating the two conditions, and the occasional merging of one into the other, simply indicates that they are not the sharply demarcated nosological entities which they have always been assumed to be? This is further suggested by the existence of intermediate forms which the French have labeled

---

*This is particularly true at the inception of psychotic illness. The sharply demarcated Kraepelinian categories are most often seen in the later stages of chronic psychoses.

"schizomanie," and which Kasanin (13) and Campbell (6) have reported as "schizo-affective psychosis."

SUMMARY

The thesis of this paper is that human behavior is the expression of a dynamic interrelationship between the individual and his environment at a particular point in time and space; that mental health and the various deviations therefrom are but expressions of varying quantitative aspects of this relationship which at certain crucial levels result in qualitative changes. The implications of this conception are discussed, and some of the preliminary conclusions reached are: (1) No person is absolutely immune to mental illness, either neurotic or psychotic. (2) Neurosis, psychopathy, and psychosis are potentially reversible, except where actual destruction of brain tissue has occurred. (3) The various forms of mental disorder merge into one another by an infinite series of gradations, and there are no sharp lines of demarcation between them. (4) The same individual can, under different conditions, suffer from a neurotic illness or psychopathy at one time, and a psychosis at another. (5) Psychosomatic disorders may occur at varying levels of mental disorder. (6) There are no truly "endogenous" mental illnesses. (7) Constitutional or hereditary factors condition the development of so-called functional mental disorders, but never in themselves determine it.

REFERENCES

1. AICHHORN, A. Wayward Youth. New York: Viking, 1945.
2. ALEXANDER, F. Fundamental concepts of psychosomatic research. Psychosom. Med. 5:205, 1943.
3. BENDER, L. Quoted in D. Levy, Maternal Overprotection. New York: Columbia University Press, 1943. P. 224.
4. BENEDICT, R. The Chrysanthemum and the Sword. Boston: Houghton Mifflin, 1946. P. 187.
5. CALDWELL, J. M. Schizophrenic psychoses. Amer. J. Psychiat. 97:1061, 1941.
6. CAMPBELL, C. M. Two cases illustrating the combination of affective and schizophrenic symptoms. Amer. J. Psychiat. 6:243, 1926.
7. FROMM-REICHMANN, F. Transference problems in schizophrenics. Psychoanal. Quart. 8:412, 1939.
8. GRINKER, R. R., and SPIEGEL, J. P. Men Under Stress. Philadelphia: Blakiston, 1945. P. 327.

9. HALLIDAY, J. L. Principles of aetiology. *Brit. J. Med. Psychol.* 19:367, 1943.
10. HOCH, P., and RACHLIN, H. L. An evaluation of manic-depressive psychosis in the light of follow-up studies. *Amer. J. Psychiat.* 97:831, 1941.
11. JUNG, C. G. Psychogenesis of schizophrenia. *J. Ment. Sci.* 85:999, 1939.
12. KARDINER, A. *The Individual and His Society.* New York: Columbia University Press, 1939. Pp. 80, 168, 266.
13. KASANIN, J. The acute schizo-affective psychosis. *Amer. J. Psychiat.* 91:97, 1933.
14. KINSEY, A. C., POMEROY, W. B., and MARTIN, C. E. *Sexual Behavior in the Human Male.* Philadelphia: Saunders, 1948.
15. LEVY, D. *Maternal Overprotection.* New York: Columbia University Press, 1943.
16. MILLER, W. R. Relationship between early schizophrenias and the neuroses. *Amer. J. Psychiat.* 96:889, 1940.
17. MYERSON, A. Neuroses and neuropsychoses. *Amer. J. Psychiat.* 93:263, 1936.
18. NOVIKOFF, A. B. Concept of integrative levels and biology. *Science* 101:209, 1945.
19. RACHLIN, H. L. Follow-up study of Hoch's benign stupor cases. *Amer. J. Psychiat.* 92:531, 1935.
20. RACHLIN, H. L. Statistical study of benign stupor in five New York State hospitals. *Psychiat. Quart.* 11:436, 1937.
21. SCHILDER, P. Psychology of schizophrenia. *Psychoanal. Rev.* 26:380, 1939.
22. SMITH, E. R. Neuroses resulting from combat. *Amer. J. Psychiat.* 100:94, 1943.
23. VAN BARK, B., and BARON, S. Neurotic elements in the Rorschach record of psychotics. *Rorschach Res. Exchange* 7:166, 1943.
24. WOLBERG, L. R. *Hypnoanalysis.* New York: Grune & Stratton, 1945.
25. ZILBOORG, G. The deeper layers of schizophrenic psychosis. *Amer. J. Psychiat.* 88:493, 1931.

3

SOME OBSERVATIONS ON
SUPERSTITION
IN CONTEMPORARY LIFE
(1954)

As man's scientific knowledge has increased, it is often naturally assumed that his irrational beliefs must be diminishing proportionately. Much of our supposed superiority in this regard, however, over earlier or more primitive societies is actually more apparent than real.

The term "superstition" should be reserved for "beliefs or practices groundless in themselves and *inconsistent with the degree of enlightenment reached by the community to which one belongs*" (15a; italics mine). An inaccurate belief which was consistent with the level of scientific development in the period during which it was held, therefore, does not merit the appellation of superstition. Thus the astrological beliefs of the Middle Ages were in harmony with existing scientific theories and were held by many intelligent and well-educated people. They were reasonable conclusions based upon inaccurate premises, and as such did not constitute superstition any more than the old practice of treating all illnesses by bloodletting did. There are many such examples. To hold to such beliefs or practices, however, after the premises upon which they were originally based have been demonstrated to be irrational, would be clearly superstitious.

It is surprising to discover how many beliefs of irrational nature persist in contemporary society despite the far-reaching advances in our technological understanding. Dr. Wayland Hand of the University of California at Los Angeles, who has been making a comprehensive compilation of the superstitious beliefs and practices still extant in the United States, conservatively estimates their number at 80,000 (7)! Most of these, of course, are limited to relatively small groups of uneducated people and can be regarded as largely the fruit of ignorance. When, however, superstitions are encountered which are not merely extremely common, but which exist with equal frequency among educated people and uneducated ones, the explanation of ignorance no longer suffices, and their source must be sought elsewhere.

Such a superstition is the widespread practice of "knocking on wood." Funk and Wagnall's *Standard Dictionary of Folklore* describes this as "one of the commonest superstitions in all lands and cultures," and "one of the few retained when others are abandoned by the sophisticated" (16, p. 585). Hardly a week goes by either in clinical practice or social relationships in which one does not observe some individual performing this ceremonial. Often, it is true, it is carried out with a defensive smile; sometimes it is merely thought, but not actually done; and occasionally it is executed in a quasi-humorous manner, as when an individual says "knock on wood" and then taps on his skull. The psychoanalytically oriented observer, however, will recognize that the intent may be as real in these symbolic acts as it is in the more direct one, even though the action is defensively masked or distorted.

The historical roots of this superstition are shrouded in obscurity. Most students of folklore trace it back to the earliest times in which men worshiped certain beneficent spirits which were believed to inhabit trees of various species (12). Certain trees were identified with certain deities. In Ancient Greece the oak was considered sacred to Zeus; in Scandinavia the ash tree was dedicated to Thor, God of Thunder; while in Egypt the sycamore was believed sacred to the Goddess Hathor. In time the cult of the oak tree became the dominant one over most of Europe. The oak was thought to be the dwelling place of the Sky and Thunder God, probably because it was the tree most commonly struck by lightning. It was believed, further, that the winds conveyed the thoughts of men to the leaves of the oak which then communicated them to the spirit god within. Thus, to avert evil through boasting, sympathetic magic in the form of touching the oak had to be employed. This meant that one would be rendered immune to the vengeance of the irritable Sky God. From the touching of the oak, the superstition evidently evolved in time to the belief that the touching of any piece of wood would ward off evil from a boasting assertion.

In the further course of time, the spirits associated with trees were represented by posts, idols or masks (15b). Altars were added and the trunk was roughly shaped to represent the superhuman occupant. This was probably the origin of idol worship. Following the death of Christ this ancient superstition is believed to have been transferred to the cult of the Holy Cross and to the practice of sanctuary, in which a hunted person touching the door of a church was regarded as under the protection of the Church and of the Holy Cross which the church signified. A similar development of a new tradition to rationalize the persistence of an ancient custom can be observed in the Holy Land, where hallowed trees are often connected with the names of saints or prophets.

The practice of knocking on wood, as is well known, is generally performed whenever any announcement signifying good health, success, or good fortune is made. Underlying this ritual, therefore, must be the assumption that such an announcement will antagonize some all-seeing or all-hearing Higher Authority. There are many folk expressions which reflect this widespread conviction. "Pride goeth before a fall" and "He that talks of happiness summons grief" are typical examples. The counterpart of this is expressed with equal frequency in the concept that God or Fate prefers man to be humble. "Blessed are the humble" and "The meek shall inherit the earth" exemplify this belief.

There are many examples in Greco-Roman mythology which illustrate the belief that the gods resent pride in mortals, or are jealous of them. The conflicts of Jupiter and Juno with their mortal rivals, and Minerva's famous contest with Arachne come to mind. Perhaps the most touching story of this kind, however, is that of Niobe, Queen of Thebes, who had "failed to learn the lesson of humility" and had the temerity to boast pridefully of her seven sons and seven daughters, and claim superiority over the goddess Latona, who had had only two children. Latona's indignation impelled her children, Apollo and Diana, to seek immediate vengeance, and one by one all of Niobe's fourteen children were struck dead by arrows sent from the clouds. Her grief-stricken husband destroyed himself, and Niobe herself was so overwhelmed by her desolation that she turned to stone, but her tears continued to flow. Thus she remained forever "a mass of rock, from which a trickling stream flows, the tribute of her never-ending grief" (1, p. 95).

It has long been recognized that the gods and goddesses involved in these examples of folklore are parent surrogates, and that these myths represent cultural projections of elements in the pattern of experience between the child and these authority figures. It is reasonable to assume, therefore, that these myths and folk beliefs concerning the jealousy of the gods and their insistence on man's humility have a significant counterpart, in the societies in which they occur, in certain basic aspects of the child's relationship with his parent.

One of the genetic sources of these beliefs in our culture must be the competitive and hostile attitude of the child to the parent of the opposite sex, which often becomes projected in the child's fantasy life as competitiveness and hostility on the part of that parent to the child. But in addition to these well-known oedipal feelings, the child in our culture also has feelings of resentment toward the parent of *either* sex who enforces the disciplinary prohibitions upon the child's wish to live by the pleasure principle. The average child in our society, however, is not free to express this hostility for fear of losing the parental love and protection which are the core of his emotional security. The basic formula involved in this aspect of the child-parent relationship can be expressed as follows: "If I am docile and submissive and acknowledge the authority of the parent, I will be loved and protected; if I am not, I will be punished."

I believe that this aspect of the parent-child relationship is a highly significant one for most people in our culture. Even where relatively "progressive" concepts of child upbringing dominate the association between parent and child, this formula still tends to be one of the most important operational factors between them. It is not limited only to the "oedipal" period, but pervades every aspect of the application of social restraints to the child's pursuit of the pleasure principle from infancy through adolescence—weaning, bowel training, keeping clean, eating properly, brushing teeth, going to sleep at a proper hour, doing homework, practicing a musical instrument, and all the countless other elements which go under the broad category of discipline or training in our society.

Despite subsequent cultural emphasis on emotional independence and self-assertiveness, traces of the earlier configurations are rarely entirely eliminated, and may find partial expression in the kind of popular superstition of which "knocking on wood" is a representative example. To the degree to which earlier dependency attitudes still exert an active influence upon ego function, any action or thought which carries with it an implication of self-sufficiency is subjectively perceived as a dangerous one. In my clinical experience, when the practice of knocking on wood is strongly present in an individual, it is invariably associated with a high degree of emotional immaturity toward authority figures.

Let me make clear at this point that I am not implying that this type of superstition is universal in our culture or that it exists with equal intensity among all who exhibit it. There are all gradations of dependence upon this practice, from those individuals in whom it is quite mild and who can forswear using it with relatively little inner tension, to those in whom any effort to control it would lead to intense anxiety. For the latter group of persons, a self-confident or boastful remark carries the unconscious implication that one might be so self-sufficient as not to require the protection of the parent or parent symbol. By knocking on wood the individual denies and undoes this "aggressive" implication, and magically propitiates the authority symbol. The psychiatrically oriented person will readily recognize this as a compulsively ritualistic act closely related in form and in unconscious dynamics to practices observed in obsessive-compulsive neuroses.

But the unconscious relationship to parental authority in the life history of the individual is probably not the only factor involved in the widespread incidence of the wood-knocking superstition. There is reason to think that rivalry factors rooted in certain specific aspects of our culture play a significant contributory role. The competitive nature of our social structure makes every person a potential rival against every other person for the goods and gratifications of life. One of the common techniques employed for warding off the envy and hostility inherent in such rivalry is to deny or minimize one's own prosperity or good fortune. We see this reflected in countless patterns of behavior and speech in contemporary society. Many individuals respond to queries concerning their health with "not bad," rather than "excellent." A businessman whose enterprise is flourishing, when asked how business is going, often conceals his success with the noncommittal comment of "could be better" or "fair." A patient who bought a new car experienced anxiety when a neighbor enviously complimented him upon it, and felt constrained to reply, "Yes, it's nice, but I don't know how I'm going to pay for it." Another, upon purchase of a luxurious new home, felt it necessary to inform everyone who admired it that he had obtained it for only a fraction of its true worth. The reticence of most people—even with intimate friends or relatives—concerning their material assets is a striking phenomenon in our culture. Many people will discuss intimate aspects of their sex lives sooner than the details of their financial structure, particularly if there are assets which might arouse envy. Not infrequently, on the other hand, persons will have no hesitancy in proclaiming their indigence or the degree of their indebtedness to all the world; they may even falsely claim poverty when they are in fact affluent.

Occasionally the maintenance of an air of misery may become one of the central character defenses of an individual. A patient, in analysis, brought out that she was deeply convinced that if she allowed herself to feel happy something bad would happen to her. A favorite poem of hers, by A. E. Housman (8), aptly expressed her characteristic approach to life:

> The thoughts of others
> Were light and fleeting,
> Of lovers meeting
> Or luck or fame.
> Mine were of trouble,
> And mine were steady,
> So I was ready
> When trouble came.

A similar defensive pattern is seen in the characteristic tendency of many people to anticipate the worst when they are engaged in some competitive pursuit, as if to claim any expectation of success would bring ill-fortune. The tendency of students before an examination to bewail their chances, and the traditional pessimism of football coaches are cases in point.

Sometimes even the assumption that one will continue living is unconsciously perceived as a dangerous piece of complacency which Fate will punish. Accordingly, disclosure of plans for the future is often tempered by the phrases "God willing," or "If I live," etc. A recent research study (9) of the beliefs of pregnant women in contemporary society revealed an interesting superstition which is related to this concept. This is the fear that many pregnant women have of buying the layette for their children prior to the seventh or eighth month of pregnancy. As one woman put it, "If you plan way in advance, something might happen." In some instances this superstition concerning the making of preparations in advance extends even to the fear of choosing a name for the child prior to its actual birth.

A related phenomenon is the fear of success which is encountered clinically. To many people success is an anxiety-provoking event because they fear it may arouse the envious retaliation of others, as well as deprive then of dependent protection. One patient, in whom knocking on wood had all the force of a compulsive ritual, and who developed severe anxiety if he attempted to restrain it, graphically expressed the dynamic significance of his fear of success by describing being successful as the equivalent of "walking around with an erection." To him success clearly meant challenging the authoritarian father figures in his life and arousing the danger of their castrative retaliation. This flight from self-assertiveness is a widespread phenomenon in our culture and has been fully discussed by Erich Fromm (6).

The question of the degree to which the factor of exposure or nonexposure to such superstitions plays a part in people's employment of them may well be raised at this point. It must be obvious that if a person were never exposed to a specific superstition the likelihood of his utilizing it would be nonexistent. The fact is, however, that few, if any, people in our culture grow up without at some time or other coming into contact with the more common superstitious beliefs. Whether or not an individual adopts such a belief once he encounters it, and the degree to which he may be governed by it, will depend to a significant extent, I believe, on some of the underlying psychodynamic factors which I have described.

However, in a deeper sense, the question of whether or not people actually exhibit the superstition of knocking on wood is secondary to the basic patterns of feeling within a society which this type of superstition reflects. Where such superstitions persist and survive they are merely indicators of underlying patterns of intrasocial hostility and envy, with consequent fears of success and self-assertiveness. These basic attitudes are far more widespread in our society than are the specific superstitions which a segment of the population utilizes as a form of magical defense against them.

Still other questions may be asked at this point. Are there not also attitudes in our culture which are directly antithetical to those described in this paper? Is there also not a striving for self-assertiveness? Are there not also strong tendencies to the ostentatious display of success and prosperity? Is not success admired as well as envied? These statements, of course, are true, but these antithetical attitudes represent the opposite side of the very same coin which we are describing. It is precisely because almost everyone in our society desires success and competes for it that there tends to be, among those who achieve it, a fear of arousing hostile envy. The simultaneous existence of these contradictory attitudes, far from being surprising, is a psychological and cultural inevitability.

A superstition very closely related to "knocking on wood," which similarly illustrates the fear of success and the warding off of competitive envy, is the custom of abjuring the "evil eye," which has its origin in a widespread ancient belief that certain persons could bewitch, harm, or even kill with a glance. In contrast to the superstition of knocking on wood, that of the "evil eye" generally (but not always) postulates a more personal and identifiable source of danger. This practice of "overlooking," as it is often called, is usually considered to be malicious. It is apt most frequently to be applied to people who are healthy, prosperous and happy. The living symbols of such happiness, such as attractive children or valuable animals, are considered especially vulnerable to the evil eye, as are also nursing mothers. The bridal veil is thought to have originated as a specific protection against overlooking, for the happy bride is thought to be a special target of the envious (16, p. 838). It is more than likely that the Mohammedan custom of keeping their women veiled has a similar historical origin (4, p.235).

Géza Róheim wrote about the evil eye in one of his last papers

(13, p. 283), and brings out a number of facts which shed additional light on this phenomenon. He points out that old women and witches (both projections of the envious mother figure) are especially apt to be possessors of the evil eye. (I cannot agree with Róheim, however, that the evil-eye superstition is always a projection of the aggression of the sucking infant onto the person of the witch-mother. Its meaning, as we shall see, is more generalized.) Some Mohammedans, Róheim points out (p. 287), believe that "to take food in the presence of some hungry looker-on is to take poison," and they "are told to serve guests the same quality of food which they themselves take, to avoid the evil eye." Also "the guest must always be served first, otherwise the evil eye, or the evil wishes of the guest will be mobilized."

In this relationship between food and envy, one can discern, as Róheim indicates, that one of the key factors in the evil-eye belief is "oral" envy and "oral" aggression.* The expressions to "devour with one's eyes" or "his eyes are bigger than his stomach" (to signify that one desires more than he can eat) are indicators of the relationship between visual envy and oral aggression, and may be a clue to the earliest psychological roots of the evil-eye concept. That is to say, when the success or good fortune of an individual is seen by the symbolic parents or siblings, they are presumably filled with envy and with a desire either to orally incorporate (possess) the good fortune themselves, or else to orally devour (destroy) it. In this way, looking with envy becomes equivalent to destroying, and must be warded off by the proper magical phrase or action.

Thus, among many peoples, praise of anything which may stimulate envy in others, particularly of fine children or animals, is followed by the statement "May the evil eye not strike it," or by the invocation of God's blessing upon it.

It is interesting to note that in Scotland the most potent charm

---

*An obvious corollary to this is the implication that success causes pain to the onlooker. A German folk saying quoted to me by a patient aptly illustrates this point:

Nicht hoch gelebt,	(Fly not high,
Nicht hoch geflogen.	Live not high.
Reiss nicht aus	Pluck not out
Des anderen augen.	The other's eye.)

against the evil eye was a branch of mountain ash (rowan wood), thus confirming the close relationship that clearly exists between the wood-touching superstition and that of the evil eye. Similar charms have been described in Norway, Sweden, Germany, and various parts of the United States.

The good luck charms and religious medals so widely worn by large groups within our population are also derivations of the amulets which were carried in ancient times as protections against the evil eye.

Róheim, in the reference cited, speculates about the possible unconscious significance of the various symbols used as countermagic against the evil eye, and suggests that they are essentially phallic symbols. The most obvious example of this is the myth of Perseus who, with his sword, destroys the evil-eye symbol of Medusa. One might draw similar inferences about the earliest meaning of tree worship, since trees often represent phallic symbols in the unconscious, although wood itself at times appears as a maternal symbol, or even a bisexual symbol (14). Such speculations, however, are only of academic interest at best, since the current meaning of a widespread practice of this kind must be sought in the cultural phenomena which perpetuate it, rather than in its possible earliest psychodynamic significance. The use of a particular amulet, for example, after thousands of years of cultural transmission, can no longer be explained in terms of its original psychological meaning.

Of much greater importance than this kind of speculation, I believe, is the relationship between these "envy superstitions" and the cultural patterns of the societies in which they are found.

It would be of great importance to know whether this kind of superstition has existed in all times and in all cultures, or whether it makes its appearance only under certain conditions. One fact stands out importantly in this regard. *There are primitive societies in which this particular kind of magic does not exist.* That is not to say that they do not employ magic. Magical practices exist in *all* cultures so far as is known. But the magic in primitive societies like the Zuñi, Trobriand, and others, although used for many purposes—e.g., to invoke the help of the gods in certain ventures, to obtain revenge for insults or injuries, to destroy a real enemy or danger, etc.—does not exhibit the particular quality of the warding off of envy or of the fear of success to which the superstitions of knocking on wood or abjuring the evil eye are related. What is the difference, if any, between the societies in which these superstitions exist and those in which they do not? Ralph Linton, the noted anthropologist, has reported a study of two closely related cultures which is extremely suggestive in this regard (11a, p. 349; 11b, p. 251).

The first of these is the Tanala, a hill tribe of Western Madagascar. Prior to about 200 years ago the economic basis of their life was the cultivation of dry rice by the cutting and burning method. This gave a good crop the first year and a moderately good one 5 to 10 years later, after which the land had to be abandoned for 20 to 25 years until there was a heavy new growth of jungle. The usual native method was to utilize as much of the original jungle as possible, with the village in the center, then to move the village each year to a new locality and begin the process again. Under these conditions there was no opportunity for individual ownership of land to develop. The village as a whole owned it. Family members all worked the land in a group, and if a family had bad luck with its crop one year, the village elders would give it an advantage the next. As a result, no marked inequalities in wealth between the joint families ever developed, and subsistence was guaranteed to all.

With the development of the cultivation of wet rice, there was a striking change in the social organization of the Tanala. Since rice terraces grew crops most of the year, the land which they occupied never really went out of use, and therefore never reverted to the village to be reassigned. Only a limited amount of land could be utilized for wet rice cultivation, and those households which had not had the energy and foresight to take up wet rice land at first soon found themselves permanently excluded. Thus over a period of 100 years there slowly grew up, within what had formerly been a classless society, a class of landowners, finally culminating around 1840 in the setting up of a definite caste system with a king and a hereditary nobility.

What interests us primarily, however, is the change that took place as a consequence in the psychology of the individual in Tanala society. The change is seen most sharply when we contrast it to the psychology of the Betsileo, a tribe of wet rice cultivators located just to the east of the Tanala. To quote Linton: "We can regard Betsileo as the Tanala culture, after all the changes consequent upon wet rice had become consolidated, organized, and institutionalized" (11b, p. 284).

Comparing superstitious beliefs among the Betsileo, then, with those among the early Tanala, what do we find? There was a striking absence of the fear of sorcery among the early Tanala. (This was less true of the later Tanala when the introduction of wet rice led to rudimentary class differentiation.) Malevolent magic did exist, but it was used as a weapon only against other lineages, never within one. Moreover, it was never used as an instrument of envy, but only for purposes of revenge for actual injuries received—for insults, for nonpayment of debts, or for refusal of a daughter requested in marriage.

Among the Betsileo, on the other hand, malevolent magic played a far greater role in the life of the individual. The approaching birth of a child was not announced, for fear of sorcery. Malevolent sorcerers, who were very scarce in old Tanala, were believed to be very numerous in Betsileo. Everyone, in fact, was suspected of being one! There was a marked increase in belief in omens, dreams and superstitions as contrasted to the Tanala, and much more general apprehension. The superstitions all indicated some fear of retaliatory misfortune. When a person died at the moment of a good harvest he was believed to have been killed by his wealth—a testimony to the power attributed to the hostile envy of others.

What conclusions can we draw concerning the cultural roots of this type of envy-superstition from this study of Linton's? It seems to suggest that a significant factor in their origin may be the development within a society of a group which controls the means of subsistence, in contrast to a group which does not. Under such circumstances the activation of "oral" envy within that culture may find expression in superstitions which reflect the anxiety of the "haves" in relationship to the "have-nots." Success, then, becomes something which, although universally sought, once achieved, is concealed as a potential target of envy and aggression from others.

It is interesting to note that sibling-rivalry and oedipal-rivalry factors alone do not seem to suffice in themselves to produce this type of superstitious belief. Although such factors exist in many primitive communal societies and are reflected in their myths and magical beliefs, the specific fear of success seems to make its appearance only where differential ownership of the sources of subsistence develops within the group. It is significant that the myth of the jealous god is found only in such relatively more differentiated societies. It is perhaps superfluous, but nonetheless important, to note also that these cultural influences do not operate in any mysterious or impersonal manner. They are conveyed to the individual originally through the medium of the family, particularly the parents, and subsequently through other interpersonal relationships, and become part of the individual's own intrapsychic equipment through the well-known mechanisms of identification and introjection. In more complex societies like our own, other media of communication, such as schools, radio, television, movies, newspapers and books, also become significant avenues of transmission of cultural attitudes.

The relationship between superstitious practices and various religious ceremonials, obsessional rituals, and even psychotic delusions has been commented upon by many observers (2, 5, 10).

It is of interest in this regard to note that the most superstitious person I have ever encountered in clinical practice was also a severe obsessional neurotic and an intensely devout person insofar as the observance of religious rituals was concerned. Both of his parents were strongly religious* and great emphasis was placed throughout his childhood on a strict observance of all of the orthodox rituals and practices of their religion. To fail in the observance of any of them was regarded as a serious breach of faith which was certain to call down the punishment of God in some manner.

As far back as the patient could remember, magical and superstitious thinking had played an important part in his life. There was no popular superstition to which he did not defer. He knocked on wood, avoided walking under ladders, feared black cats, broken

---

*In any of the comments concerning religion which follow, I am referring only to its authoritarian, idolatrous, magical or ritualistic aspects, not to its ethical aspects, which have nothing in common with superstition.

mirrors, the number 13, etc., and any unavoidable breach of these superstitions and many others was attended by intense anxiety. He manifested a strong conviction of the magical omnipotence of thought, and any mention of disaster-laden words such as death, disease, or injury, or of certain key numbers, was absolutely taboo in his presence.

When each of his parents died he reacted with intense guilt and blamed their deaths on some minor transgressions on his part. In each instance he tried to expiate his guilt partially by a rigid observance of all of the orthodox religious rituals required of him. More than twenty years after his father's death, any failure on the patient's part to perform the required rituals on the anniversary of the death was attended by severe anxiety and self-recrimination.

Without going into an exposition of the complex psychodynamics of this patient (which would require a separate paper in itself), it is clear that his superstitions, obsessional and religious rituals all represented efforts at dealing with anxiety by regression to that phase of magical, omnipotent thinking through which children in our culture pass when they become aware of their helplessness in the face of frustration (3). The purpose of this regressive thinking is to enlist the support of, or to ward off the anticipated hostility of, the omnipotent parent symbol variously designated as God, Fate, or Luck. The ritual employed, whether religious, obsessional or superstitious, is a form of magic, the unconscious dynamics of which are no different essentially from those underlying the magical practices of ancient or primitive peoples.*

In summary, in this paper we have attempted to explore the psychological and cultural roots of one of the commonest of modern superstitions—the practice of knocking on wood. We have postulated that it represents an unconscious effort to achieve protection against envy and hostility from two potential sources, those representing parental or authority symbols, and those representing sibling symbols. The assumption that pride, success or self-confidence will arouse

---

*This does not negate, however, the integrative value which religious rituals have for many individuals in our society. Where practices have widespread social sanction, as in religion, their ego-syntonic value is, of course, far greater than that of practices which the society regards as deviant.

the antagonism or envy of the authority symbol is seen as being in part a genetic derivation of earlier parent-child relationships in our culture—a projection of the child's envy of and hostility to the parents and siblings, as well as a perpetuation of the archaic childhood conception that to be loved by the authority figure it is necessary to be humble, submissive and compliant. We have seen, however, that an additional factor, which apparently has also to be present for this type of superstition to develop in a culture, is the kind of socioeconomic system which results in strong intrasocial competitiveness, hostility and envy.

An important implication of these facts is that we cannot expect that such superstitious practices will disappear or even diminish merely with further advances in man's scientific or technological knowledge, since their existence depends more on unconscious emotional factors than on conscious intellectual ones. Only as the personal and cultural sources of man's unconscious feelings of helplessness and insecurity are resolved will his dependence on magic diminish.

REFERENCES

1. BULFINCH, THOMAS. *Bulfinch's Mythology.* Modern Lib., New York, 1934.
2. CAMPBELL, CHARLES MACFIE. *Delusion and Belief,* p. 8. Harvard Univ. Press, Cambridge, 1927.
3. FERENCZI, SANDOR. "Stages in the Development of the Sense of Reality" (1913), in *Sex and Psychoanalysis,* p. 213. Basic Books, New York, 1950.
4. FIELDING, WILLIAM J. *Strange Superstitions and Magical Practices.* Blakiston, Philadelphia, 1945.
5. FREUD, S. "Obsessive Acts and Religious Practices," in *Collected Papers,* Vol. 2, p. 25. Hogarth Press, London, 1907.
6. FROMM, ERICH. *Escape from Freedom.* Farrar & Rinehart, New York, 1941.
7. HAND, WAYLAND. Personal communication.
8. HOUSMAN, A. E. *Collected Poems,* p. 165. Henry Holt, New York, 1940.
9. KAUFMAN, LORRAINE. Personal communication concerning her doctoral thesis, Department of Anthropology and Sociology, Univ. of California, Los Angeles.
10. KAUFMAN, M. RALPH. *Religious Delusions in Schizophrenia.* Internat. J. Psychoanal., 20: 1939.
11. LINTON, RALPH. (a) *The Study of Man.* Appleton-Century, New York, 1936. (b) Also in Abram Kardiner. *The Individual and His Society.* Columbia Univ. Press, New York, 1939.
12. RADFORD, E. and M. A. *Encyclopedia of Superstitions,* pp. 243–244. Rider, London, 1947.

13. RÓHEIM, GÉZA. "The Evil Eye," in *Yearbook of Psychoanalysis*, Vol. 9. Internat. Univ. Press, New York, 1953.
14. SAUL, LEON J. *Wood as a Bisexual Symbol.* Psychoanal. Quart., 20: 616, 1951.
15. *Encyclopaedia Britannica.* (14th ed.) (a) Vol. 21, p. 577. (b) Vol. 22, p. 446. New York and London, 1929.
16. *Standard Dictionary of Folklore, Mythology and Legend,* Vol. 2, Funk & Wagnalls, New York, 1950.

4

THE INDIVIDUAL, THE FAMILY

AND THE COMMUNITY

(1959)

As a consequence of increasing interdisciplinary communication among psychiatry, psychology, sociology and anthropology, there has been a growing awareness in recent years of their complex interrelatedness and interdependence. Social anthropologists, who used to deal chiefly with descriptions of the external trappings of various cultures, have become progressively concerned with understanding the origins and the meanings of diverse cultural institutions and their relationship to individual and family life within the culture. Conversely, psychiatrists and clinical psychologists have begun to realize that no awareness of individual psychodynamics truly can be complete without an understanding of the complex interpenetration of individual personality development with family structure, community organization and cultural mores. This is not to imply that these various disciplines are merging and losing their distinctive orientations, but, like specialists in the field of medicine, each is learning that its own complexities can be understood best only by a full awareness of all its interrelationships.

In the remarks which follow I shall endeavor to explore some present-day aspects of the intricate interdependency that exists among individual, family and community in America. We are living in an era of extraordinary change—change which is occurring at a tempo that probably has no previous parallel in the entire history of man. The technologic innovations which scientists predict within the next 10 to 25 years in the uses of atomic energy, in automation, in techniques of communication, in transportation over and under the surface of our planet and in travel into space, to mention but a few, stagger the imagination. What changes these ultimately will bring with them in the patterns of family life and in the personality of man can only be guessed at and perhaps, for the time being, are best left to the creative imaginations of the science fiction writers.

Indeed, if we try to survey the transformations that are going on even in contemporary community and family life the task is almost equally difficult. This is not merely because the rapidly changing scene is apt to make our conclusions obsolete almost before they are reached but also because ours is a particularly complex society. There is much less of the uniformity here that characterizes some of the societies of the Old World; and although the sharp cutting down the stream of immigration in the past four decades has resulted in the melting pot of American life being stirred into greater homogeneity than ever before, the subcultural variations in mores are still quite considerable among different classes, races and ethnic groups within our country.

Therefore, generally, when social scientists talk about "the American family," they are discussing an abstraction—one based primarily on the native-born, white, urban middle class, which constitutes the largest single subcultural group within our country, and the one whose standards and aspirations form the prevailing ethos toward which most other groups tend to gravitate. With the understanding, then, that this is our focus also, let us turn to the consideration of the effects of the contemporary community on the prototypal American family and its individual members.

It is necessary at the outset that we clarify the specific sense in which we are using the term "community," since it is a vague concept which can refer to anything from a county to a continent. However, we shall use it in a much more limited sense to refer to *neighborhood*— the immediate physical and subcultural environment in which any particular family finds itself. In this sense the community traditionally always has been an important intermediary between the culture at large and the family, acting on both and, in turn, being acted upon by both.

The significant fact about the contemporary American community is that its specific influence on family life has been diminishing steadily over the past several decades. The chief reasons for this are to be found in the progressive changes that have taken place in communication and transportation. In earlier days people living together in a community were inevitably linked closely together by their geographic proximity. The barriers that stood in the way of communication with people in other areas, as well as the difficulties in transportation, held the members of the community together in bonds of mutual interest. They worked together, played together and prayed together. The community thus tended to have a high degree of stability and homogeneity which strengthened its ability to maintain social control. Each neighbor was known to every other one, and their mutual interdependency made it important to retain one another's good will, thus enhancing the pattern of mutual regulation. The social and the religious activities, the marriages, the births and the deaths were all shared experiences which led to common traditions and consistent community standards.

Today, however, the prototypal community is no longer the integrated unit that it once was. The development of the telephone, the automobile, rapid transit and air transportation have dissolved almost completely the geographic barriers which once gave the community its stability. As often as not, especially in the large urban areas and upper-middle-class suburban centers, people have no more than a nodding acquaintance with their neighbors. Their friends often live in widely separated areas, and the social, economic and recreational life of the family is no longer rooted in the geographic community.

The effect of this social fragmentation upon patterns of family life has been important and far-reaching. By making each family a relatively isolated unit in the community, it has contributed significantly to the deep inner feeling of isolation, the sense of loneliness within the crowd, that seems to characterize so many people in our time. This tendency towards isolation of the family, together with the overall trend towards smaller family groups in recent decades, also has favored the development of intensified intrafamilial dependency patterns. "Family romances" and oedipal ties, overprotectiveness, and "smother-love" all tend to flourish luxuriantly in the hothouse atmosphere of the isolated family. I believe that this has been a significant factor in the increased incidence of passive-dependent, immature personalities who are so often encountered in present-day psychiatric practice.

The dependency of today's child upon his parents is further accentuated by the actual physical aspects of modern community life. The street is no longer a safe place for play, and the growing scarcity of land in urban residential areas has led to the disappearance of the numerous neighborhood "vacant lots" which used to provide easily accessible and natural playgrounds for children. Playmates for the child often have to be specially arranged for by his parents and even imported from other neighborhoods.* As a result, the child's life, outside of school, tends often to be a relatively isolated one. Thus the modern middle-class American child seems to be in danger of losing one of the important values that used to be derived from community living—the learning process that comes from belonging to a group of peers and acquiring a social identity in the course of growing up with them. The lessons of social competition, social adaptation, leadership and submission often were learned far more effectively in the peer society of the local commuity than anywhere else.

Still another effect of the isolation of the family within the fragmented community is the loss of the sense of trust toward others that an integrated community used to foster. A man's word is no longer considered his bond. Almost everyone outside of the family circle is regarded as a stranger, and the stranger is not to be trusted. A gesture of friendship, an act of kindness, is apt to be met with the suspicious inner feeling of "I wonder what he *wants* from me," or "What's in it for him?" The traditional American motto of "In God we trust," now tends to carry the cynical addendum "All others pay cash!" and the Golden Rule of "Do unto others as you would have them do unto you" is often replaced by the brassier one of "Do others before they do you!"

Despite the fact that the community was an important instrument of local social control, it also was a significant factor in individuation. Mark Twain's Hannibal, Missouri, Sherwood Anderson's Winesburg, Ohio, and Edgar Lee Masters' Spoon River all left their distinctive

---

*This, of course, is not true in small towns, or in lower or lower middle class urban neighborhoods. (J. M., 1973)

imprints upon their inhabitants. With the loss of cohesion of community life, people's personalities bear less and less of the stamp of the relatively individualized community subculture but instead become more and more responsive to the influences of the culture at large. One of the consequences of this has been the growing trend toward conformity, which numerous students of the current scene have noted with concern. Erich Fromm has described it in the context of "escape from freedom" and "alienation from the self," David Riesman has done so in terms of the tendency to "other-directedness," William Whyte, Jr., in terms of "the organization man," and Erik Erikson in terms of the "loss of personal identity," but they are all describing the same phenomenon. People all over the country read the same magazines and books, see the same movies and TV programs, hear the same broadcasts. They wear the same clothes, drive the same kinds of cars, strive to live in the same kinds of houses with the same kinds of appliances and furnishings. Indeed, even many of the differentiating aspects of urban and rural living which used to distinguish the "city slicker" from the "hayseed" are in the process of disappearing, as today's farmer is exposed to more and more of the same communication media as is the city dweller, and rapid transportation brings him nearer and nearer to the influences of urban life.

The fact that the pressures in our culture toward conformity grow steadily stronger is no accidental occurrence. They grow naturally out of the conditions of intensified industrialization and automation of our economy and represent the kind of "social character" which an increasingly complex technologic society requires. The artisan, the ruggedly independent individual who took pride in the product that he fashioned from beginning to end and who was known to and patronized by his neighbors, is a rapidly disappearing phenomenon. In his place is the anonymous cog in the vast assembly line of production, where things are produced infinitely more efficiently and cheaply but necessarily alike. To fit into the assembly line, whether it be at the level of production or distribution, whether in the factory, in the clerical or the managerial ranks, or in the advertising apparatuses designed to create the needs that keep the assembly lines rolling, the human individual must submerge his individuality and his unique personal identity in terms of the group needs of the apparatus. The ideal of the inner-directed Renaissance Man has gradually given way to that of the other-directed Organization Man.

The remarkable rise in productive efficiency in contemporary American society has led to increasing emphasis on the need for increased domestic consumption to absorb the ever-increasing national product. To accomplish this, the techniques of advertising and merchandising have reached levels of efficiency previously undreamed of. The manner in which they have employed all of the knowledge of human motivation provided by modern individual and group psychology has been ably documented by Vance Packard in his book *The Hidden Persuaders* (1). An important consequence of this societal need has been a significant change in the Protestant Ethic which had been the social character required by earlier industrial societies and dominated community life of the past. In a society of abundance, the social emphasis necessarily shifts from being thrifty to spending more and more. It is now more important to have credit at the bank than money in it. In our increasingly automated society, the emphasis is shifting from the sanctification of hard work to the glorification of leisure-time activities in the support of which large industries have developed. As one of the high priests of the new marketing ethic, Dr. Ernest Dichter, has put it, "We are now confronted with the problem of permitting the average American to feel moral . . . even when he is spending, even when he is not saving, even when he is taking two vacations a year and buying a second and third car. One of the basic problems of this prosperity . . . is to give people the sanction and the justification to enjoy it and to demonstrate that the hedonistic approach to this life is a moral, not an immoral one" (2).

However, as one might gather from Dr. Dichter's remarks, this shift has not been achieved without inner cost to the individual. The residuals of religious teachings and old identifications create much guilt and conflict in many of those who try to conform to the new ethic of the Abundant Society. Although the conflict may not be conscious, their reactions at times seem to suggest, in the words of Elinor Wylie, that in "the Puritan marrow of (their) bones, there's something in this richness that (they) hate." The frenetic quality of the acquisitiveness and the pleasure-seeking that characterizes many modern Americans, like the forced gaiety of a New Year's Eve party, suggests a reaction-formation to deny the unconscious guilt, the emotional insecurity and the loss of personal identity that lie behind it.

The development of automation with its diminished need for huge labor forces, plus the increasing prosperity of the middle class, has led to another striking phenomenon which is having an important effect on family life—namely, the increasing move out of the large urban centers into the suburbs. Spectorsky (3) has described a syndrome which characterizes many families in the suburbs, to which he has given the name Destination Sickness. He describes it as "the constellation of physical and psychic disorders and discomforts which ensue on the artificial and premature attainment of deceptive and inadequate goals." The prototypal suburbanite whom he describes is surrounded by all the latest consumer gadgets and appliances—all bought on time. His house and car are mortgaged to the hilt but represent the best he can manage—on credit—in his and his wife's frantic effort to keep up with the Jones's. His work is in an organization in which he performs a specialized, fragmentary function which gives him little satisfaction and no real opportunity for self-expression. His inner emptiness, plus the tensions from which he suffers in the process of trying to support the pyramid of possessions which he has been driven to purchase, leave him little capacity to enjoy the leisure which our society allows him. His weekends are apt to be a torment of boredom and emptiness, and he looks forward with relief to his assembly-line activities Monday morning. At least he knows what to do with himself then. His wife, too, suffers from a similar emptiness which she seeks to fill by acquiring new possessions. She makes a career of haunting the department stores, following the "sales," and daily adding to the conglomeration of possessions, many of which are never even used. Possession for possession's sake—the accumulation of things as symbols of security—is a passion which obsesses countless modern American families. The "conspicuous consumption" which Thorstein Veblen once attributed to the small, rich "leisure class" has become the dominant goal of American society as a whole.

How do these facets of contemporary life become transmitted to the personality of the individual in our society? One of the most important ways is through the pattern of unconscious identification with the parents, by means of which much of the child's image of himself and his world is formed. In almost all societies parents are the most significant purveyors to their children of the values and mores of the culture. Parents who are anxious, confused, unsure of what they believe or do not believe, concerned only with social approval and material possessions, cannot help passing these attitudes on to their children. In an age of conformity, children learn very early from their parents that the most important thing in life is not to be one's self but rather "to be liked," to win the approval of others. As Riesman has put it: "Approval itself, irrespective of content, becomes almost the only unequivocal good in this situation: one makes good when one is approved of. Thus all power, not merely some power, is in the hands of the actual or imaginary approving group, and the child learns from his parents' reactions to him that nothing in his character, no possession he owns, no inheritance of name or talent, no work he has done is valued for itself, but only for its effect on others" (4).

Success—and particularly material success—becomes the only criterion often of one's adequacy. Children grow up in an atmosphere of social competitiveness in which the home, the furniture and the family car become the measures by which they evaluate the status of their parents and themselves. Marital conflicts and tensions tend increasingly to revolve around these same issues. The "success" of a marriage, from the modern American woman's standpoint, often is gauged by the material status of her husband, rather than by his worth as a human being. By the same token, the man is apt to appraise the worth of his own marital selection in terms of either the material status or the beauty of his wife, both external "marketing" values which bring him the approval of others, rather than her intrinsic worth as a human being, companion and mate. As motivation researcher Louis Cheskin has suggested, the contemporary American makes his selection of a mate on the basis of the size, shape and wrapping of the package instead of on its contents! Little wonder, when the factors that determine marital choice are so lacking in inner values and relatedness, that the process of communication breaks down or indeed never genuinely develops within the family.

Of course, there are other factors involved. The working life of today's father is generally alien both to his wife and children in contrast with what it was in artisan days. In turn, the father usually has little real contact with the daily life of his wife or children. Thus, except for discussions of the trivia of everyday living, husband and wife, and parents and children, often have almost nothing to say to each other, and countless family evenings are spent in the semi-autism of television viewing. It would seem to be only a matter of time before each family member will have his own television set and be able to watch his own program in splendid isolation!

Admittedly, this is a rather extreme and bleak picture of the direction in which contemporary American family life seems to be moving. However, fortunately, this is not the entire picture. Just as in the individual neurosis regressive and reparative trends may exist side by side, the same seems to hold true at a sociologic level.

Social fragmentation creates inner feelings of loneliness and anxiety, and these in turn set into action strong motivational forces within the individual designed to counteract these feelings. Whether the social needs of human beings stem from biologically rooted "herd instincts," or whether they grow out of the early social conditioning dependent on the prolonged helplessness of the human infant, may be a debatable issue, but that these social needs exist and are powerful sources of human motivation is unquestionable. In the face of the decay of community influence and the trend towards family isolation that has ensued, there are indications that the group needs of people in our society are reasserting themselves in new ways.

Some of these indications in the postwar era have been the steady lowering of age at marriage, the decline in numbers of single adults, and the increase in birth rates. There are many others. For example, the widespread move to the suburbs that has been taking place in most large urban areas is not simply an automatic consequence of better transportation facilities. It also represents a genuine striving on the part of countless Americans to recapture the values of community living which they felt they were losing in the impersonal chaos of the big city. Indeed, to some extent, they do. If they fail, as often happens, it is not because their intentions were not good but because the community itself is no longer what it used to be.

The competitive strivings and the pressures towards conformity pursue the suburban family even more fiercely than they did in the city, and the more leisurely pace of living which the family sought turns out to be an illusion. Between keeping the home and the garden up to the community's standards, and afternoons and evenings spent on boards, committees, PTA's, scout meetings, church work, entertaining the "right" people, etc., the suburban mother and father may get so submerged in their strivings for "belong-ingness" that they find themselves with even less leisure time than they had in the city, and the sense of inner emptiness may be even greater than ever.

Still another evidence of reparative strivings on the part of contemporary Americans has been the remarkable rise in the number and the influence of churches and synagogues in this country in the past 15 or 20 years. This is undoubtedly an overdetermined phenomenon, with a number of different factors involved. For some people, membership in a religious group seems to represent a search for emotional security in an age of uncertainties and anxieties. For others, it seems to reflect a rebellion against the overwhelming materialism and "marketing orientation" of our society and a search for spiritual, ethical, and moral values that would restore the inner dignity of man and give his life a meaningfulness that it seems to have lost. However, for many, the modern church or synagogue represents a center for group activities, group relationships and group values which can take the place once held by the community in this respect. The religious center of today is less and less a place where people merely gather together to worship their God. More and more it has become a social and educational center. The religious school has become an increasingly important instrument for teaching children not merely religious values and rituals but also the group identifications and group mores which the family and the community have become less able to transmit. Similarly, the social functions of the church—the dances, the picnics, the men's clubs, the women's circles and sisterhoods, the teen-age groups and the little children's groups—embrace all members of the family and provide new centers for group-belongingness to combat the vacuum and loneliness that the disorganization of community influence has created.

There have been many other searchings for group membership in recent times—hobby clubs, fraternal and sororal lodges and organizations, country clubs and community centers, and while all have grown, none seems to have the vitality of the current religious revival.*

Of course, in a broad sense, the entire trend toward what has been called "togetherness" represents not only an aspect of the "social character" which an increasingly complex technologic society requires of its membership but also reflects an inner striving for emotional security from *within* the individual in such a society; and the tendency to frown upon patterns of behavior associated with lower and upperclass mores—violence, eccentricity, irresponsibility—is part of this striving. Still another reflection of it is the postwar decline of all extremist political movements, both on the left and on the right. The values of the "beat generation" with its angry and despairing rejection of the material values of our time have found no significant answering echoes in the college youth of today.†

The ego-reparative strivings of the individual in contemporary American society reflect themselves in many other ways also—some of them constructive, others not. The extraordinary popularity which self-help books in the area of mental health—from "dianetics" to the "power of positive thinking"—have enjoyed in the past decade is one of these. Other phenomena are indicative of efforts at the narcotization of loneliness and anxiety, notably the progressive rise in the consumption of alcohol. Less obvious but probably equally significant indications of this are the steady increase in cigarette smoking, cancer scares notwithstanding, and the enormous consumption of tranquilizing drugs.

Thus far we have directed our comments to the prototypal middle-class family primarily. However, no discussion of the relationship between community and family life in contemporary Ameri-

---

*In the 1960's and 70's one would also add the remarkable proliferation of Esalen-type "encounter groups" as another evidence of the widespread search for relief from feelings of alienation. (J. M., 1973)

†This was written during the Eisenhower era, before American youth were catalyzed into a new wave of social activism by the charismatic leadership of John F. Kennedy—and more recently into a rejection of conventional social values in the trend which Charles Reich, in *The Greening of America*, has labeled "Consciousness III." (J. M., 1973)

ca can ignore the problem of the urban lower class and the impact of its community and family life upon some of our present social problems.

The natural history of the modern industrial city follows a fairly characteristic pattern. Leaving out that increase of population due to the surplus of births over deaths, its chief other source of growth is through the migration of unskilled persons who come from rural areas and smaller cities, and from other countries. Most of these come in at the bottom of the industrial totem pole and are apt to settle in the cheapest residential districts, the slum and semi-slum areas. *One of the most significant facts about these slum communities is that their imprint upon their inhabitants tends to be the same regardless of the nature of the groups which occupy them.* This is not to imply that different groups do not leave different imprints on such neighborhoods but merely to emphasize that the major effect seems to be in the reverse direction. Consider the example of juvenile delinquency. Its incidence varies markedly according to the community. Slum sections, inhabited by the lowest paid working people, have the highest rates. On the other hand, as one moves outward towards the middle- and upper-class residential communities, there is a progressive drop in delinquency rate. This drop cannot be explained in terms of different racial or ethnic origins of the groups involved. Studies have shown that delinquency and crime rates in large urban centers for such groups as German, Irish, Scandinavian, Italian, Slavic, Mexican, Negro and Puerto Rican groups have all been high when these groups occupied slum neighborhoods at various periods in their history, and all decreased when they moved to better residential districts. Although the delinquency rates for each national or racial group within the same areas were not identical, the *variation between these groups was much less than the variation between areas.* A study by Stoffler (5) revealed that the homicide rate of a particular group was low among first generation European immigrants, high in the second generation, low again in the third. This would seem to indicate that the generation whose personalities developed in the stable communities of the Old World had healthy superegos; but that their children, raised in the slum communities to which they migrated, were much more prone to violent aggression. On the other hand, as the third generation began to improve its status and move out of the slums, the homicide rate again decreased. Therefore, it is clear that the behavioral patterns of these groups are influenced significantly by their community experiences and change when they move to other areas in which the aspects of community life and mores are different.

What is it about slum life that has this influence upon the individuals within it? The answer to this question is not a simple one and has many facets—social, economic and psychological. Sociologists used to attribute much of the area's problems to the assumption that the slums were essentially disorganized communities which lacked the inner cohesiveness and group sanctions which created social controls in other kinds of communities. More recent studies (6) have thrown doubt upon this assumption. The problem of the slum district often is not that it lacks organization but rather that its own organization and group standards fail to mesh with those of the dominant middle-class society around it. Since the slum's inhabitants are people who are regarded as inferiors and often exposed to discrimination by the rest of the community, it is not surprising that they develop group patterns of defensiveness and hostility. In addition, ignorance and prejudice often contribute to intense intracommunity hostilities between different racial, ethnic or religious groups within the slum area.

The effect on family life of such a community is a disorganizing one. Parents, deprived of their traditional settings and values, find themselves confused in their relationship to their children in their new setting. In many underprivileged homes the influence of the father is seriously undermined by the circumstances of his life. If he is not working, his authority and status within the home suffer, and he is either bitter or defeated. If he is employed, his work is apt to be hard, long and unrewarding, and he returns home exhausted or incapable of evincing any interest or control over his children—or else, bitter, tired and irritable, he may make them the scapegoats for the frustrations and indignities which he may have had to endure during the day. Often he stems from an authoritarian tradition which endeavors to impose harsh and strict disciplines upon the children. However, the absence of the group sanctions which existed in his original environment, plus the fact that in the new community he not only lacks social and economic status but may also be looked down on by his children as a foreigner, all serve to negate his efforts at such authoritarian control and to foster defiance and rebelliousness in his children.

On the other hand, the mother often has to work also in order to supplement the family's meager income; or else, as is frequently the case in lower income groups, she is harassed by a large brood of children and is weighed down by a never-ending mass of routine duties. In either event she often is unable to give any individual child the emotional guidance and warmth that he needs.

Under these circumstances, it is not surprising that the "gang" on the corner becomes one of the centrally significant community institutions in the life of the child growing up in a slum district. The gang is the outlet through which his hurts and his hostilities, personal and social, can be discharged. It becomes his surrogate family, with its leader his surrogate father or big brother. It is to this group that he turns for acceptance, guidance and companionship. The goals and the sanctions of the gang become the most important guideposts in his development. It is little wonder, then, if the complex social and economic pressures within the community are such as to make racketeering, vandalism, narcotics or other forms of antisocial acting-out important patterns of gang behavior, that the young individual in the slum area will tend to become involved in these patterns, as a necessary means of achieving prestige and acceptance within his group.

Here, then, we see another pattern of community life, one, unhappily, whose influence is not diminishing upon the families who reside within it, with profoundly serious consequences for society as a whole. Clearly, a recognition of the importance of community-family-individual interaction in the genesis of juvenile delinquency, narcotics and crime problems of our time is essential in endeavoring to find constructive solutions for them.

In conclusion, then, I have tried to indicate how in recent decades, as a result of vastly improved means of communication and transportation, the geographic barriers which once gave some degree of stability and homogeneity to neighborhood communities have broken down. As a consequence, neighborhood relationships have become more tenuous, and the individual family a relatively isolated unit, with resultant intensification of intrafamilial dependency patterns, and increased patterns of distrust, suspiciousness and insecurity extrafamilially. At the same time, through mass communication media and the needs of an increasingly complex technology, the social pressures towards conformity have accelerated tremendously, leading to loss of individuation and to inner feelings of emptiness and boredom. The frenetic drive towards the acquisition of material goods is seen as one consequence of this psychological void, with the old Protestant Ethic and its emphasis on work, thrift and reward in the hereafter giving way to a new Age-of-Anxiety Ethic, in which leisure, spending and pleasure in the here-and-now have become the goals of living.

However, that these new idols are failing to relieve the inner tensions of people is indicated by their almost frantic grasping at anything which promises relief from anxiety—from self-help books to tranquilizing drugs.* It is speculated that the resurgence of religion in contemporary American life represents, in part at least, another aspect of this search for inner peace and meaningfulness.

What the society of the future will be like is difficult, if not impossible, to predict at this time. Indeed there is reason for some concern in this age of the nuclear bomb as to whether or not there will be *any* human society on this planet in decades to come. But one thing is certain—if man is to survive as a *human being,* he will have to devise social techniques which will enable community, family and individual to interact in such a way as to preserve and enhance the uniqueness and dignity of the individual, instead of submerging or degrading it. If we fail to accomplish that, nothing else will matter.

---

*At the time this was written the enormous expansion of illicit drug use, from marijuana to heroin, with all of its widespread ramifications, particularly among young people, had not yet taken place. (J. M., 1973)

REFERENCES

1. PACKARD, VANCE: *The Hidden Persuaders,* New York, David McKay Co., Inc., 1957.
2. Quoted from Whyte, W. H. Jr.: *The Organization Man,* p. 19, New York, Simon & Schuster, Inc., 1956.
3. SPECTORSKY, A. C.: *Destination Sickness* in *What's New,* No. 204, 1958.
4. RIESMAN, DAVID: *The Lonely Crowd,* New Haven, Yale Univ. Press, p. 66, 1953.
5. STOFFLER, E. H.: "A Study of National and Cultural Differences in Criminal Tendency," Arch. Psychol., N.Y.; No. 185, pp. 1–60, 1935.
6. WHYTE, W. F.: *Street Corner Society,* ed. 2, Chicago, Univ. Chicago Press, 1955.

5

THE CANCER PATIENT AND HIS FAMILY
(1963)

The problem of the psychological impact of cancer upon the patient and his family is but a fragment of a much broader problem, that of the attitude of human beings to the reality of death. This is something with which man has probably been struggling since the dawn of reason. The fact that the religion or mythology of all peoples invariably contains some wishful assumption of an afterlife or an immortal "soul" is eloquent evidence of the universal reluctance of human beings to accept the finality of death. In the words of Sigmund Freud, "Our own death is indeed unimaginable, and whenever we make the attempt to imagine it, we can perceive that we really survive as spectators . . . In the unconscious, everyone of us is convinced of his own immortality."

FEARS OF DEATH

Despite this general aversion to facing the inevitability of death, it is a striking phenomenon that human beings who are living effective and satisfying lives are rarely particularly concerned with or troubled by thoughts of dying. A categorical assumption may be made that whenever one encounters an individual who is obsessively preoccupied with death or the fear of death, one finds a person who is having difficulty in dealing with life. The neurotic fear of death generally rests upon two underlying attitudes. The first of these is often conscious or preconscious and is frequently verbalized by the individual himself; it consists of an awareness that he is getting no pleasure out of living and a fear that death will cheat him before he has a chance to achieve some of his desired satisfactions. The second attitude is a deeper one and is usually unconscious; it consists of a repressed wish to escape from the conflicts and responsibilities with which the individual is struggling into the blissful Nirvana of an endless untroubled sleep. Where this wish is particularly strong, it is as though the individual is unconsciously wishing he were dead—a wish, however, which his conscious self rejects with horror. Thus, as is often the case in phobias, the denied unconscious wish, "I wish I were dead," is expressed in the conscious fear, "I am afraid I am going to die."

This does not mean, however, that the psychologically healthy person has no qualms about dying. On the contrary, he loves life and usually clings to it with incredible tenacity, even in the face of extraordinary pain or suffering.

PSYCHOLOGICAL IMPLICATIONS OF CANCER

It falls to the lot of the physician, as he fights disease and death, to be a particularly frequent observer of the dramatic struggle for life in which human beings engage. Not the least of these struggles is that which centers around cancer, a disease which in the popular mind still tends to be practically synonymous with death. There are few other diseases which carry as much menace for the average person. It is probable that one important reason for this is inherent in the fact that most people regard cancer as a foreign agent, an alien thing within the body which, if neglected, inexorably destroys the human being who harbors it. Most other diseases are part of ourselves; it is we who are sick. But cancer is a thing apart from us which "eats us up." There is something in the unconscious psychological perception of cancer which sees it as a devouring process and thus related to one of the most primitive and archaic fears of childhood, that of being eaten up. The big bad wolf of the "Three Little Pigs" and "Little Red Riding Hood," the old witch of "Hansel and Gretel," to say nothing of the whale that swallowed Jonah, are a few of the variations on this theme in mythology which reflect this infantile unconscious fear.

Varying Psychological Reactions to Cancer

Despite the pervasiveness of this fear, however, it is a common observation that different individuals react very differently to the knowledge of having cancer. There are those who face it with great objectivity and courage, others who are thrown into panic or depression, and still others who refuse to accept it at all. Are there any guideposts which the physician can use in predicting the kind of reaction his patient is apt to have to the disclosure of the presence of a cancer?

Any approach to this problem must first take into consideration the fact that when we talk of cancer we are not speaking about a unitary thing. Cancers vary enormously in their origins and life histories. The location and type of the cancer, its relative benignancy or malignancy, and the stage at which it is discovered, all have a bearing upon the question. Obviously it makes a considerable difference if the lesion under consideration is a relatively superficial and benign one that can be eradicated completely and permanently. To be able to couple the telling of a patient that he has a cancer with the assurance that it can and will be completely eradicated is quite a different matter from presenting a patient with the diagnosis of a cancer the outcome of which is going to be definitely fatal, or at best uncertain. In the remarks which follow it shall be assumed that we are dealing with the lethal type, since it is in this circumstance that the professional conscience of the physician is most apt to be perplexed.

The ability of a patient to face this kind of a situation depends, among other things, on his psychological capacity to adapt to stress. Individuals with a high ego-integrative capacity (ego strength) may show a remarkable ability to face the certainty of death from cancer with objectivity and calm. Most physicians can recall an example, either from their clinical practices or personal acquaintanceships, of a person who has continued courageously as long as possible upon his occupational, social, and personal life in spite of the certain knowledge of having an incurable cancer.

Such a placid acceptance of death, however, is not always evidence of ego strength. Occasionally it may be a reflection of a repressed wish to retreat from life's problems and responsibilities, or it may reflect satisfaction of unconscious self-destructive impulses stemming from deeply buried guilt feelings. In still other instances the secondary gain from the illness in terms of the increased attention, affection, and solicitude received from friends and relatives may actually outweigh the threat of death itself. Dr. Ruth Weston, writing in *When Doctors are Patients,* described exactly such a reaction: "I was still lonely, still needing approval and affection, so that when I received both in quite overwhelming amounts at the time of my operation for cancer of the breast, it meant far more to me than the dangers and discomforts involved in the diagnosis and the surgery . . . I found that . . . a part of me . . . welcomed the idea, even of dying, as long as I could get attention and be relieved of guilt during the process. . . ."

On the other hand, the physician not infrequently encounters patients who clearly indicate that they cannot and do not wish to face the fact that they have an incurable cancer. Even in the face of the most obvious evidence they continue to cling to the conviction that they are suffering from something else.

A highly intelligent professional woman had one year previously undergone a radical mastectomy for a malignant mammary carcinoma and was now in a state of terminal cachexia, suffering from multiple bony metastases. Although it was incredible that this educated and sophisticated woman did not suspect that she was suffering from recurrence of her cancer, she clung firmly to the conviction that her persistent symptoms were due to "arthritis," as her physician had told her. When asked whether she ever worried that they might be due to the former cancer, she replied emphatically, "Oh, no, that was completely cured!"

Dr. Leo Bartemeier tells the story of a 54-year-old obstetrician who told a neurosurgical colleague of his that he was having trouble with his back and that he would like him to look at the x-ray films and express his opinion. As they both looked at the pictures, the neurosurgeon immediately realized that any third-year medical student would have easily identified the metastases that were plainly visible. Yet the well-trained and experienced obstetrician had obviously "blocked out" any recognition of them.

This pattern of nonrecognition, termed "denial," is a defensive mechanism employed by the ego to protect itself against overwhelming, catastrophic anxiety. One of the things we have learned in psychiatry is to respect such defenses when we encounter them. To attempt to ride roughshod over them can sometimes precipitate a severe panic, psychosis, or even a suicidal reaction.

Between the extremes of complete acceptance, on the one hand, and total denial, on the other, one may find variations. A common reaction on the part of patients to the discovery that they have a cancer is an initial response of shock, depression, and a tendency toward denial. Within a matter of days or weeks, however, they are usually able to bring themselves to face the facts of their illness more and more realistically. Renneker and Cutler, in a study of a group of 50 patients with cancer of the breast, stated that all of them knew they had cancer even if not told by their physicians.

I recall a man who was dying of a gastric cancer which had been represented to him as chronic pancreatitis whispering to me, "I know it's a cancer, but the family feels better if they think I don't know."

This underlines a rather common observation, that not infrequently the families of cancer patients take the news of the disease far harder than do the patients themselves.

THE IMPORTANCE OF HOPE

One of the most significant, and in some ways tragic, aspects of this problem is the way in which doomed cancer patients and their families will grasp at the faintest spark of hope that death may be postponed. They will often go from doctor to doctor seeking one who will fan such a spark to life with easy promises. This makes them fair prey for callous charlatans who do not hesitate to exploit these hopes for profit.

For the ethical physician, however, there is a lesson in such situations which ought not to be ignored, namely, the fundamental importance of *never taking a totally hopeless attitude toward a patient with cancer.* This does not imply that it is either ethical or desirable to promise an improbable cure. But every physician knows of instances in which a hopeless prognosis was given to a patient, who then proceeded to survive long beyond the predicted time limit. On that basis alone, the physician is not only justified but even obligated never to close the door of hope completely, neither for the patient nor his family but particularly for the patient. The possibility that he may have even one chance in a thousand may be the decisive factor in an individual's capacity to endure psychologically what might otherwise be an intolerable situation. Moreover, the very will to live in itself often depends on this persistence of hope. Many a patient has clung tenaciously to life on this basis long beyond the time expected. On the other hand, patients who are shorn of hope and the will to carry on often give up the struggle for life far more quickly than their condition warrants. For these reasons, even if the physician is himself totally convinced that a malignancy is therapeutically hopeless, it is his legitimate function to continue active treatment. Although such procedure may not affect the cancer, it does benefit the ego of the patient, who desperately needs to feel helped and supported to the very end.

WHAT SHALL WE TELL THE FAMILY?

What, then, shall we tell the cancer patient and his relatives? Most physicians agree that on medicolegal grounds alone it is essential that responsible members of the patient's family always be told the truth, regardless of what is said to the patient. One may get varied reactions, again ranging from total denial to calm acceptance of the facts, depending upon the ego strength of the individuals involved and the nature of their interpersonal relationship with the cancer patient. Sometimes the physician becomes the target of an irrational hostility from the family, as if the tragic facts were of his making. In such situations, it behooves the doctor to remain objective and understanding, since at such a time the emotionally upset family members become his patients too, so to speak. Keeping hope alive, assuring the family that everything humanly possible that might help will be done, and calling in consultants whenever it is felt that it might be reassuring are among the measures that make it easier for a family to absorb the impact of the situation. Where a family member, like a patient, tends to deny the reality of a cancer, it is for similar reasons: the anxiety is too great for him to cope with all at once. The wise physician will not force the issue and will allow for time to enable the relative gradually to digest the painful reality. In some situations, reassurance of relatives that they are not responsible through inattention or neglect for the patient's illness may be an important ingredient in enabling them to face it. It is an ironic fact that the most violent reactions of anguish in family members to the impact of such a disease do not necessarily bespeak the greatest love for the patient. Such reactions, like those of the loudest mourners at a funeral, are often overcompensatory denials of unconscious guilt or hostility feelings toward the patient.

WHAT SHALL WE TELL THE PATIENT?

One encounters much difference of opinion among doctors concerning the question of what the cancer patient should be told. These differences depend on the personality of the physician, on the specialty of medicine which he practices, and on the extent of his psychiatric knowledge.

The personality of the doctor has a great bearing on his ability to discuss the diagnosis of cancer with a patient. Such a situation makes enormous demands on the emotions of the physician. If the physician himself has a deep fear of the disease or of death, consciously or unconsciously, it is bound to affect his attitude toward the patient with cancer. It is little wonder, therefore, that many physicians find it easier not to tell the patient the truth and then to rationalize their decision as being based on what is best for the patient, even though surveys have shown that most patients want to be told if they have cancer.

The specialty of the doctor, and consequently the kind of cancer which he encounters in his practice, also has a bearing on his attitude. A survey by Fitts and Ravdin among Philadelphia physicians revealed that 94 per cent of dermatologists favored telling their patients they had a cancer, in contrast to 41 per cent of surgeons and 30 per cent of certified general practitioners. The higher figure among dermatologists undoubtedly reflects the more favorable prognosis in skin cancer; it is much easier to tell a patient the truth when the outlook is an optimistic one.

The degree of psychiatric awareness possessed by the doctor also has a bearing upon his decision. The common assumption that most patients will respond with a serious emotional break or suicide if they learn they have a cancer is simply not borne out by the facts. It is true that the initial reaction of many patients to a diagnosis of cancer is one of shock or depression. The severity of such a reaction is related not only to the inner dynamics of the patient's personality but also to the degree to which such knowledge comes to him as a surprise. In most instances, patients begin to know or suspect that they may have a cancer either from the nature of their symptoms or in the course of the physician's diagnostic work-up. As a consequence, their psychological defenses have been mobilized and they are better able to adapt to the diagnosis of cancer when it finally comes. In the occasional instance in which the discovery of cancer comes as a complete surprise, the absence of prior mobilization of psychological defenses results in a greater initial shock reaction. In most cases, however, this initial shock reaction is a transitory one, and in a matter of days or weeks, the patient will gradually begin to adapt to the reality of the situation.

The assumption that suicide is a frequent reaction to the knowledge of cancer is a common misconception. Litin and Wilmer of the Mayo Clinic, in a survey of all suicides which took place in Olmstead County over a seventeen-year period, found only one suicide that had any temporal relationship to the diagnosis of cancer.

Much of the reluctance among certain medical authorities to tell patients they have a cancer seems to stem from the assumption that such a pronouncement is equivalent to a death sentence. This is no longer unequivocally so, and is becoming less and less so with every passing year as newer techniques of treatment are perfected. It is both ethically and scientifically reasonable and justifiable never to completely close the door of hope for any cancer patient.

To summarize, then, there are cogent reasons for telling most patients the truth. By this I mean telling them that they have a cancer and enlisting their cooperation in taking whatever measures may be necessary to deal with it. *No patient, however, should be told his disease is hopeless.* The reasons for such an approach can be outlined as follows:

1) The patient has a legal right to know the truth.
2) Surveys (Harpole; Kelly and Friesen) indicate that the large

majority of patients—from 82 to 97 per cent—want to be told if they have a cancer.

3) Patients who have cancers which are cured should know what they had so that they can encourage other people and help combat the myth of cancer's incurability.

4) Patients who know what they have are apt to be more cooperative in follow-up care and treatment.

5) Patients with certain kinds of cancer, notably breast cancer, cannot help knowing or suspecting the truth in the light of the surgery that has been performed. To attempt to deny the obvious in such instances may actually intensify their anxiety by making them feel that the truth is too terrible to be mentioned. An honest facing of the facts without removing hope is the fairest way of meeting such situations.

6) Patients are entitled to know if their life expectancy is limited, so they can arrange their affairs and do the things they may wish to do in the limited span of time left to them.

7) Patients often take the news of cancer far better than doctors anticipate. A not uncommon observation is that ocassionally a highly neurotic individual will react to such catastrophic news with surprising emotional maturity, and actually seem to grow in the face of it. The power of human beings to adapt themselves to the inevitable should not be underestimated.

Granting the cogency of these points, however, how can the physician recognize that minority of cases in which telling the patient that he has a cancer may prove harmful? The most important signpost is the degree of denial which the patient manifests to the suspicion of cancer during diagnostic studies. The patient who obviously avoids any mention of the possibility of cancer, or who recoils with panic at even the faintest suggestion of it, is showing defensive tendencies toward denial which should be respected in the interest of his mental equilibrium. The fact that he cannot tolerate even a tentative consideration of the disease is an indication that he is not yet ready to face it as a certainty. A consistently supportive and encouraging attitude on the part of the doctor, however, may, over a period of time, make it possible for even some of these patients gradually to mobilize their adaptive strengths and face their problems more realistically. Somewhat analogous situations are encountered in other areas of medical practice in the reactions of patients to the information that they have tuberculosis, or will require an amputation, or even that they will have to undergo psychoanalysis!

A basic therapeutic hopefulness is an essential attribute of a good physician in all aspects of medical practice, but in relation to the cancer patient, it is a sine qua non.

REFERENCES

FITTS, W. T., and RAVDIN, I. S.: What Philadelphia Physicians Tell Patients with Cancer. *J.A.M.A.* 153:901, 1953.

HARPOLE, B. P.: To Tell or Not to Tell. *Current Medical Digest,* April, 1955.

KELLY, W. D., and FRIESEN, S. R.: Do Cancer Patients Want to be Told? *Surgery* 27:822, 1950.

RENNEKER, R., and CUTLER, M.: Psychological Problems of Adjustment to Cancer of the Breast. *J.A.M.A.* 148:833, 1952.

SYMPOSIUM: What Shall We Tell the Cancer Patient? *Proc. Mayo Clin.* 35:239, 1960.

6

THE CRISIS OF MIDDLE AGE
(1967)

In recent years the concept of crisis has occupied an increasingly important position in psychiatric theory as a period in which an individual, subject to stress, reaches a crucial point of tension from which either adaptive integration or maladaptive disorganization must eventuate. The significance of crisis, psychotherapeutically, is that at such periods of stress, properly presented interventions can be of maximum efficacy.

Erikson (1) originally introduced the concept of *developmental crisis* in relationship to his well-known "eight stages of man." There are indeed many developmental crises throughout human existence, beginning with the process of birth itself. Others include: the crucial first year of life—which lays the groundwork for basic security in interpersonal relationships; the acculturation stresses of the second and third years of life—of fundamental importance in connection with the development of inner and outer control mechanisms and relationships to authority symbols; the crisis of the oedipal period— with all of its fateful implications; the separation crises involved in the first school attendance and the first extended departure from home; adolescence; the first employment and heterosexual experiences; marriage; and parenthood.

The purpose of this communication is to focus upon still another period of life—the middle years—as a particularly important developmental crisis which, apart from our concern with the gross psychopathologies of menopause, has not received sufficient attention as an inevitable aspect of the aging process in our society.

What makes middle age a crisis period? There are four major factors—somatic, cultural, economic, and psychological.

71

1. As individuals reach the middle years of life, the *somatic* evidences of the aging process can no longer be ignored. There comes a moment in the life of every man and woman when the decreased elasticity of the skin, the accumulating wrinkles, and the coarsening of the features force themselves into awareness in a way that can no longer be denied by the psychologically healthy person. There is the inevitable fateful day when reading glasses are prescribed for the first time, or when a man, catching sight of the back of his head in a three-way mirror, realizes that the balding person at whom he is looking is no other than himself. For the woman there is the sagging of breasts once proudly firm, the beginning of irregularity of menstruation, and then the finality of its cessation. For both men and women there is the slackening of muscular activity and the tendency toward increase in weight, with the never-ending subsequent struggle between oral craving and oral frustration. I am purposely omitting discussion of actual somatic pathologies. My point is that quite apart from any specific pathological syndromes, the *normal* somatic changes that accompany the middle years constitute a series of critical emotional stresses for all people, the significance and impact of which, however, vary in different individuals for reasons that I shall presently discuss.

2. The second important area of stress is the *cultural* one. This is especially relevant in the United States, where youth and physical vigor are particularly valued. One might speculate that the high valuation of these patterns in American culture may be a carry-over of our frontier history where such physical attributes were indeed essential for survival. Regardless of its source, however, it is worth noting that this is a peculiarly potent aspect of American cultural life which does not exist to the same degree for older European and Asian cultures, where middle-aged people are still considered attractive and desirable and where the elderly receive considerably more respect and appreciation. Consequently, in the context of American culture, the beginning loss of youth and vigor is a relatively severer narcissistic injury.

Still another relevant factor in American cultural life is the great value placed upon individual success, whether it be in terms of prestige, wealth, or power. The failure to have achieved such success by the time middle age has arrived also, as we shall see, constitutes a significant stress in our milieu.

3. The middle years of life also carry with them many increased *economic* stresses. There still exists a prejudice against hiring older people, particularly in the white- and blue-collar areas; indeed, the increasing advent of automation may increase this discrimination rather than decrease it. Moreover, children in a complex technology require more extended support due to their prolonged training needs. In addition, the middle-aged person often is faced with the heavy economic burden of supporting aging and ailing relatives. It is possible that this latter burden now will be somewhat eased with the advent of Medicare, but the steady increase of their own medical costs may well continue to represent a serious economic threat to many people in the middle years of life. The insidious diminution in purchasing power which the steady progress of inflation has brought with it in recent decades constitutes an additional source of strain to most people in this age group.

4. Most important, however, for the middle years, are the *psychological* stresses, not only in response to the above mentioned somatic and environmental pressures, but also to specific emotional factors. *Separation loss* is a key and recurring psychological stress during this period: the loss of one's youthful self-image, the increased frequency of illness and death among relatives and friends, the loss of children who leave home, and the loss of love in the "tired" marriage where intimacy has been replaced by mutual toleration and sex takes place without passion or tenderness.

Most significantly stressful, however, are two additional factors which are usually unconscious, and which affect all middle-aged people. The first of these—already touched upon—involves the *loss of the fantasy hopes of youth:* the hopes of fame, of accomplishment, of wealth, and of romance. One of the fundamental adjustments that most people have to make in the middle years, if these fantasies have not been achieved, is the facing of the hard fact that their fulfillment has become improbable. This involves a profound problem in self-acceptance and in the willingness and ability to make compromises with inexorable realities.

The second factor, and perhaps even a more challenging one, is the fact that the somatic changes of middle age carry with them an inescapable *confrontation with the fact of mortality.* The defenses which have worked so well in youth—the illusion of immortality and the denial of one's own ultimate death—can no longer be maintained. The result is a marked increase in what has come to be known as "existential anxiety" (2), the anxiety that is derived from fully facing both the limits of existence and our ultimate nonexistence.

An interesting fact, however, is that all of these stresses operate differentially in men and women. In the middle years of life women manifest psychiatric disorders three to four times as frequently as men do. Why is this so? It is certainly not due to a greater physiological vulnerability to the aging process. If anything, modern American women maintain their youthful appearance at least as well as men do; indeed, the artifices of the cosmetic industry help them to maintain the illusion of youth far better than men. The evidence strongly suggests, rather, that the reasons for this difference in morbidity are cultural and psychological. First, there is much greater emphasis in our culture on the importance of beauty and youth in women as compared to men. Second, the cessation of menses is an obvious narcissistic injury as compared to the more insidious, less visible diminution of virility in aging men. Third, the woman's loss of reproductive capacity at menopause is in direct contrast to the preservation of this capacity in men. Finally, the majority of women in our society still form their identities as mothers and wives, within the family, rather than as persons in the outside world. In middle age, however, the functional role of a woman as a mother and a wife assumes less importance, with children becoming less dependent and the husband less attentive. Consequently many middle-aged women are apt to feel as though they are being discarded and retired to a cultural ash-heap, while their husbands are still able to feel relatively needed and involved in the outside world. (Ironically this functional difference is reversed in the sixties and the seventies when the woman is apt to find herself much more useful and needed, in the grandmother role, than is the man of comparable age!)

Despite these cultural variables, the manner in which these normal stresses of middle life are dealt with in any individual man or woman depends upon factors which are highly personal and idiosyncratic. These factors, for both men and women are:

1. The basic ego-integrative capacity of the individual—the capacity for flexible adaptation in contrast to emotional rigidity;
2. The nature of interpersonal relationships—the character of the

marriage and of the relationship to children, other relatives, and friends;

3. The sense of continuing usefulness, which depends on the extent of the individual's functional relationships, and the degree of self-fulfillment that they afford; and

4. The breadth of interests in the outside world.

Generally speaking, the weaker the ego-adaptive capacity, the more limited the base of interpersonal relationships, the narrower the foundation of the sense of usefulness and of the interest in the outside world—the more critical will be the impact of the middle-years' stresses.

In general, four major patterns of response to the stresses of middle life can be distinguished,* each, of course, subject to considerable idiosyncratic variations and blendings. They are not mutually exclusive. (1) *Denial by escape.* Here we see people trying to avoid facing their inner anxieties by patterns of compulsive activity. This is why so many middle-aged couples fear being alone with themselves or one another, and are constantly escaping into the wasteland of TV, or to movies, card games, and parties. The formula that dominates their lives is "What are we doing tonight?" Another common defense is that of (2) *denial by overcompensation* with efforts to recapture the lost feelings of youth. Not for nothing are these years sometimes characterized as "the dangerous forties"! The woman utilizing this defense is apt to embark on a desperate search for the romance and the love that has gone out of her marriage; while the man seeks to refurbish his tarnishing narcissistic self-image by pursuing a chain of sexual conquests. As might be expected, this is a crisis period for marriages, and the incidence of divorce reaches a high peak.

If these commonly used defenses fail to work, then we may see various forms of (3) *decompensation,* with anxiety states, depressive reactions, apathetic surrender, or feelings of rage.** These patterns

---

*It should be emphasized that these reactions are typical of contemporary American life, and are not universal for all times and all cultures. Obviously, patterns of adaptation and maladaptation are strongly affected by the mores, the outlets, and the technology of the sociocultural milieu—viz. McLuhan's challenging concepts in *Understanding Media* (3).

**Viz: Dylan Thomas' anguished cry: "Rage, rage against the dying of the light!"

of decompensation make up what are commonly recognized as the psychological "disorders of the menopause."

On the other hand, if the individual is able to meet the critical developmental stresses of the middle years and deal with them successfully, then the outcome is (4) a state of higher *integration* than he or she has previously achieved—an integration that means an added dimension of emotional maturity; a heightened awareness of self and of others; a lessening of narcissistic self-involvement and an increase in the capacity to cathect service to others; a greater ability to find pleasure in the achievement of our children, our students, and our youth in general; a renewed capacity for productivity and creativity; and, finally, a deeper appreciation of the complexity and the rich bittersweetness that characterize our temporary sojourn on this planet of laughter and tears.

> *For age is opportunity no less*
> *Than youth itself, though in another dress.*
> Longfellow

REFERENCES

1. ERIKSON, E. H. *Childhood and Society.* New York: W. W. Norton & Co., 1950.
2. MAY, R., ANGEL, E., and ELLENBERGER, H. F. (eds.), *Existence.* New York: Basic Books, 1958.
3. McLUHAN, M. *Understanding Media.* New York: McGraw Hill, 1964.

7

"NORMAL" AND "DEVIANT" SEXUAL
BEHAVIOR
(1971)

It is difficult to approach the topic of human sexuality with the same kind of dispassionate scientific objectivity that can be applied to functions such as speech, digestion, or locomotion. Sexual behavior is so intimately entwined with moral issues, religious and cultural value systems, and even aesthetic reactions, that those who attempt to deal with it too open-mindedly are likely to be charged by their contemporaries with being immoral or amoral, if not illegal. Sigmund Freud's efforts at the turn of the 19th century to bring the "problems of the bedroom" under scientific scrutiny caused both colleagues and friends to turn away from him in embarrassment, and even sixty years later, in the relatively enlightened second half of the 20th century, the meticulous physiological studies of Masters and Johnson stimulated cries of outrage in many quarters and titters of embarrassment in others.

Nevertheless, no discussion of human sexual behavior can be truly objective if one does not attempt to stand outside of the narrow framework of one's own cultural bias to see how the raw data of human sexual biology are shaped by and shape the infinitely varied mosaics of human experience in different places and at different times.

Historical Considerations

Even a cursory look at the recorded history of human sexuality makes it abundantly clear that patterns of sexual behavior and

77

morality have taken many diverse forms over the centuries. Far from being "natural" and inevitable, our contemporary sexual codes and mores, seen in historical perspective, would appear no less grotesque to people of other eras than theirs appear to us. Our attitudes concerning nudity, virginity, fidelity, love, marriage, and "proper" sexual behavior are meaningful only within the context of our own cultural and religious mores. Thus, in the first millennium of the Christian era, in many parts of what is now Europe, public nudity was no cause for shame (as is still true in some aboriginal settings), virginity was not prized, marriage was usually a temporary arrangement, and extramarital relations were taken for granted. Frank and open sexuality was the rule, and incest was frequent. Women were open aggressors in inviting sexual intercourse. Bastardy was a mark of distinction because it often implied that some important person had slept with one's mother. In early feudal times new brides were usually deflowered by the feudal lord (jus primae noctis). In other early societies all the wedding guests would copulate with the bride. Far from being considered a source of concern to the husband, these practices were considered a way of strengthening the marriage in that the pain of the initial coitus would not be associated with the husband.

It was not until the Medieval Church was able to strengthen and extend its control over the peoples of Europe that guilt about sexuality began to be a cardinal feature of Western life. Even the early Hebraic laws against adultery had nothing to do with fidelity but were primarily concerned with protecting the property rights of another man (the wife being considered property). Married men were free to maintain concubines or, if they preferred, multiple wives; also, there was no ban in the Old Testament on premarital sex. The Medieval Church, however, exalted celibacy and virginity. In its efforts to make license in sexual intercourse as difficult as possible, it sanctioned it only for procreative purposes and ordained laws against abortion—laws that had not existed among the Greeks, Romans, or Jews. At one time it went so far as to make sexual intercourse between married couples illegal on Sundays, Wednesdays, and Fridays, as well as for forty days before Easter and forty days before Christmas, and also from the time of conception to forty days after parturition. (By contrast, Mohammedan law considered it grounds for divorce if intercourse did not take place at least once a week.)

Moreover, when the sexual taboos of the Medieval Church began to be widely enforced by cruel sanctions, a veritable epidemic of sexual pathology ensued—sodomy, flagellation, hysterical "possession" by witches and devils, incubi, succubi, phantom pregnancies, stigmata, and the like. In contrast, it is worth noting that in societies in which access to sexuality was open and guilt-free—the early Greeks, Europe prior to the Middle Ages and most "primitive" societies—the so-called sexual perversions tended not to be present. The homosexuality of the early Greeks, incidentally, was not an exclusive homosexuality, but part of a pattern of bisexuality in which homosexual feelings were considered to be as natural as heterosexual ones.

The ideals of romantic love and marriage for love which are taken for granted today are a relatively late development in Western history and did not make their appearance until the 12th century AD (1). Clearly, there is nothing about our current sexual attitudes and practices that can be assumed to be either sacrosanct or immutable. They have been subject to much change and evolution in the past, and they will undoubtedly be different in the future.

Biological and Cultural Considerations

Before we can proceed, it is necessary to clarify certain fundamental questions about the nature of human sexuality that have a bearing on the problem of sexual deviation. What is the biological core of human sexuality? Is it exclusively heterosexual, or does it have a bisexual composition? Is man "naturally" polygamous? Is woman naturally monoandrous? Are most "perversions" "unnatural"? What form does natural sexuality take in children?

Zoological and cross-cultural studies in recent years clearly demonstrate that the issue of sexual behavior goes far beyond its reproductive functions. Caspari's definition of the sexual process as "the exchange of nuclear material between cells of mating types or sexes" may have validity for relatively primitive forms of life, but as we ascend the phylogenetic scale this definition becomes manifestly inadequate. Patterns of sexual behavior evolve with the species, and at higher mammalian levels there is an increasing emphasis on various sex-related activities rather than on purely reproductive ones.

Sex in human beings is usually spoken of as being an "instinct." By this we mean that it is a fundamental behavioral pattern dependent on internal biological factors but capable of being triggered by external cues. Either may create a state of disequilibrium experienced as urgency or tension; this tension then leads to behavior that has the effect of restoring the previous state of balance, with an accompanying sense of subjective gratification. It is important to remember, however, that such a reaction takes quite a different form in human beings than it does in lower animals, even though the term instinct is used equally for both. The lower in the scale of evolution an animal is, the more totally developed and less modifiable are such instinctual patterns; but as one moves up the evolutionary scale inherited instinctual patterns tend to become less preformed and more subject to modification by learning. This development reaches its highest point in man, whose instinctual patterns at birth tend to be relatively unfocused biological drives, subject to enormous modifiability by learning and experience. This is a major factor in the extraordinary range of human adaptability.

This essentially unfocused quality of man's sexual drive in infancy is what Hampson and Hampson (2) have referred to as man's inherent "psychosexual neutrality" at birth—a neutrality that "permits the development and perpetuation of diverse patterns of psychosexual orientaton and functioning in accordance with the life experiences each individual may encounter and transact." This concept of psychosexual neutrality does not, as some have mistakenly inferred, mean a "driveless" state, but rather an inborn biological drive with no specific inborn object, but with the potential for adapting its gratifactory needs to whatever objects the environment makes available to it. The term "psychosexual multipotentiality" probably expresses this more adequately than does "psychosexual neutrality."

In human sexual behavior, situational and learning factors are of major importance in arousal and response. In the absence of heterosexual objects, human beings (as well as many lower animals) may ultimately seek gratification in homosexual objects, or if no human object is available, in relations with animals of other species, or even by contact with inanimate objects. Even the physiological route of gratification, whether through the genitals or some other erogenous zone, or via patterns of behavior which seem to have no inherent elements of erogenicity in them at all, are subject to conditioning by specific experiences or associations. Other factors in sexual responsiveness include age, health, fatigue, nutritional state, and recency of drive fulfillment.

Freud believed that the bisexual anlage which can be observed in the human embryo is subsequently reflected in a universal bisexual tendency at a psychological level. The evidences of such psychic bisexuality, in this view, are seen in "latent homosexual" manifestations such as affectionate feelings for members of one's own sex and in patterns of behavior or interest that are usually (in our culture) considered to be characteristic of the opposite sex. Examples of these would be artistic or culinary interests or "passive" attitudes in males, or athletic or scientific interests or "aggressive" attitudes in females.

This hypothesis was first challenged in the psychoanalytic literature by Rado (3) who pointed out that "in the final shaping of the normal individual the double embryological origin of the genital system does not result in any physiological duality of reproductive functioning." More than this, we now know that with the exception of the relatively uncommon individuals with sexual chromosome abnormalities, in almost all human beings biological sex is clearly differentiated at the moment of conception by the XX and XY chromosomal patterns. Nevertheless, the theory of psychic bisexuality is sometimes still defended on the basis that both "male" and "female" sex hormones—androgens and estrogens—can be found in the blood of both sexes. However, although the biological activity of these hormones is essential for the growth and maturation of the primary genital apparatus in both sexes and for the development of secondary sexual characteristics, there is no evidence in humans that these hormones affect the direction of human sexuality or that they determine psychological "masculinity" or "femininity" (4). As Money has put it,

There is no primary genetic or other innate mechanism to preordain the masculinity or femininity of psychosexual differentiation. . . . The analogy is with language. Genetics and

innate determinants ordain only that language can develop . . .
but not whether the language will be Nahuatl, Arabic, English,
or any other. (5)

Psychological and behavioral patterns of masculinity or femininity
constitute what is meant by "gender role," and are not necessarily
synonymous with an individual's biological sex. As the Hampsons
have pointed out:

> The psychologic phenomenon which we have termed gender
> role, or psychosexual orientation, evolves gradually in the course
> of growing up and cannot be assigned or discarded at will.
> The components of gender role are neither static nor universal.
> They change with the times and are an integral part of each
> culture and subculture. Thus one may expect important dif-
> ferences in what is to be considered typical and appropriate
> masculine or feminine gender roles as displayed by a native
> of Thailand and a native of Maryland . . . (2)

Opler, in the same vein, comments that

> a Navajo Indian may be a he-man, a gambler, and a philanderer
> while dressing in bright blouses adorned with jeweled belts,
> necklaces, and bracelets. French courtiers in the retinues of effete
> monarchs were equally philanderers, though rouged, powdered,
> and bedecked with fine lace. The Andaman Islanders like to
> have the man sit on his wife's lap in fond greetings, and friends
> and relatives, of the same or opposite sex, greet one another
> in the same manner after absences, crying in the affected manner
> of the mid-Victorian woman. . . . Obviously, the style of social
> and sexual behavior is something of an amalgam and is culturally
> influenced. (6)

The fact is that the patterning of human sexual behavior begins
at birth. From the moment a child is identified as either boy or
girl, it begins to be shaped by multitudinous cues which communicate
certain gender role expectations to it over the suceeding years. This
results in a "core gender identity" of either maleness or femaleness,
which becomes so profoundly fixed by the age of three, that efforts
to reverse this identity after that time are almost always doomed
to failure (2).

Within every society, the process of acculturation that takes place during these critical years begins to condition the child's behavior so as to enable it to conform to the mores of its environment—how and what it should eat, where and when it may urinate and defecate, what and whom it may play with, how it should think and express itself, and how and toward whom it may express its sexual needs. The so-called "polymorphous-perverse" sexual behavior of young children described by Freud in his *Three Contributions to the Theory of Sex* constitutes the normal behavior of children before the acculturation processes of our society have funneled their sexual patterns into "proper channels." From it we can infer what form the "natural sexuality" of man would probably take if no cultural taboos or restrictions at all existed in this sphere. Freud obviously was not unaware of this when he wrote that "it is absolutely impossible not to recognize in the uniform predisposition to all perversions. . . . a universal and primitive human tendency" (7).

Developmental Factors

In his libido theory, Freud hypothesized that the sexual instinct followed a phylogenetically predestined evolutionary pathway. In the first year of life, the primary erotogenic focus was the oral zone, in the second and third years, the anal zone, and in the fourth and fifth years, the phallic zone. From the sixth year to puberty, the sexual drive then underwent an involutional process—the "latency period"—during which the "sexual energy" was deflected from sexual goals and "sublimated." With puberty, the sexual drive was again unleashed and now directed toward the ultimate adult goal of full genital gratification.

With the shift in psychoanalytic theory from an instinct-psychology to an ego-psychology, the unfolding of human sexuality may be viewed in a somewhat different light. The infant's sexual needs are seen as rather primitive and undifferentiated at birth. Such as they are, they find expression in the exercise of the child's relatively undeveloped ego functions—in sucking, in body movements, and in experiencing cutaneous and kinesthetic sensations. In the course of its adaptive development the child discovers sucking its thumb and handling its genitals as special sources of somatic pleasure, and if not discouraged, will utilize these as accessory sources of gratification. Indeed, infantile masturbation may be regarded as one of the earliest experiences of autonomy in normal development. When the child discovers erogenous zones within himself that he can stimulate to give himself pleasure, he has achieved a significant step in ego mastery. Such masturbation is analogous to the behavioral patterns described by Olds (8) in his experimental rats when they discovered their ability to stimulate a "pleasure area" in their hypothalamus.

This author has never been convinced that the shift to "anal erogenicity" during the second year is either as clear-cut or as inevitable as Freud believed. Where it does seem to occur, it may well be the consequence of the emphasis on bowel training which takes place at this time in our culture, and which often becomes the locus for an emotionally laden transaction between child and mother. Moreover, the struggle at this point is not so much over the issue of the child's wish for anal-zone pleasure per se, as it is over the child's wish to move its bowels whenever and wherever it wishes. Thus the issue is not anality, but the broader one of the pleasure-principle versus the reality-principle—the basic battle-ground of every acculturation process.

It is probably not accidental also that phallic-zone interest develops when it does. The third year of life corresponds with the shift in cultural emphasis from bowel sphincter training to the development of urinary control. Simultaneously, the developing and intrusive ego of the child at this age begins to perceive, and concern itself with, the shame-ridden issues of the anatomical differences between the sexes, where babies come from, and how much fun it is to play with the forbidden genitals. This is the period of the "polymorphous-perverse."

That a latency period should occur in our culture after this kind of behavior should not come as a surprise. Freud believed this period to be "organically determined," but the absence of such a reaction of latency in cultures where there are no prohibitions to the free expression of sexuality in children, clearly indicates that this is not so. Sexual latency, when it occurs, is obviously the result of repression in a culture that strongly indoctrinates the child with the conviction that its "polymorphous and perverse" sexual interests are dirty, shameful, and sinful. Under this pressure, with threats of physical punishment and loss of love (both "castration" threats), many children in our society repress their sexuality until the imperative thrust of puberty brings it to the fore again. It is worth noting, however, that there has been evidence in recent years that increasing numbers of children in their prepubertal years continue to be sexually active and interested. This is a reflection of the more accepting attitudes toward sexuality that have been emerging in our culture in recent decades.

The subsequent vicissitudes of adult sexuality also take many forms. Monogamy as a compulsory pattern of mateship, for example, occurs in only a minority of human societies—only 16% of 185 societies studied by Ford and Beach (9). (Even in that 16%, less than one third wholly disapproved of both premarital and extramarital liaisons.) Strict monogamy, however, is not necessarily a mark of advanced civilization—some extremely primitive societies are strongly monogamous.

Patterns of monogamy and polygamy (or polyandry) are usually dependent on economic factors. Even in societies where multiple mateships are permitted, only the well-to-do usually are able to exercise this option, and single mateships, although not required, are the rule.

Rules governing premarital and extramarital relations also vary widely in different cultures. There are numerous societies in which extramarital sex is permitted and expected, and in which there is no censure of adultery. Indeed, among the polyandrous Toda of India, there is no word in their language for adultery, and moral opprobrium is attached to the man who begrudges his wife to another! It is interesting to note also that in societies that have no double standard in sexual matters and in which liaisons are freely permitted, women avail themselves of their opportunities as eagerly as men, a fact that casts serious doubts on the popular assumption that females are, by nature, less sexually assertive than males.

Definition of Sexual Deviation

How then can one define sexual deviations? It is clear from our preceding discussion that an adequate definition cannot be based on any assumption of the biological "naturalness" of any particular pattern of sexual behavior in man. What is evaluated as psychologically healthy in one era or culture may not be so in another. The normal sexual behavior of an adolescent girl among the Marquesans or Trobrianders would be considered nymphomanic or delinquent in our society. Homosexual behavior is regarded as deviant in many cultures, including our own, but was not so adjudged in ancient Greece and pre-Meiji Japan, or among the Tanalans of Madagascar, the Siwanis of Africa, the Aranda of Australia, the Keraki of New Guinea, and many others.

It is sometimes argued that this kind of culture-oriented relativistic concept of normalcy is fallacious because it fails to recognize that there is an "optimal" conception of health that transcends all cultural norms. The difficulty with this argument is that the concept of optimal itself is culture-bound. Even granting that within any culture a concept such as personality homeostasis or self-realization has validity, the content of such concepts still varies in different times and places. A definition of psychological health in psychoanalytic terms implies the ability of the "ego" to effectively handle and integrate its relationships with the "id," the "superego," and the outer world. Such definition could undoubtedly be used cross-culturally. But again, its content will vary in different cultural contexts since the nature of the "normal" superego and of the outer world are culture-dependent.

COMMENT

It seems, therefore, that there is no way in which the concepts of normal and deviant sexual behavior can be divorced from the value systems of our society; and since such value systems are always in the process of evolution and change, we must be prepared to face the possibility that some patterns currently considered deviant may not always be so regarded. The fact that we now refer to sexual "deviations" rather than to "perversions" already represents an evolutionary change within our culture toward a more objective and scientific approach to these problems, in contrast to the highly moralistic and pejorative approach of the previous generation. Perhaps some day we shall talk simply of "variations" in sexual object choice.

Such a relativistic approach to normalcy should not, however, be mistaken for a nihilistic one. We are all products of our culture, and within the context of our current Western cultural value system there are indeed certain patterns that can be regarded as psychologically optimal and healthy.

Although there is a wide spectrum of variations in human sexual motivation and behavior—most human beings, in the privacy of their bedrooms, in one way or another, and at one time or another, violate the rigid conventional standards of "proper" sexual behavior—there are nevertheless certain more widely deviant patterns of sexual behavior that in all likelihood would be considered abnormal in every society. For example, practices that involve serious injury to one of the participants in the sexual relationship could hardly be considered adaptive in any society since they would ultimately jeopardize its survival.

One way of defining a large category of sexual practices that is considered deviant in our culture is that they involve the habitual and preferential use of nongenital outlets for sexual release. The emphasis in this definition is on the terms "habitual" and "preferential," since extragenital gratification may be a part of normal sexual foreplay, or of variations in sexual experiences between perfectly normal adults. When, however, such variant activity becomes an habitual end in itself, it almost always, in the context of our culture, means some disturbance in personality functioning.

It should be noted that the above definition is a psychiatric not a legal one. Statutes in most of the United States regard *any* use of nongenital outlets for sexual release as illegal. Kinsey and his co-workers, after their extensive surveys of sexual practices of males and females, concluded that there are probably very few adults who have not technically violated such statutes at one time or another.

Other major forms of sexual behavior that are defined as deviant in our society involve activity that is homosexual, or sexual activity with immature partners of either sex (pedophilia), animals (bestiality), dead people (necrophilia), or inanimate objects (fetishism).

Although sexual deviations are commonly separated in terms of their outstanding clinical manifestations, in actuality they are far from discrete phenomena. There is frequent overlapping among them and it is not uncommon for an individual to present simultaneous evidence of more than one of these manifestations. Thus, a fetishist may also be an exhibitionist and a voyeur; a transvestite may also be involved in sadomasochistic practices; incest and pedophilia may be associated in the same person, and so forth.

The reason for this overlapping rests in the underlying psychodynamics that are common to all sexual deviations in our society. The deviant is in almost all instances an individual who has difficulty in achieving normal or satisfactory sexual relations with a mature partner of the opposite sex. Thus his deviant practices represent alternative ways of attempting to achieve sexual gratification; they are displacement phenomena and in many instances the displacement mechanism may operate in more than one direction. Some deviants exhibit polymorphous-perverse patterns of sexual behavior akin to that of very young children who have not yet been adequately acculturated. In this sense they may be considered to have been "fixated" at an early stage of psychosexual development, or to have "regressed" to this stage.

The choice of deviant pattern, like the choice of symptom in neurosis, is dependent on complex determinants which have to be ferreted out by a painstaking history and psychodynamic evaluation in each individual case. Disturbances in core family relationships, impairment in gender identity development, poor ego development, and specific conditioning experiences are all involved.

Apart from such clearly definable deviant patterns, human sexual relationships are often complicated by unconscious motivations of fear, hate, or guilt, which leave their stamps on the quality of the sexual transactions between partners. In our culture, a key distinguishing factor between what is regarded as healthy or unhealthy sexual behavior is whether such behavior is motivated by feelings of love or whether it becomes a vehicle for the discharge of anxiety, hostility, or guilt. Healthy sexuality seeks erotic pleasure in the context of tenderness and affection; pathologic sexuality is motivated by needs for reassurance or relief from nonsexual sources of tension. Healthy sexuality seeks both to give and receive pleasure; neurotic forms are unbalanced toward excessive giving or taking. Healthy sexuality is discriminating as to partner; neurotic patterns often tend to be nondiscriminating. The periodicity of healthy sexuality is determined primarily by recurrent erotic tensions in the context of affection. Neurotic sexual drives, on the other hand, are triggered less by erotic needs than by nonerotic tensions and are therefore more apt to be compulsive in their patterns of occurrence.

A sharp line of distinction, however, cannot always be drawn between healthy and neurotic sexuality. Since patterns of sexual behavior always reflect personality patterns and problems, and since no one in our complex society is totally exempt from individual idiosyncracies, tensions, and anxieties, these will be manifested in sexual patterns no less than in other areas of interpersonal transactions. No human being is perfect, and nowhere is the humanity of man more transparent than in the varied patterns of his sexual relationships.

REFERENCES

1. TAYLOR, G. R.: *Sex in History.* New York, Vanguard Press, 1954.
2. HAMPSON, J. L., HAMPSON, JOAN G.: The ontogenesis of sexual behavior in man, in Young, W. C. (ed): *Sex and Internal Secretions.* Baltimore, Williams & Wilkins, 1961, vol. 2, ed. 3.
3. RADO, S.: *Psychoanalysis of Behavior.* New York, Grune & Stratton, 1956, vol. 1.
4. PERLOFF, W. H.: Hormones and homosexuality, in Marmor, J. (ed): *Sexual Inversion: The Multiple Roots of Homosexuality.* New York, Basic Books, 1965, pp. 44–69.
5. MONEY, J.: Developmental differentiation of femininity and masculinity compared, in Farber, S. M., Wilson, R. H. L. (eds): *Man and Civilization.* New York, McGraw Hill Book Co., 1963, pp. 56–57.
6. OPLER, M. K.: Anthropological and cross-cultural aspects of homosexuality, in Marmor, J. (ed): *Sexual Inversion: The Multiple Roots of Homosexuality.* New York, Basic Books, 1965, pp. 108–123.
7. FREUD, S.: *Three Essays on the Theory of Sexuality.* J. Strachey (trans, 1905), New York, Basic Books, 1962.
8. OLDS, J.: Self stimulation of the brain. *Science* 127:315–324, 1958.
9. FORD, C. S., BEACH, F. A.: *Patterns of Sexual Behavior.* New York, Harper & Bros, 1952.

Part II

PSYCHOANALYSIS

8

THE THEORY AND PRACTICE OF
PSYCHOANALYSIS
(1946)

Psychoanalysis has occupied an anomalous position among liberals and Marxists for many years. On the one hand, attracted by its dynamic conception of mental illness, its objective approach to sex, and its scientific-materialistic approach to religion, these groups have been among its staunchest supporters. On the other hand, there has been a tendency among some advanced liberals and particularly among Marxists to view psychoanalysis with suspicion and disfavor. This unfavorable attitude has been based on a number of factors, of which two have been chiefly conspicuous. The first was the preoccupation of Freudian psychoanalysis with the so-called instinctual and sex life of the individual, and the consequent tendency to minimize the importance of socioeconomic forces in the etiology of mental illness. The second was the tendency to regard the structure of society and its institutions as expressions of individual vicissitudes, thus leading to naive sociological pronouncements—for instance, that wars are caused by explosive outbursts of instinctual aggressions; that all radicals are neurotics who hate their fathers and, ergo, revolutions are expressions of an unresolved Oedipus complex in the revolting group; that cooperative societies—socialist states—can never really work because instinctually all human beings are selfish, aggressive, and mutually competitive with one another, and "you can't change human nature." (It was largely on account of this reactionary sociological orientation, both explicit and implicit in some of Freud's writings, that Freudianism was so summarily rejected in the Soviet Union after the Russian revolution.)

Two examples of this distrust of psychoanalysis by left wing critics have been articles by Francis Bartlett (1) and Joseph Wortis (2). Both of these articles contain a number of fundamental errors and reveal a lack of understanding of certain aspects of modern psychoanalysis. It is important that the misconceptions expressed by these authors be clarified lest they seriously influence liberal opinion and cut off large numbers of people from an understanding and utilization of what still remains one of the most powerful instruments that we have in the therapy of the neuroses.

A great deal of the confusion prevailing in discussions about psychoanalysis lies in the fact that in the course of the past few decades there have emerged a number of different "schools" of psychoanalysis representing various degrees of divergence from orthodox Freudian theory. Many of the objections which are raised by current critics of Freudian theory and practice have been raised much earlier by progressive analysts themselves, who have been continuously revising both their theoretical views and their techniques in the light of newer ideas. Many people lose sight of the fact that psychoanalysis, no less than other scientific disciplines, is in a constant state of flux, and both its theory and practice are being progressively modified with new advances in the realms of anthropology, sociology, medicine, and psychology.

Much of the impression of the rigidity and unchangeability of psychoanalysis is unfortunately due to some Freudians themselves who insist that nothing new or significant has emerged in psychoanalysis since Freud laid down its basic premises, thus negating the value of such significant contributions to psychoanalytic thought as those of Ferenczi, Adler, Wilhelm Reich, Kardiner, Rado, and Horney, to mention only a few. Like fundamentalists of another sphere, such Freudians are convinced that "it's all writ in the Bible," and the coup de grace in any discussion between such devotees usually consists of quoting chapter and verse from one of Freud's books.

Psychoanalysis today, however, although it still rests on the broad foundations of Freud's basic discoveries, encompasses a wide variety of theoretical and practical viewpoints. It will help to clarify much of the discussion that follows if it is kept in mind that the term psychoanalysis is generally used in two broadly different ways: (1)

it is applied to a body of theory about normal and abnormal human behavior; and (2) to a technique of therapy for abnormal human behavior. For the sake of simplicity these two aspects of psychoanalysis will be discussed separately, although in practice they are interdependent.

I. PSYCHOANALYSIS AS A BODY OF THEORY

The following remarks about Freudian theory are intended not as a comprehensive or cohesive presentation, which would be beyond the limits of this paper, but merely as a brief sampling of some of its outstanding derivations. Freud believed that adult personality was determined by the vicissitudes experienced by the individual's instinctual drives, chiefly those concerned with sexual gratification, inasmuch as these were the ones which inevitably encounter taboos and repression. This repression in turn leads to castration anxiety, which is the basis of superego development and consequently of character formation. The sexual instinct supposedly goes through a phylogenetically predetermined series of stages (oral, anal, phallic, and genital) and fixation at or regression to one of these earlier levels is presumed to be the source of neurotic or psychotic behavior in later life. Character traits such as greed, ambition, miserliness and obstinacy are considered reflections of these pregenital fixations. The human unconscious, or that part of it known as the id, is a "caldron of seething excitement" and animal emotions. It is immutable and unchanging and the best that society can hope to do is to cover it with a veneer of repression and sublimation which will prevent these animal instincts from gaining the ascendancy. Consequently any unselfish sentiments such as generosity or cooperativeness are really sublimations of, or reaction formations against, underlying feelings of selfishness or aggression. Graphic art is a sublimation of sexual voyeurism; dancing or acting, of sexual exhibitionism; thirst for knowledge, of sexual curiosity; surgery, of unconscious sadism, etc. Thus the relationship between the individual and society is seen as one of conflicting interests; and mental health at best is merely a compromise which the individual achieves between his inner needs and the restrictions of society. Under conditions of great stress or danger the thin veneer imposed by culture is supposedly stripped away, exposing in all its pristine ugliness the essential animal nature of man. Since man is by nature a beast, all efforts at creating a cooperative commonwealth are inevitably doomed to failure, for they deny to man the necessary aggressive outlets offered by capitalist society. Woman's personality is specifically and inevitably influenced by her biologically-rooted envy of man's penis, which is presumed to be inherently superior and more desirable than a vagina. Many "feminine" traits are presumed to be resultants of this basic "penis envy." Feminine modesty is thus an outgrowth of woman's desire to conceal her genital defect, her vanity a compensation for her sense of inadequacy, and even the art of weaving is conjectured to have been developed by woman as a result of this same inner need to hide her defect.

Not all Freudians of today, however, believe or propound all of these ideas. One of the striking developments of recent years has been the growing awareness among Freudians themselves that they have been too preoccupied with the instinct life of the individual and that character analysis ("ego psychology") deserves greater importance than they have previously given it. As a result of this there has been increasing interest among them in the problems of character structure (3) and many of them, although adhering formally to Freudian theory, actually discard much of it in their practical work with patients.

The most progressive proponents of psychoanalysis today, however, have definitely repudiated the instinct theories of Freud and operate upon new theoretical concepts which provide more satisfactory, effective explanations for the manifold complexities of human behavior. It cannot be too strongly emphasized, however, that even the most advanced psychoanalytic thinking today still rests strongly on certain revolutionary propositions of Freud which are as valid now as they were fifty years ago. It is worth pointing out what these are since in a body they form the basic groundwork which distinguishes psychoanalysis of all varieties from other forms of psychotherapy. Briefly these may be summarized as follows:

1. *The concept of psychic determinism.* Cause and effect are as valid in the field of psychological phenomena as they are in the field of physical phenomena. In other words, all thoughts, sequences

of thoughts, dreams, fantasies and slips of the tongue must have logical and reasonable explanations. These may not always be obvious or apparent but they must nonetheless exist.

2. *The existence of unconscious mental activity.* Although a dialectician may justifiably criticize the concept of "an unconscious" as a separate and discrete unit of mental life, it is nevertheless a demonstrable fact that unconscious mental activity does exist in all degrees from barely preconscious ideas to others of which an individual is totally unaware. The former can easily be brought to the level of consciousness by the individual's simply directing his attention to them. The latter, however, can be recovered by the individual only with great difficulty and only by overcoming strong resistances within himself to facing them. He may often deny their existence and is amazed by the evidences of their influence upon his thought and behavior. This is a fact of the utmost significance and one which every practicing analyst can demonstrate daily in his office. It has also been demonstrated experimentally, as in Luria's well known experiments (4) in the creation of unconscious "complexes" by hypnosis and in Erickson's hypnotic experiments along similar lines (5).

3. *The significance of dreams.* This is a corollary of psychic determinism and is an important aid in all psychoanalytic therapy. Although, depending on their theoretical bias, different schools of analysts may differ to some extent on what any particular dream signifies, all analysts agree that dreams have meaning and that they are valid expressions of certain aspects of the individual's mental life. This is equally true of fantasies and daydreams.

4. *The significance of free association.* This, too, is a corollary of psychic determinism. The assumption here is that when thoughts are freely expressed and completely uncensored there will be a logical thread in the sequence of ideas which in experienced hands permits insight into unconscious mental processes. The uninhibited expression of all thoughts also has the effect of widening the field of consciousness for the individual himself.

5. *The significance of inner conflict.* This involves the basic concept of neuroses as products of dynamic conflicting forces within the individual. Although Freud visualized this conflict as deriving exclusively from frustration of libidinal urges of the individual, while

progressive analysts construe it as deriving more frequently in our present-day culture from the thwarting of non-instinctual security needs, all analysts recognize inner conflict as basic in the development of neuroses.

6. *Mental mechanisms of repression, projection, compensation and reaction formation.* These are used as operational concepts by almost all psychoanalysts although here, too, there are considerable differences of opinion about the nature of these mechanisms.

7. *The importance of "transference."* Although here, too, there are significant differences of opinion among psychoanalysts concerning the exact nature of the transference phenomenon, the technique of coping with it is a particularly unique psychoanalytic tool which distinguishes all varieties of psychoanalysis from other forms of psychotherapy. This phenomenon will be discussed at greater length later in this article.

These fundamental discoveries of Freud assure his position as the outstanding genius of psychoanalysis regardless of how completely his metapsychological theories have come to be rejected with the passing of time. It should not be forgotten that Freud himself did not regard these theories of his as inviolable and designated them as the "mythology" of psychoanalysis (6). It is important that progressives should not lose sight of the fact that in his time Freud's discoveries were decidedly revolutionary and that they have greatly advanced and furthered not only our understanding of mental illness but also the liberalization of sex education, social case work, and the mental hygiene and child guidance movements of today. The fact that political reactionaries often try to utilize some of Freud's theories for their own purpose must not lead progressives to reject what is good and useful in Freud's contributions.

The question may be raised, then: In what way does the theoretical basis of the most progressive viewpoint of psychoanalysis today differ from that of Freud? Briefly, it rejects any mechanistic division of human personality development into well defined "stages" (oral, anal, phallic and genital) as well as any compartmentalizing of the human personality (id, ego, superego). Instead it conceives of human development as a continuous stream of biosocial interrelationships in which each phase of development merges insensibly into the next one and dialectically influences its character. It rejects any fixed conception of human nature based upon instincts, but instead recognizes that the "nature of man" is a resultant of the interaction between his biological and social inheritances and is therefore variable and mutable (7). (In other words, human nature *can* be changed, and a better society can change it for the better.) It recognizes the overwhelming importance of basic biological drives and needs which man has in common with all other animals—needs for food, sexual gratification, and protection from the elements—but it insists that the aims of these drives in humans and the objects toward which they are expressed depend on the specific socioeconomic relationships to which the human being has been exposed. It recognizes that neurotic patterns are resultants of the culture in which they develop (8), and that they consequently change with changes in that culture. For instance, it is a matter of common observation among psychiatrists that the patterns of neurosis have been undergoing a gradual but definite change even within the past fifty years. The major hysterias which abounded in psychiatric literature before the turn of the century are now becoming relatively rare, while diffuse anxiety states, psychosomatic conditions, and obsessive-compulsive disorders seem to be more common. Even in the span of the first and second World Wars, it has been noted that whereas cardiac syndrome ("soldier's heart") was the common disease of World War I, in World War II it has been relatively rare and has been replaced by a predominance of functional gastrointestinal disorders (9).

Thus, progressive psychoanalysis sees the relationship between the individual and society as a dialectical one and denies that any basic conflict of interests inevitably exists between the two. It continues to recognize the historical importance of childhood experiences in the development of neurotic character but it does not deny the potentiality of change throughout the life of the individual. It is in early childhood, however, that basic character patterns are set down which tend to become the child's "frame of reference" in relation to his later experiences and life relationships. Where these character patterns are of a neurotic nature (for instance in the attitude that "to be loved I must be submissive and obedient," or "people are not to be trusted or depended on") they tend to become more and more strongly reinforced as the individual develops. Thus a person who suffers from a deep conviction that he is unlovable withdraws from people into a defensive shell; by so doing he actually prevents people from loving him, which reinforces his basic conviction and leads to further withdrawal. In this manner a vicious cycle is set up from which there is sometimes no release except through the medium of psychotherapy. It is for this reason that we speak of the neurotic character as being relatively rigid, in contrast to the more plastic and flexible character structure of the normal individual, who by reason of his more accurate perception of reality is able to alter his behavior as the needs of reality demand. The importance of early parental attitudes in the laying down of many elements of individual character structure can be demonstrated clinically, and is undeniable. But it is not in their biological or mechanical role as parents, but rather in their position as chief purveyors and reflectors to the growing child of the contradictory patterns in our culture (ethical concepts, class position, sexual taboos, competitiveness, insecurity, ambitions, prejudices, fears and superstitions), that they exercise their powerful influence. The neurotic envy of men which so many women in our culture reveal in analysis is also regarded as a resultant of certain aspects of our culture (10), rather than as springing from an innate recognition of the "biological superiority of the penis" (a concept which reflects the unconscious male chauvinism of Freud and his time). It is significant in this regard that as our culture has gradually offered greater opportunities to women, particularly since the first World War, this specific symptom is coming to play a diminishing role in feminine neuroses.

The foregoing does not pretend to be an exhaustive account of the modern viewpoint in psychoanalysis but it does, we hope, point out some of the major ways in which it differs from the extreme Freudian approach. Some of these differences will be elucidated further in the paragraphs that follow.

Apart from the theoretical basis of psychoanalysis there are three technical adjuvants to it which have become fixed in the popular mind. First among these is the practice of lying on a couch; second is the necessity for daily visits; and third, the impression that the analyst sits passively aloof and rarely speaks to the patient.

It should be emphasized that progressive psychoanalysis today does not encompass any rigid adherence to these formalistic rituals. What distinguishes psychoanalysis from other forms of psychotherapy is its concern with liberating the basic unconscious conflicts underlying the neurosis, in contrast to more superficial techniques of persuasion, suggestion, or milieu therapy. But whether these unconscious conflicts are dispelled with the patient in the prone, sitting, or erect posture is relatively unimportant so long as the analytic work proceeds satisfactorily. There is a popular idea, sometimes fostered by rigid Freudians, that if the patient doesn't lie on the couch he isn't being psychoanalyzed. It should be remembered, however, that one of Freud's chief reasons for insisting on this technique was a purely personal one—namely, that he could not "bear to be gazed at for eight hours a day (or more)" (11). However, what is most comfortable for the analyst is not always what is best for the patient, and modern psychoanalysts tend to be more flexible about this rule (12). That is not to say that the technique of lying on the couch is without any point. On the contrary, for many individuals this position makes possible the achievement of greater relaxation and greater freedom in associations; particularly for dependent, compliant personalities who guide their every word by anxiously watching the expression on the analyst's face for approval or disapproval, the partial separation from the analyst offered by the couch is of great value. On the other hand, for the emotionally detached patient who avoids any intimate human contact, the couch offers a refuge into which he can withdraw even further; and for such patients it may be of the utmost importance therapeutically to work in a more direct face-to-face manner. In short, the progressive analyst adapts his techniques to the needs of the patient.

Similarly with the frequency of consultations: although daily visits often make the analytic work easier and preserve its continuity more adequately, this does not mean that analysis cannot be performed with less frequent visits. Whether this can be done successfully depends not merely on how severe and acute is the neurotic disturbance but also on the intelligence and cooperativeness of the patient and the degree to which he "works on" the analysis between visits and maintains its thread of continuity.

Finally, the concept of the analyst as a completely emotionless and passive figure is also rapidly disappearing. More and more it is being recognized that the psychoanalytic relationship is an interpersonal relationship between the patient and analyst, and that the effectiveness of the therapeutic process hinges in large measure on how this relationship is handled by the psychoanalyst. An attitude of human warmth and genuine interest on the part of the analyst is one of the active ingredients of the therapeutic process, and any artificial aloofness or coldness is not only without value but may at times be positively harmful to an anxious patient. This does not imply that the progressive analyst does all the talking; on the contrary, he must still know when to be silent, but instead of being an impersonal "mirror" in front of which the patient performs, he is an active participant in a dynamic human relationship.*

II. THE NATURE OF PSYCHOANALYTIC THERAPY

Our second question is: How does psychoanalytic therapy work? It is important to state at the very outset that there are definite indications and contraindications for psychoanalytic therapy and that psychoanalysts do not recommend or utilize psychoanalysis for all forms of neurotic disturbances. There are many mild neurotic reactions, situational neuroses, or mild depressive reactions which are easily handled in a few interviews or by some positive recommendation on the part of the therapist. There are great numbers of mild neurotic reactions, moreover, which never reach any therapist but which are spontaneously resolved in the crucible of daily life. It should be borne in mind, therefore, that the following remarks about psychoanalytic therapy apply to the handling of severe psychoneuroses and character disturbances of long standing which are impervious to superficial techniques of psychotherapy or to "spontaneous" cure.

---

*The "rule of silence" which Freud imposed on psychoanalytic technique was a scientifically valuable and necessary one when psychoanalysis was still young and in an investigatory phase. Today, "with increased experience, insight, and skill in the practical utilization of psychoanalysis, it is frequently possible to proceed quickly towards the same goal by an utterly unconventional, direct and precise questioning." See Frieda Fromm-Reichmann (12, p.278).

It is a common error to assume (as Bartlett and Wortis do) (13) that psychoanalytic treatment consists merely of a "painstaking unravelling of mental symptoms and personal problems" but that in itself it does not lead to any corrective line of action. As a result of that erroneous assumption, Wortis concludes that "analysis in other words is a preliminary to treatment and is not in itself a treatment." Such a statement reveals a lack of knowledge of the actual dynamics of psychoanalytic therapy. A change in the activity of the patient is an inevitable accompaniment of any successful psychoanalytic therapy, and an integral part of it. The acquisition of insight into the nature of unconscious conflicts is only one aspect of analytic therapy. Insight in itself, it is true, often constitutes a remarkable liberating force which enables the individual without further ado to change his reactions and overcome his inhibitions. Not infrequently, however, insight may be acquired relatively early in analysis, yet the analysis proceeds for many months thereafter. It is in the application of these insights to actual behavior in real life that the neurotic's "resistance to change" or "clinging to illness" usually becomes evident, and it is in the analyst's efforts to help the neurotic to overcome these resistances, in the analysis of his defenses, and in the mobilizing of all his effective resources towards the goal of changing his behavior, that the real struggle of the analytic treatment takes place. Freud called this period the "working through" period and said of it: "This 'working through' of the resistances may in practice amount to an arduous task for the patient and a trial of patience for the analyst. Nevertheless it is the part of the work that effects the greatest changes in the patient and that distinguishes analytic treatment from every kind of suggestive treatment" (14).

In his earlier works Freud first expressed the belief that neurosis was caused by a single traumatic experience early in childhood, usually sexual in character, and that the bringing to consciousness of the repressed memory of this experience would cause a violent emotional discharge ("abreaction"), after which the patient would be cured. In the light of his later experiences, however, he discarded this idea, yet it has remained fixed in the popular mind, probably because of its dramatic potentialities and the magical suddenness of the promised cure. Traces of this early psychoanalytical belief are still manifest in the avidity with which some Freudians pursue infantile memories. The earlier the memory the greater the value they tend to attribute to it. The manner in which this pursuit of infantile memories sometimes becomes an end in itself is illustrated by Horney's amusing example of the patient who gave as the reason for wishing to resume analysis the fact that she still had an amnesia for the first five years of her life (15).

The progressive analyst, too, seeks to unravel the experiences of childhood; not as an end in itself, however, but rather as a means of helping the patient to understand more fully the roots and origins of his present character structure. This understanding is therapeutically very helpful to the patient in that it gives him an historical perspective on his difficulties and thus assists him to throw off the hopelessness which often accompanies his feeling that he has "always been this way."

Actually the cure of a neurosis or neurotic character disturbance is in most instances neither simple, dramatic, nor sudden. It is a long and complex procedure in which the analyst pits all of his knowledge and influence against the protean defenses and resistances of the patient's character structure. In this struggle the decisive factor is played by the so-called transference situation. The transference consists of the application to the analyst by the patient of the irrational and distorted aspects of his character structure. Thus a patient who is dominated by a deep distrust and fear of people will reflect these attitudes irrationally in his relationship with the analyst. The therapeutic process consists not only in analyzing the origins of this distrust and giving the patient insight into it, but also in the living interpersonal relationships between the analyst and patient in which the analyst demonstrates repeatedly the falsity of the patient's concepts. Time and again the patient "tests" the analyst, sometimes consciously, more often unconsciously. Often such tests are based on unreasonable expectations, analysis of which leads the patient to a deeper understanding of the nature of his difficulty. The clarifying of these attitudes in relation to the analyst opens the patient's eyes to similar expectations and reactions which he has toward other individuals, reactions which explain much of his interpersonal conflicts and difficulties. Finally, even after much insight has been achieved, the patient may occasionally still say in despair to the analyst: "I see what I must do very clearly and I understand why I am afraid to do it, but I am still afraid." At this point the quiet, steady, and implicit emotional support of the analyst enables the patient to cope with his despair and to take the initial steps in the "testing of reality" which the application of insight involves. The dynamic consequences of each step forward in his readjustment, together with the ever-recurring resistances, are persistently interpreted, and with the resultant fresh insights the patient is enabled to move step by step forward along the new path of an altered relationship to himself and his fellow men.

A few remarks may be made at this point about differences in therapeutic techniques between classic Freudians and progressive psychoanalysts. It is perfectly true that theory and practice are interrelated and that the practice which is based on the most accurate theory will prove to have the greatest effectiveness and widest applicability in the long run. But it would be a mistake to assume from what has been said that Freudian analysts are incapable of treating and curing neurotic patients. As a matter of verifiable fact, they treat most severe neurotics more effectively than the average non-analytic psychiatrist can. How do they do this? The following example may help to clarify this point.

Freud pointed out that the Oedipus complex is the nuclear complex of all neuroses. By this he meant that the average male neurotic when deeply analyzed is found to be suffering from the effects of an incestuous attachment to his mother and an unresolved fear and hatred of his father. On the basis of this theory, the ultimate goal of an orthodox Freudian analysis is to free the patient from his incestuous mother-attachment and his neurotic fear and hatred of his father. This is done by pointing out over and over again, in countless examples, associations, and dreams, all the facets of these "infantile" attitudes and enabling the patient to become free of them—that is, to form independent object-attachments instead of clinging to various "mother-surrogates," and to develop healthier and more realistic relationships to the "father-representatives" in his life. In the course of such therapy, the ego defenses, resistances, character formations, and transference reactions of the patient are interpreted and analyzed. Thus, in spite of the faulty theoretical basis on which this treatment rests, its ultimate result in skillful hands is to create a more independent and more effective personality. The reason for this is that like so many of Freud's theoretical formulations, the theory of the Oedipus complex contains within it the germ of a very important truth. That truth is that the central problem of many neurotic personalities in our culture revolves around problems of passive dependent attitudes (read "incestuous mother-attachment") with resultant compulsive needs for affection and protection on the one hand, and on the other, around problems relating to difficulties in coping with authority (read "fear and hatred of father") with resultant submissiveness and repressed hostilities. The progressive psychoanalyst works with the same problems, but his conception of what goes on in the patient is a more complicated and dialectical one. Thus, while the progressive analyst realizes the importance of early parental attitudes and childhood relationships, he sees that what happens to the child as a result is that a certain type of character structure develops—a series of deeply ingrained attitudes toward people and toward himself—which then acquires a dynamic quality of its own. These attitudes lead to a kind of behavior which results in their perpetuation so that the pattern of behavior tends to repeat itself over and over again. Freud called this "repetition-compulsion," but thought that it arose out of some mysterious biological propensity of matter rather than out of the dynamics of the character constellation itself. Some of the outstanding differences between the Freudian and modern approach to the Oedipus complex in a neurotic male may be represented very schematically in the accompanying table.

It will be seen from this schematic picture that the Freudian sees the Oedipus complex as being biologically rooted, and therefore inevitable in any culture, and conceives of the supposed incestuous desire for the mother and "consequent" fear of the father as being the cause of neurotic character formation; the adult neurotic patterns, moreover, are seen as direct repetitive expressions of the early childhood patterns. The progressive analyst, on the other hand, views the Oedipus complex as a resultant of a particular type of family setting in a particular type of culture; out of it develops a dynamic character structure with adult patterns which, although indirectly derived from childhood patterns, are not simple repetitions of them; and the incestuous fantasies and castration fears occasion-

FREUDIAN THEORY

Childhood Behavior → *Unconscious Adult Behavior Patterns*

Biologically rooted
{
Love for mother (incestuous) → "Infantile" attachment to mother-surrogates → {Passive dependent attitudes; compulsive need for affection; incest dreams and fantasies

Fear of father (fear of castration) → "Infantile" fear of father-surrogates → {Submissiveness; repressed hostilities; "castration anxieties"
}

PROGRESSIVE THEORY

Childhood Behavior → *Unconscious Adult Behavior Patterns*

Arising in a given society*
{
Attachment to mother
Competition with father
} Passive dependent character structure → {
Fear of responsibility
Compulsive need for affection
Repressed hostilities
Submissiveness
Fear and resentment of authority
} → {*May* be expressed symbolically in incest fantasies and dreams and in "castration anxiety"

*I.e., in a specific family setting within a patriarchal, monogamous, competitive culture.

ally expressed in such neuroses are seen as symbolic expressions and resultants of the neurotic character structure rather than as causes of it.

Thus the newer psychoanalytic technique gives the patient a more dynamic and more accurate conception of why he acts as he does but both techniques endeavor to help the patient to achieve greater emotional independence, a rational attitude towards authority and the ability to assume responsibility. It should be clear that for many patients it may make little practical difference as to which technique is applied; what is important is the repeated analysis and demonstration through interpretation of his practical activities, his dreams, his free associations, his resistances, and his transference reactions, of the irrational basis of his interpersonal relationships and of the dynamics of his character structure. The Freudian lays greater emphasis on the supposed sexual origins of the patient's difficulties and on the goal of normal sexual activity, but since the latter represents the most intimate kind of interpersonal relationship, the skillful Freudian must inevitably come to grips with the patient's character structure and must work at improving his interpersonal relationships. The progressive analyst, on the other hand, focuses on helping the total personality structure, and in so doing inevitably improves sexual functioning; moreover, by greater efficiency and more direct approach to the seat of the problem, his method tends to avoid much waste of time.

There are certain instances, however, in which the differences in theory are of such a nature that they must lead to important divergences in practice. For example, one of the frequent conflicts in women of today is that between the obligations and impulses towards domestic life and motherhood on the one hand and their desires, on the other hand, to fulfill themselves creatively in the world outside of the home. To the rigid Freudian this conflict is often posed in the form of a conflict between "femininity" and neurotic "penis envy"; and the therapeutic emphasis is thus inevitably laid upon efforts to have the woman "accept her femininity," which implies resigning herself to a passive dependent role and renouncing her "neurotic" impulses. That this solution is never really satisfactory was admitted by Freud himself in one of his last papers (16), in which he confessed to a certain hopelessness in relation to therapy of women, stating: "In no phase of one's analytic work does one suffer more from the oppressive feeling that all one's efforts have been in vain and from the suspicion that one is 'talking to the winds' than when one tries to persuade a female patient to abandon her wish for a penis as impossible . . . Our women patients feel an inner conviction that the analysis will avail them nothing and they will be none the better for it. We can only agree with them when we discover that their strongest motive in coming for treatment was the hope that they might somehow still obtain a male organ . . . ."

To the analyst, however, who is not bound by a theoretical conviction that passive dependency in women is biologically rooted and therefore normal and desirable, the problem may assume quite a different aspect. He recognizes that it is both reasonable and desirable for woman as well as for man to seek to play a constructive and creative role in society; that her objections to being bound to the reactionary program of "Kinder, Kuche, and Kirche" are well founded and valid, and that the customary subjugation of women in our society is not a biological necessity but a reflection of our culture. Consequently such an analyst would concede a certain validity in the woman's distaste for a career of housekeeping, and would endeavor to help her work out solutions leading to a constructive participation in the broader currents of life while meeting the essential obligations of her domestic existence. Erich Fromm (17) has aptly described this difference in orientation between the two viewpoints when he indicates that had Nora of Ibsen's *A Doll's House* come to a rigid Freudian analyst for treatment, he would have tended to focus on the problem of her "neurotic rebelliousness" against her husband's authority, while a progressive analyst would be inclined to approach her problem with the inquiry as to why she had for so long been willing to negate her individuality.

Another example of how such theoretical differences may lead to significant divergences in practice is indicated by the approach to a politically radical patient. Many progressives have grown to suspect psychoanalysis because so often radicals undergoing psychoanalytic treatment have emerged from it with their radical fervor lost or seriously impaired. This occurrence is fostered by the tendency of the conservative Freudian to aim at a therapeutic goal of "social adaptation" and to interpret all radical activity as being neurotic in origin. Consequently the energy of such an analysis tends to be focused on the endeavor to have the patient renounce his "neurotic rebelliousness" and learn to "accept authority."

The progressive analyst, on the other hand, while not blind to the fact that some individuals who are radical are indeed neurotically rebellious to all authority, nevertheless is not bound by theory to assume that all radicals fall into this category, and therefore to attack any evidence of radicalism per se as neurotic. In such hands, therefore, the problem of the radical patient can be approached in an entirely different light—e.g., what are the intrapsychic conflicts, anxieties, and inhibitions which are limiting the effectiveness of his work and of his social protest activities?

III. THE INDIVIDUAL NEUROTIC AND OUR SOCIETY

Francis Bartlett, whose monograph on Sigmund Freud (18) presented a valid and (in this writer's opinion) an unusually brilliant analysis of the ideological weakness of some of Freud's theories, has, as we have noted, more recently attempted to evaluate some of the newer theories of psychoanalysis as well as its value as a therapeutic procedure. In this later article (19) he makes a number of penetrating comments, but they are so interspersed with misconceptions that their positive value is considerably reduced.

A criticism which Bartlett makes jointly with Wortis is that analysis is concerned only with the "understanding of [the patient's] defects" and has nothing to do with action on the part of the patient. This charge only reveals a lack of direct clinical experience with psychoanalysis on the part of these critics, for it is precisely around the problem of action, and the patient's inner resistances to translating his understanding into constructive action, that the major portion of analytic time is consumed. This was clearly indicated earlier in this article. Nevertheless the liberating power of real insight—of a genuine understanding by the patient, not only of the nature of his neurotic mechanisms, but of all of their disastrous implications for his personality—should not be underestimated. Such an understanding is an essential condition for enabling the patient to overcome his powerful inner resistances to change. Without it psychotherapy becomes reduced to the technique of authoritative suggestion and persuasion which characterized it before Freud's revolutionary discoveries. To assume as do Bartlett and Wortis that "the mere activity of participation in cooperative work for socially useful ends is therapeutic" for the average severe neurotic is contrary to fact. All experienced psychiatrists, and most lay people for that matter, know of many individuals who, although actively engaged in socially useful or progressive causes, are nevertheless extremely neurotic and unhappy. What Bartlett and Wortis overlook is the fact that the neurotic's rigid character structure and distorted perceptions usually prevent him at the very outset either from entering into a constructive situation or, if in one, from benefiting from it. Symptoms of neurotic envy, competitiveness, power drives, and the like, exist among radicals as well as among conservatives, and a neurotic character structure will manifest itself in a progressive medium as well as in a reactionary one.

In another part of his article Bartlett imputes to Horney the belief that a person may be "unconsciously anxious without any physiological response at all" and to Freud the assumption that an "instinct could be presumed to operate 24 hours a day, whether appropriate bodily processes occur or not." Since Bartlett does not quote the sources for his conclusions, I shall not argue as to whether or not Horney or Freud ever actually made statements that warranted such an interpretation. I seriously question, however, whether Horney ever really conceived of unconscious anxiety as being without a physiological basis, or Freud of instinct as functioning in any such manner as indicated. I am certain that I am on solid ground when I state that very few practicing analysts today can be validly accused of holding to such an idealistic concept. One of the cornerstones of all modern psychiatric thinking, whether analytic or non-analytic, is the concept of psychobiological unity. No emotion or idea, whether conscious or unconscious, is presumed to exist without some corresponding physiological basis. "Unconscious anxiety" never exists merely as an "idea"; it is always reflected in muscular tension, psychosomatic disturbances, behavior distortions, or dream activities.

On the basis of this misconception Bartlett then proceeds to attack the concept of "abstract emotion." He states: "What is basic in

personality is not an abstract emotional force but the totality of
conflicting attitudes, convictions, prejudices and deeply rooted principles which have grown out of habitual participation in social life
. . . . But emotions do not and cannot exist apart from that character
as abstract forces." This is an admirable statement, and one with
which no progressive psychoanalyst would disagree. But with whom
is Bartlett arguing? I know of no dominant point of view in
psychoanalysis today that would take issue with that statement.
Bartlett is annihilating a straw man set up by himself.

As a matter of fact, Bartlett comes dangerously close in parts
of his article to making the very error he is attacking, namely, to
setting up an artificial dichotomy between ideas and emotions. He
speaks of "profound convictions" and "one-sided attitudes" almost
as though they are pure intellectual abstractions devoid of emotional
content. Actually, emotions and ideas are so indissolubly fused in
the character structure that they cannot be separated from one
another without changing their essential nature. A simple example
will illustrate this elementary fact. If a soldier were induced by
repeated experiences to anticipate danger whenever he heard the
whistle of an approaching shell, he might exhibit a definite fear
reaction each time he heard a similar sound. What is the nature
of this reaction? Is it a profound intellectual conviction or "idea"
that he is going to be hurt? Or is it an "abstract" fear with no
ideational content whatever? The answer is that it is neither; that
the ideational content and emotional response are fused into a single
unit, and it is precisely this interpenetration which the repeated
experiences have effected.

To say, therefore, as Bartlett does, that such "deep-seated convictions" as the sense of being alone, powerless, and insecure in a
potentially hostile world are "not emotions at all" but just "ideas"
is to reduce human reactions to a kind of cold intellectual rationalism
which does not correspond to fact. His neurotic individual is a person
caught in a conflict between opposing sets of "ideas" devoid of
emotional content, while his normal person is one who is "guided
by correct theories" and reacts "directly to the most complex social
situations without deviating a hair's breadth from what is reasonable."
Shades of eighteenth-century rationalism! Where in all this cold
intellectual world do feelings come in? Where do "love and appreciation of others, and the desire to do one's part regardless of personal

consequences" enter? Where are the strivings for security and gratification?

Let us carry this point further. Bartlett has a perfectly valid conception when he asserts that somewhere in the background of all human emotional reactions are certain conscious or unconscious attitudes or convictions. His error is in attempting to divorce these ideas from their attendant emotional reactions instead of recognizing their dialectical unity with one another. Thus he tends to minimize the tremendous role of emotion in the neurotic conflict. To do this is to strip the neurosis of skin and flesh and leave only the bones. Luria has demonstrated experimentally the dynamic tie-up of emotions and ideas in neurosis in his creation of artificial "complexes," which he significantly designates as "affective complexes." The entire concept of repression, which is one of the cornerstones of dynamic psychiatry, depends on this close bond between painful affect and ideas. It is precisely this fusion, as a result of various life experiences, of painful affect (anxiety) with specific ideas which leads to the act of "putting the ideas out of one's mind."

In his example of the foreman who develops conflicts over his contradictory class role, Bartlett seems to give further evidence of a belief that neurosis develops purely out of conflicts in the present to which the individual is "passively" exposed, while he completely ignores the historical soil which produces the specific potency of these conflicts in the individual. To attribute a neurosis like the foreman's purely to his ambivalence about his job is like attributing World War I to the shooting of the Austrian archduke at Sarajevo, or World War II to Hitler's invasion of Poland. Any student of historical materialism would recognize at once that a genuine understanding of such events must include a thorough knowledge of the historical socioeconomic background of these incidents which made their occurrence at a particular moment in time and space so explosive. Bartlett's "explanation" of the neurosis of his foreman commits the same error. It completely neglects the personal historical background of the foreman which made the particular situation so traumatic for him. The situation in itself cannot be the total explanation, for if it were, all foremen would develop such a neurosis. (It might be fair to assume that many foremen may have feelings of conflict as a result of their contradictory class role, but they obviously do not all develop severe neurotic reactions such as Bartlett describes.) An analogy might be seen in the example of a worker who, following an accidental injury at work, develops a neurosis—a so-called traumatic hysteria. To attempt to "explain" his neurosis in terms of his insecurity under capitalism or his resentment of his exploited status—while such statements might in themselves be entirely valid—would shed no light on why this particular worker developed the specific symptoms which he did, for not all workers who suffer injuries at work develop traumatic hysterias. Only by analyzing this worker's individual life history can we completely elucidate all the forces which produced his neurotic symptom at that particular point in time and space.

This error of Bartlett's deserves further elucidation, for it brings up the entire question of the manner in which individual and socioeconomic forces are dialectically interrelated in the formation of character structure. The progressive psychoanalyst of today takes full cognizance of socioeconomic forces in the formation of character and neurosis in our society. Our forms of production; the structure of the family; the pervasive sense of insecurity; class position; the contradictions between our Christian ethics of brotherhood, truth, justice, and fair play, in contrast with the ruthless, competitive nature of our society which pays premiums for aggressiveness, deceit, hypocrisy and individualistic self-aggrandizement; all of these factors and many more leave their indelible impress on the personality and character structure of every person subjected to them. So true is this that psychoanalysts commonly agree that, strictly speaking, there are no unneurotic people in our culture, just differences in degree of neuroticism.

But such socioeconomic analyses, although they offer valid explanations for the *general* character of people in our society, cannot be used to explain *individual* neuroses and character differences, as Bartlett seems to be trying to do. Despite certain general similarities and trends which can be observed in all neuroses in our culture, and which derive from certain forces in that culture, there are nevertheless infinite variations in individual neurotic patterns, in the choice of symptoms, and in the degree of character disturbance which can be understood only in the light of the individual's personal life history. It makes a profound difference, for example, in the development of any individual character structure—*regardless of the individual's class position*—whether the mother and father were loving and permissive or hostile and repressive; whether the family ties were close and affectionate or loose and unfriendly; whether the parents were happily married, separated or divorced; whether siblings were present or absent and what their relationship to one another was.

This does not mean that the individual's life history is studied in a vacuum. It is most fully understood, indeed, only in the context of the cultural medium in which it has developed. But the study of the medium alone cannot explain individual differences, as Bartlett seems to imply. Just as Freud made the error of directly transferring his findings about individual patients to social groups (thus ignoring the sound dialectical doctrine that a group is more than just the sum of its individual components and has a movement and quality of its own), so Bartlett is making the equally dangerous error of attempting to psychologize about individuals merely by analyzing their class position. This is a kind of pseudo-Marxism which reduces Marxist theory to an absurdity. The psychology of the individual has a history, movement, and series of laws of its own, and only by understanding them adequately can the complex dialectical interrelationship between the individual and society be adequately comprehended. Statements such as the labeling of the individual's character structure as being simply "the outcome of his class position," or "the terms aggression and anxiety become . . . therapeutically useless if they are not articulated in terms of current political and economic trends" are examples of this type of distorted Marxist approach.*

---

*Cf. Engels' letter to Joseph Bloch, in which he expounds the significance, among other forces, of "individual wills," determined in part by "physical constitution" and "personal circumstances," as important contributors to the historical process, and states that "if someone twists this [the materialist conception of history] into the statement that the economic element is the *only* determining one, he transforms it into a meaningless, abstract and absurd phrase." Engels goes on to state: "Marx and I are ourselves partly to blame for the fact that younger writers sometimes lay more stress on the economic side than is due to it. We had to emphasize this main principle in opposition to our adversaries, who denied it, and we had not always the time, the place, or the opportunity to allow the other elements involved in the interaction to come into their rights."

This tendency to negate the dynamics of individual forces in the interaction with social forces leads to a conception of the individual as a relatively passive agent in the interaction. Such an attitude appears in Bartlett's repeated statements in his article that the individual "passively receives ideas and beliefs from his culture." This sounds very much like Locke's old conception of the tabula rasa. While I cannot believe that Bartlett really adheres to such a conception, the tendency to this kind of formulation results from his minimization of individual dynamics in the sociopsychological "parallelogram of forces." The individual is never a passive figure in the dialectical interrelationship with society. Driven as he is by powerful inner biosocial needs for security and satisfaction, he is always an active force in the interrelationship, even when his surface reactions are apparently "passive."

One of Bartlett's chief points, however, is a valid one and worth emphasizing. In Horney's theory of neurosis, he remarks, the constructive forces of the individual "are regarded as existing apart from the neurotic structure instead of being . . . essential to the formation of the basic conflicts." This is a point well taken. Horney conceives of neurosis as springing out of conflicts between mutually incompatible neurotic trends, such as the "neurotic need for affection" on the one hand and the "neurotic need for power" on the other. This conception of Horney's, in the writer's opinion also, leaves out something extremely important and essential, namely, the significant dynamic role of constructive forces in the actual genesis of the neurotic conflict. The need for affection, for example, is not necessarily neurotic; it is so only when it is indiscriminate or exaggerated. Within normal limits it is one of those socially constructive forces in the individual which seek to bind him in close and friendly ties with other people. As such it exerts a powerful influence on the individual, and the person who finds himself gradually becoming more and more isolated from others by virtue, say, of the neurotic need to dominate, develops conflicts precisely because his constructive goals become threatened by the effects of the neurotic trend.

Similarly, other needs of the individual in our society, needs for self-expression, for emotional growth and creativeness, for recognition by one's fellow men, for someone to share one's life with, all are powerful constructive forces in the life of the individual, the thwarting of which, by neurotic trends, may cause neurotic conflicts. In the deepest sense these conflicts are expressions of the contradictory currents in our present culture as they reflect themselves in the personal life experiences of the individual. By considering the sources of neurotic conflict as exclusively confined to opposing neurotic trends, Horney fails to recognize the role which the constructive forces in the individual constantly play in the dynamics of the character structure and of the neurotic conflict, and by thus isolating the constructive forces from the arena of conflict, her conception of the neurotic character structure becomes a dualistic instead of a monistic one. The constructive forces within the individual are not only responsible for the struggle against the neurotic trends; they drive him to seek help when necessary, and they are the decisive factors in the ultimate achievement of mental health.

REFERENCES

1. FRANCIS BARTLETT, "Recent Trends in Psychoanalysis," *Science & Society,* IX (Summer, 1945).
2. JOSEPH WORTIS, "Freudianism and the Psychoanalytic Tradition," *American Journal of Psychiatry,* XXV (May, 1945).
3. See ANNA FREUD, *The Ego and the Mechanisms of Defense* (London, 1937), and WILHELM REICH, *Character-Analysis* (New York, 1945).
4. A. R. LURIA, *The Nature of Human Conflicts* (New York, 1932).
5. MILTON H. ERICKSON, "Experimental Demonstration of the Psychopathology of Everyday Life," *Psychoanalytical Quarterly,* VIII (1939), p. 338; "Demonstration of Mental Mechanisms by Hypnosis," *Archives for Neurology and Psychiatry,* XLII (1939), p. 367; "A Study of Hypnotically Induced Complexes by Means of the Luria Technique," *Journal of Genetic Psychology,* XXX (1934), p. 65.
6. SIGMUND FREUD, *New Introductory Lectures* (New York, 1944), p. 131.
7. J. MARMOR, "The Role of Instinct in Human Behavior," *Psychiatry,* (1942), p. 509. (Chapter 1, this volume)
8. KAREN HORNEY, *The Neurotic Personality of Our Time* (New York, 1937), also ABRAM KARDINER, *The Individual and His Society* (New York, 1939) and *The Psychological Frontiers of Society* (New York, 1945).
9. GRINKER and SPIEGEL, *Men Under Stress* (Philadelphia, 1945), p. 254.
10. KAREN HORNEY, *New Ways in Psychoanalysis* (New York, 1939), ch. 6, and also CLARA THOMPSON, "The Role of Women in This Culture," *Psychiatry,* IV (1941), p. 1, and "Penis-Envy in Women," *ibid.,* VI (1943), p. 123.
11. SIGMUND FREUD, *Collected Papers,* II (London, 1933), p. 354.

12. FRIEDA FROMM-REICHMANN, "Psychoanalytic Psychotherapy with Psychotics," *Psychiatry*, VI (1943), p. 277.
13. See references 1 and 2.
14. SIGMUND FREUD, *Collected Papers*, II, p. 376.
15. KAREN HORNEY, *New Ways in Psychoanalysis*, p. 140.
16. SIGMUND FREUD, "Analysis, Terminable and Interminable," *International Journal of Psychoanalysis*, XVIII (1937).
17. ERICH FROMM, "The Social Philosophy of Will Therapy," *Psychiatry*, II (1939), p. 229.
18. FRANCIS BARTLETT, *Sigmund Freud* (London, 1938).
19. See reference 1.

9

PSYCHOANALYSIS AND DIALECTICAL
MATERIALISM
(1949)

Over the years the influence of psychoanalysis has slowly spread, and has left its mark not only upon psychology and medicine, but also upon anthropology, sociology, and every phase of art and literature. In America it has begun to find its way into the curricula of the hitherto hostile medical schools, some of which are for the first time now offering full postgraduate psychoanalytic training courses; and the autonomous psychoanalytic institutes are besieged as never before by constantly growing numbers of young psychiatrists, eager for specialized instruction.

Criticisms of psychoanalysis, however, although perhaps less widespread than formerly, are persistent. A growing group of scientifically oriented thinkers has criticized the theoretical concepts of classical psychoanalysis as being at variance with the concepts of modern materialism. This criticism cannot lightly be charged to ignorance, bias, or inner "resistance" in the critics. Much in classical psychoanalytic theory is open to objection on such grounds. It is the contention of this writer, however, that psychoanalysis, stripped of its debatable superstructure and reduced to its *basic concepts,* is fully in accord with the principles of modern materialism; that its instinctivistic and mechanistic aspects are subject to increasing criticism within its own ranks; and that psychoanalytic theory, no less than the theory of any of the other basic social sciences, reflects its historical and socioeconomic mileu, and is consequently changing and adapting itself to the progress of scientific knowledge.

119

Contrary to popular belief, there is no close unity among psychoanalysts today either in theory or in practice. For a long time there
was a considerable tendency among the more classical followers
of Freud to insist on such unity among professed psychoanalysts;
but as Ernest Jones, dean of British psychoanalysts and one of Freud's
earliest followers, has said:

> The impossibility of this ideal is being recognized and it is
> being replaced by the more practicable, though difficult enough,
> endeavor to distinguish between what constitute the essential
> characteristics of psychoanalysis and what are superimposed and
> more varying features. Here we cannot do better than follow
> Freud's own definition. Psychoanalysis is simply the study of
> mental processes of which we are unaware, of what for the
> sake of brevity we call the unconscious. The psychoanalytic
> method of carrying out this study is that characterized by the
> free association technique of analyzing the observable phenomena
> of transference and resistance. As Freud himself said, anyone
> following this path is practicing psychoanalysis even if he comes
> to conclusions different from Freud's . . . and it is plain that
> we should be forsaking the sphere of science for that of theology
> were we to regard these conclusions . . . as being sacrosanct
> and eternal. (1)

Let us examine the elements upon which this basic definition
of psychoanalysis as given by Freud rests. They are "the study
of mental processes of which we are unaware," "the free association
technique," and "the phenomena of transference and resistance."
These elements are by no means separate and distinct from one
another. Historically and practically they are closely interrelated
and form a unified, dynamic concept of certain aspects of mental
activity which is the cornerstone of all psychoanalytic theory and
practice, regardless of the extent to which this theory and practice
may vary in other respects among analysts.

That mental processes of which we are unaware exist is no longer
a debatable matter. One may properly question, as some critics do,
the validity of designating such processes in terms of a particular
"area" of the mind known as "the unconscious," but the reality
of the processes has been conclusively demonstrated not only clinically
but experimentally. The experimental evidence is crucial, for out

of it, as we shall see, comes the confirmation also of the validity of the free association technique and of the concepts of repression and resistance. Let us first, however, briefly review the historical development of these basic concepts.

Prior to Freud, not only was psychiatry itself static and purely descriptive, but also experimental investigations of human personality, will and emotion, without an adequate guiding theory, were largely fruitless. Freud started his practice in 1886 utilizing electrotherapy, suggestion, and hypnosis, the accepted therapeutic methods of the day. But he learned very early that these tools were unsatisfactory. In all severe cases, he saw "the suggestions which had been applied crumble away again; and then the disease or some substitute for it returned" (2). Some years before, an older colleague, Dr. Breuer, had told Freud of his discovery that under hypnosis a "widening of consciousness" seemed to take place, which enabled his patient (the famous Anna O.) to recall many experiences which were not accessible to her in a normal state. Recalling this, Freud began to use hypnosis in investigating the historical antecedents of his patients' neurotic illnesses, and confirmed Breuer's finding that memories, thoughts, and impulses which had previously dropped out of consciousness could thus be brought out, revealing significant connections between the recollections and the character of the symptoms.

Freud next asked himself why it was so difficult to bring to consciousness these dynamically charged ideas and emotions. It seemed logical to assume that they could not become conscious because a certain force was operating in opposition to them. He became acutely aware of this when his inability to hypnotize many of his patients compelled him to seek other means of widening the sphere of their awareness. No amount of direct questioning or urging achieved this desired result. Finally he evolved the method of asking his patients to tell him everything that came to their minds without rejecting anything, and regardless of whether the material seemed relevant or not. By this technique, to which he gave the name of "free association," Freud discovered that patients were actually able to recover many thoughts, impulses, and memories which had hitherto been accessible only through hypnosis. This represented an important technical advance, of which he wrote,

"The history of psychoanalysis proper . . . begins with the new technique that dispenses with hypnosis" (3). But while by this technique patients were able to bring previously unconscious ideas into consciousness, Freud observed that they succeeded only in the face of considerable inner resistance. The reluctance of the patient to express certain thoughts, the slips of the tongue, the significant gaps in memory, the "accidental" omissions and inaccuracies all pointed unmistakably to the existence of emotional conflict. It seemed apparent that the impulses and ideas which were unconscious had become so because they were incompatible with other aspects of the patient's personality, and that they had been kept out of awareness as an economical measure to protect the personality from the pain of persistent conscious conflict. Out of this clinical observation Freud developed the concept of repression, which

> is the foundation stone on which the structure of psychoanalysis rests, the most essential part of it, and yet it is nothing but a theoretical formulation of a phenomenon which may be observed to recur as often as one undertakes an analysis of a neurotic without resorting to hypnosis. (4)

It is worth noting that the free associational technique which led to this theoretical advance rests upon a basic assumption which is thoroughly in accord with modern scientific thinking—the assumption that all psychic phenomena, far from being accidental and haphazard, are strictly determined. This is the concept of *psychic determination*—that cause and effect relationships hold true for psychological phenomena as for all other phenomena. There must be, Freud assumed, a rational explanation for even the minutest psychological event or process, whether it be a dream, fantasy, slip of the tongue, lapse of memory, or merely the sequence in which one thought follows another. He took as his working basis the assumption that the patient's thoughts were not haphazard, but were influenced by his repressed attitudes and impulses, and to a certain extent were derived from them.*

---

*It was this assumption which laid the groundwork for Freud's monumental discoveries about the nature of dreams. It is worth noting that no system of psychology, other than the psychoanalytic, has offered a rational explanation

The earliest confirmation of this assumption—"the first bridge between experimental psychology and psychoanalysis" (5)—was in the word association test which Jung adapted from Wundt. In this test Jung showed that, whenever the response to a word stimulus was greatly retarded or was otherwise unusual in character, it could be demonstrated that the word stimulus was associated in the subject's mind with some repressed complex. The experiments, however, could not in themselves be considered decisive, since the complex itself, being unknown to both subject and experimenter, could not be adequately controlled during the experiment. Luria observes:

> The psychologist, as compared with the physicist and the chemist, finds himself in a very unfavorable position; even with the best possible experimentation he usually has to admit regretfully that a great many of the facts he analyses are beyond his control, not capable of being recorded . . .
>
> The ideal for the psychological experimenter has become the possibility to reconstruct artificially the phenomenon under examination, because only this enables one to keep it entirely under control . . .
>
> It is quite comprehensible, therefore, that only an artificial insertion of an affective complex into the psyche of the subject, which complex is known in all details, can create for the psychologist a situation where it would be easier for him to record all the factors forming the affective reaction.

This decisive experiment was performed by Luria himself in 1924–1925:

> We suggested to the person under test, while in a sufficiently deep hypnotic state, a certain situation . . . in which he was playing a rôle irreconcilable with his habits and contrary to his usual behavior. We made those suggestions imperatively, and forced the person under hypnotism to feel the situation suggested

of dream material. While individual analysts, depending upon their theoretical orientation, often differ as to the meaning of certain dream patterns, all analysts accept and utilize Freud's brilliant concepts of the *mechanisms* involved in the formation of dreams—the so-called "dream work" of symbolization, condensation, displacement, etc. These discoveries of Freud have taken dreams once and for all out of the realm of mysticism and related them to the world of reality.

with sufficient painfulness; we thus obtained an actual and rather sharply expressed acute affect. After awakening the person under test . . . we had a subject who was "loaded" with certain definite affective complexes, which mostly remained unknown to himself, but which were recorded by us in almost all important details.

[The patients] all were subjected to the following standard operation: the person under test was put to sleep, and a traumatic situation previously prepared was suggested to him. After the suggestion was made, an amnesia was suggested to the person (in control cases the amnesia was not suggested and we observed a natural post-hypnotic amnesia) and he was awakened. Before the hypnosis, we used a number of word-stimuli—a part of them having a direct bearing on the complex which later was suggested to him; and we obtained the usual series of associated answers with connected motor reactions.* Simultaneously we recorded a free number of chain associations,† which were connected with the respective motor pressures. That operation was repeated a second time after the suggestion was made to the person in his post-hypnotic states; after this the subject was again put to sleep and the suggestion made was countermanded. After his second awakening, he was tested again in the same way.

Luria was impressed by "the entire elimination from the consciousness of what had occurred" and by the fact that "only a few signs, like a heavy feeling, a general anxiousness, etc., remain as symptoms of the fact that in the subject's past there is concealed some severe trauma . . . A strong emotion is hidden here in the past . . . removed from consciousness, though apparently it is still active."

He then went on to test the word associations and connected motor reactions of his subjects, and found that "every time the subject responds to the words connected with the complex with

---

*"Motor reactions" refers to Luria's method of recording motor responses in his subjects during the word association test. At the instant of response the subject must press a bulb with the fingers of his right hand, a motion which is recorded as a curve on a chart. Normally the curve is regular and occurs simultaneously with the word-response. In the presence of emotional disturbances the curve becomes stronger, irregular, or rises and falls before and after the word-response. Luria also recorded the breathing responses of his subjects, and noted similar irregularities in the breathing pattern when emotional disturbances occurred.

†That is, free-associational word-chains.

distinct retardation and shows a curve of pressure reaching almost to the limit." But even more striking were the free-associational word reactions. In these he noticed that "the subject reconstructs quite unintentionally the [suggested] situation . . . in the chain series, not knowing why that situation has come to her mind, and not being able to explain its contents." His conclusion is identical with Freud's assumption: *"The affective complex constructed by us, though not yet being conscious, creates an affective state and determines the flow of the free associative series."*

These decisive experiments by a noted materialist psychologist—repeated, confirmed, and extended by Erickson in the United States (6)—thus confirm in the laboratory the facts which Freud noted clinically: that psychic conflict could result in the development of "affective complexes"* which, though concealed from the consciousness of the individual by some defensive functional mechanism, nevertheless continued to exert a significant effect upon his thoughts and actions. The repressive mechanism, says Luria, "seems to be the mechanism which saves the personality from the over-excitement and from the disorganisation connected with an open appearance of the conflict" (7). The existence of conflict, repression, resistance, and unconscious mental activity, and the validity of the free-association technique are all confirmed in these experiments.

There remains but one other basic assumption of psychoanalysis to consider at this point—the phenomenon of transference. Transference was not "invented" by Freud. It is merely a term which he applied to an incontrovertible clinical fact—namely, that neurotic patients frequently react to the therapist in an irrational fashion, inconsistent with the reality situation. The more neurotic the patient, the more marked is such a reaction apt to be. Unfortunately the concept of transference is often used loosely to include all attitudes that a patient has towards his therapist. If the patient likes the therapist, that is a "positive transference." If he dislikes him, that

---

*There has been considerable difference of opinion among progressive analysts in recent years as to whether affects are ever actually subject to repression. Some contend that only memories, thoughts, and ideas can be repressed, but that affects themselves are always appropriate to the way in which the individual sees reality. Full discussion of the pros and cons of the problem, however, would take us beyond the limitations of this paper.

is a "negative transference." Such a use of the concept leaves no room for rational judgment on the part of the patient and becomes meaningless. If a patient likes a therapist who is friendly and warm, and dislikes one who is surly or uninterested, this is not necessarily a transference reaction. It may be, and often is, a perfectly valid and realistic judgment on the part of the patient. It would probably be better to use the terms "rapport" and "lack of rapport" for such realistic reactions. Freud himself specifically restricted "transference" to irrational attitudes on the part of the patient. His explanation of these attitudes was that the patient was reacting to the analyst with an identical repetition of behavior that had previously been manifested to an emotionally significant figure in the patient's infantile past, e.g., father, mother or sibling; that he was in effect "transferring" to the analyst these attitudes as though the analyst actually represented this emotionally charged figure.

This explanation is considered overly mechanistic by progressive psychoanalysts; but the observations themselves are indisputable and of the greatest significance. The modern tendency is to regard the transference phenomenon not as a mechanical "repetition-compulsion" of earlier attitudes, but as a dynamic expression of certain attitudes, faulty perceptions, or distorted "frames of reference" which have their roots, it is true, in earlier experiences but are not identical with them. Thus a neurotic patient who in early life has been severely traumatized by parental rejection may develop a belief that he is unlovable; and his subsequent relations with people, being colored by this conviction, will be dominated by an unrealistic suspiciousness, hostility, and withdrawal from them. These unrealistic attitudes are also manifested in relation to the analyst to whom he comes for help. From a practical therapeutic standpoint it may at times be of minor importance whether one states that the patient "sees the analyst as the rejecting parent" or whether one states that the patient has developed out of his early experiences a conviction that he is unlovable, with consequent attitudes that manifest themselves in all of his significant interpersonal relationships. To some patients both statements may be equally meaningful and useful. From the philosophical standpoint, however, the first statement is a mechanistic one, while the second is dialectical and has a wider field of reference.

Another basic idea which is implicit in the concept of transference is that of the historical origin of neurotic difficulties. This parallels in the psychological field the concept of historical materialism in the field of sociology and economics. It is "the historical principle as applied to the development of human consciousness" (8). It rests on the assumption that what an individual is at any given moment (i.e., his character structure) is determined by the interaction of his biological inheritance with the sum total of his past experience. For this reason psychoanalysis, like historical materialism, has been frequently attacked by philosophical idealists as denying the existence of "free will." Insofar as psychoanalysis affirms that man's behavior is not mystically independent of his environment, the charge is true. But the affirmation is often corrupted by its critics to mean that psychoanalysis therefore denies the possibility of man's being free to alter his behavior. This is a corruption of psychoanalysis just as the corresponding charge against historical materialism is a corruption of the latter. Like the latter, psychoanalysis affirms that the more men understand about themselves and the world in which they live, the freer they can be in dealing with their environment. This assumption in fact is the rationale behind the very existence of psychoanalytic therapy. Hegel's phrase that "necessity is blind only insofar as it is not understood" may be paraphrased to say that "human impulses are blind only insofar as they are not understood."

Now it will be remembered that one of the distinguishing characteristics of psychoanalysis is that it not only recognizes the phenomenon of transference but utilizes it in the therapeutic process itself. A full discussion of how this is done would require an article in itself; but very briefly we may say that transference manifestations may be utilized in a psychotherapeutic relationship in one of two main ways. One method aims at cure by making the patient aware of his unrealistic attitudes and helping him to study the mode and circumstances of their operation, their relationship to external events, and the consequences of their activity, so that they eventually become modified through insight. This is the method of psychoanalysis. The other method is to use the unrealistic authority with which the patient endows the therapist to influence the patient to better forms of behavior; this essentially is the operational basis for most forms of non-analytic psychotherapy—suggestion, guidance, etc.

Contrary to the misconceptions of some critics (9), the psychoanalytic technique is not a prelude to action on the part of the patient, but is closely integrated with what goes on in the patient's daily life. "A change in the activity of the patient is an inevitable accompaniment of any successful psychoanalytic therapy, and an integral part of it" (10).

So much then for the basic assumptions of psychoanalysis: the concept of unconscious mental activity, with its corollary concepts of conflict, repression, and resistance; the concept of psychic determinism, with its corollary assumption of the validity of free association and the significance of dreams; and finally, the concept of transference with its corollary recognition of the historical determination of behavior. All these are functional dynamic concepts, and none is at variance with modern scientific materialism. Insofar as they represent correct observations of psychological reality, any theory of human behavior which goes beyond restating them in other terms* to negate them must of necessity be incomplete or inaccurate.

Now we come to the problem of examining that considerable superstructure of psychoanalytic theory which constitutes Freud's theory of instincts and its numerous derivatives. At the very outset, however, we are faced with a manifest difficulty. When dealing with a collection of writings as voluminous as Freud's, it is possible, as with the Bible, to lift individual sentences out of context and thereby demonstrate almost anything one is seeking to prove. It has not been at all difficult, for example, for some exponents of Freud (13) to "prove" by repeated isolated quotations from his works that he was a thoroughgoing dialectical materialist. If we are to

---

*McGill and Welch (11), for example, have made an effort to explain many psychoanalytic concepts in purely behavioral terms. While such efforts are both valuable and useful, they do not, in my opinion, negate the validity and predictive value of these basic psychoanalytic concepts. As McGill himself has said in another connection: "What is not always appreciated is that inferences enter into the interpretation of all the data of science. The only question is whether the inferences are valid and whether they facilitate prediction" (12). One of the difficulties attendant upon a purely behavioral approach to mental disorder is that often the disorder finds its chief mode of expression in disturbances of thought—e.g., schizophrenic thinking—which can be dealt with adequately only at a conceptual level. Similarly, no purely behavioral approach, so far as the writer knows, has been able to cope effectively with the problem of dream interpretation.

evaluate Freud's thinking properly from the philosophical stand-point, however, we cannot lay undue emphasis on such isolated statements, but must be guided by the main currents of it, by the overwhelming preponderance of its direction. If we do this we cannot escape the conclusion that the theoretical superstructure which Freud erected upon the scientific nucleus already discussed represents a combination of mechanical materialistic with entelechistic* thinking. In justice to Freud, however, it should be pointed out that although he emphatically insisted upon the validity of his concept of repression and resistance as "a theoretic inference legitimately drawn from innumerable observations" (14) he made no such claim for his theory of the instincts, which he characterized as the "mythology" (15) of psychoanalysis. Further evidence of his inner uncertainty about this aspect of his work is furnished by the fact that throughout his lifetime he constantly struggled with it, making repeated revisions in it in an effort to make it more effectively fit the observable phenomena of human behavior.

For Freud the human being was first and foremost a biological organism, and in following man's vicissitudes he was primarily interested in what happened to man's biological needs in the course of his growth and development. All of his subsequent needs were conceived of as outgrowths, reflections, or "sublimations" of these basic biological "instinctual" drives. Although Freud did not ignore the significance of cultural institutions in influencing the drives, the basic, major determinant in his opinion was the Oedipus complex which arose out of the child's attraction to the parent of the opposite sex and the fear of retribution from the parent of the same sex. Freud regarded this conflict as essentially biological in origin and hence universal to all human beings. "This probably holds true," he felt, "not only in the life of individuals but also in the history of the human species as a whole" (16). Moreover, he considered the "reactions against the instinctual demands of the Oedipus complex" as the prime source of human achievement and the chief basis for the development of the social institutions in every culture—religion, morality, art, literature, etc.

---

*"Entelechy" and "entelechism," as used in this article, refer to Freud's concept of instincts as having an autonomous character, which is fundamentally unalterable by the environment.

In some respects Freud's thinking is strikingly similar to Hobbes's. Like Hobbes, he believed that man's "innate" tendencies were essentially selfish, animalistic, and antisocial. The chief function of society (and education) was to "inhibit, forbid, and suppress" these impulses which would otherwise destroy it. For this reason Freud was pessimistic about the possibility of success of any cooperative commonwealth, because it would be contrary to "human nature" to expect human beings to be anything but selfishly individualistic. In his concept of human nature as something fixed and ineradicable, which social influences could modify or conceal but never genuinely alter,* Freud clearly discloses both his entelechism and his mechanistic materialism. Like parts of a machine, the individual and society impinge upon each other, and changes take place at the periphery; but the basic character of man remains unaltered, to emerge in pristine ugliness in time of war or other stress. This unalterable "essential nature" of man, however, is an entelechistic concept.†

Fenichel, Osborn, and other upholders of Freud's instinct theory

---

*Ludwig Jekels, one of Freud's early pupils and associates, presents this concept dramatically when, in disputing the thesis that the nature of man can change, he says: "This being, prostrate by the burden of heredity and constitution, driven either by his urges or by tormenting anxiety, nailed to his ego by his narcissism . . . seems unlikely to promise such changeability, and there is little chance for him to become the demiurge of an entirely new world" (17). Note the similarity of this concept to the doctrine of original sin. It is of interest to note also a remark of A. A. Brill, dean of classical American analysts, quoted in the *New York Times* of July 23, 1947: "We admit with the Bible that the imagination of the human heart is evil from the beginning, but we do not blame the child for its feelings and actions. We feel it is born that way."

†Bartlett in his essay on Freud (18) has ably elaborated upon the similarity of the Freudian id to the "isolated individual" or "natural man" of Hobbes and Rousseau, and shown the relationship of all three concepts to the productive relations which exist in contemporary capitalist society. However, he seems to me to make a serious error in interpreting Freud's use of entelechies as idealism. Strictly speaking, "the fundamental principle of idealism is that matter, the actual material world we find ourselves a part of, is not the final reality" (19). If there is any one thread that may be said to run consistently through all of Freud's writings it is his oft-asserted conviction that all of man's mental and emotional life was firmly rooted in material, biological origins. The "instincts" as conceived of by Freud are strictly materialistic phenomena with somatic sources. The fact that they are entelechistic concepts does not warrant characterizing them as idealistic. An entelechy may be either an idealistic or a mechanical

have often claimed that it is a misinterpretation of Freud's views to state that he overemphasized the significance of biological forces in man's adaptation to his environment.

> Man [says Fenichel] is guided by certain basic biological drives which are not at all rigid patterns but are formed and developed according to satisfying and frustrating experiences, which means through social forces. . . . According to Freud the human being becomes a human being (an "ego") by entering into "interrelations" with other human beings. . . . Social relations can only "form individuals" because of a certain biological structure of man; and the study of this biological basis and of what happens to this basis under different social circumstances . . . makes it understandable how social relations form individuals. . . . The statement that a biological substratum is molded by institutions does in no way imply an underestimation of the influence of the institutions. (20)

These statements of Fenichel deserve careful analysis, not only because he was one of the most erudite and brilliant exponents of Freud's classical theories, but also because he was aware of the importance of social forces and of the contradictions within our modern capitalist economy. Yet his comments illustrate one of the basic fallacies of classical Freudian thinking. It is not that Freud (or Fenichel and others) ignores or necessarily underestimates the significance of social influences upon the individual, but that he interprets this influence *mechanistically* instead of *dialectically*. The Freudian view is that man is a biological animal "molded" by his

---

materialistic concept. That Freud's entelechistic thinking is an outgrowth of his mechanistic materialism and has nothing to do with philosophic idealism is amply demonstrated by the preponderant weight of evidence in his writings. Bartlett's efforts to "prove" Freud's idealism by lifting an occasional sentence out of context are as manifestly lacking in objectivity as the contrary efforts to "prove" him to be a dialectical materialist. On the other hand, there is no denying that the derivations of entelechistic thinking often lead to conceptions of society which *serve the interests* of the philosophic idealists. This is true, for example, of Freud's conception of a fixed "human nature" and of his explanation of social institutions as instinct derivatives. To classify him on this basis as an idealist, however, is incorrect. Freud's theoretical limitations, as we shall see, flow not from any tendency to idealism, but from the fact that his materialism was mechanistic instead of dialectical.

environment, but that the basic "biological substratum" in the form of the reservoir of "instinctual" impulses remains essentially unaltered. Their *external manifestations* are, it is true, transformed by social influences, but their basic *inner nature* remains unaltered— compare Fenichel's statement almost in the same breath as his previous one, that "character traits . . . are not at all adaptations made by the ego, but things which happen to the ego against its will by instinctual forces which return from the repressed" (21). The modern dialectical view, however, is that out of the interrelationship between man's biological inheritance and his social environment a new *unity* is formed, a fusion in which *the biological as such no longer exists in man's psychological expressions;* it cannot any longer be separated from the social. The development of the human cortex, with its language and association functions, represents the physiological expression of this unity. A human body without a human brain is no longer human; it is something else but no longer "man." The needs of man can consequently no longer be expressed in simple biological terms; even the basic needs of hunger and sex cannot be isolated from the social influence of the cerebral cortex.

This conception is expressed on a physiological level in the holistic concept of brain activity. Few modern neurophysiologists would assert that subcortical structures have an activity of their own, independent of the activity of the cortex. The living brain functions as a unit; no cortical or subcortical activity takes place that is not at every moment relative to and dependent on the activity of the rest of the nervous system. One could, it is true, study the activity of the isolated subcortex by decorticating the brain; but then one would be dealing with a different unit which could not be validly compared with the subcortex which is integrated in a total living brain. In short, it would no longer be a "human" subcortex. By the same token one might conceivably study the sexual drive or hunger drive in a person who had been totally isolated from social contacts all his life, but then one would not be studying man as we know him but something totally different. What we call "human nature" grows out of man's social relationships and cannot be separated therefrom (22).

This viewpoint is not, as some classical Freudians insist, an antibiological one, or an overemphasis on environment, or a denial of the great importance of man's biological needs. It is merely a dialectical conception of how these needs operate in contrast to a mechanistic one. I have elsewhere stated the problem as follows:

> The old conflicts of heredity versus environment or biology versus culture become meaningless when viewed from the organismic approach of modern psychology. Even in the lower forms of animal life, the organism is immersed in an environment from the very beginning of the life cycle. Each stage of development is determined by the cooperation of heredity and environmental forces. Since the earlier stages influence the character of the development of the later stages, the hereditary and environmental factors become more and more interpenetrated as development proceeds. Nowhere is this more true than in humans, where the cultural factors become indissolubly interrelated with organic processes through the laying down of language patterns in the association centers of the cortex. Thus there develops a new unity which is qualitatively unique in the animal world—a sociobiological unity—called human nature. This interpenetration is so complex and so complete that one cannot separate the hereditary from the environmental factors in man without destroying the specific quality which constitutes the nature of man, just as water cannot be separated into hydrogen and oxygen without destroying that quality which constitutes water. (23)

It is around this same problem that the modern critics of Freud's emphasis upon sexuality rest their arguments. It is not necessary to deny the great importance of the sexual drives, or to question the existence of infantile sexuality, in order to take issue with Freud on this point. The tremendous part which sexual needs play in the life of every person is a phenomenon which any honest student of the human personality can find for himself if he does not close his mind to the observable facts; the same is true of the existence of infantile sexuality. But to assume, as Freud does, that these sexual needs are the prime determinants of character is quite another matter, and one which the modern materialists correctly criticize as one-sided. It is not being "antibiological" to see the sexual needs of human beings as but one vector in the complex series of forces which determine human behavior. Certainly the modes of production whereby men live, their social and economic status, and their security needs for sustenance and shelter all play equally significant roles in the molding of personality. Modern anthropological researches (24) have thoroughly exploded the fiction of the universality of the Oedipus complex and have effectively demonstrated that "human nature" differs significantly in different cultures. The personality of man in our western culture differs sharply from that of the Zuñi Indian, for example, not primarily because of the difference in the fate of their sexual impulses, but because of the total difference in their respective socioeconomic organizations and institutions, which themselves are responsible for the difference in sexual attitudes (25).

Consider further Freud's concept of instinctual aggression. Few doctrines are so thoroughly ingrained in classical psychoanalytic thinking as this theory. It is a particularly persuasive doctrine, for who can look about him in our western culture without finding apparent evidence of its universal existence, from childhood to the grave? The question, however, whether this apparently universal aggression is instinctive and a primary inherited expression of "human nature" in all cultures and in all times, or whether it constitutes secondary or derived behavior, is crucial both scientifically and philosophically; for much of the pessimism of Freud and of some of his classical followers concerning the potentialities of man derives from this concept. Moreover, it has been used repeatedly by political defenders of the status quo to justify many of the inequities of our economic order as being inevitable reflections of "human nature." The chief arguments marshaled by the classical Freudian in the defense of this thesis are: its apparent universality; the fact that animals are apparently innately aggressive; the apparently universal selfishness and destructiveness of young children; and the predominance of aggresssion in "primitive" tribes (which Freud considered to be the phylogenetic precursors of our own civilization).

Maslow has summarized the modern evidence against these arguments as follows:

a) Not only are not all animals aggressive but even among those which are, the higher one rises in the phyletic scale, the more one finds that aggression becomes less and less primary and more and more derived, more and more functional, more and more a reasonable understandable reaction to a totality of motivation. . . . The chimpanzee, that animal of all animals which is closest to the human being [is] actually more cooperative, more friendly and less aggressive than the average human being.

b) Studies of children show them to be as frequently generous and cooperative as they are hostile and destructive:

The child who is insecure, . . . thwarted or threatened in his needs for safety, love, belongingness and self-esteem, is the child who will show more selfishness, hatred, aggression and destructiveness.

c) Studies of comparative cultures show great variations in the degree of aggressiveness and hostility displayed, and not a few so-called primitive tribes are remarkable for the almost complete absence of these traits among their people (26).

Despite these facts the classical Freudian is apt to argue that aggression is instinctual nevertheless, and that its apparent absence in some children or some cultures merely means that it is repressed. The very statement of the problem in these terms, however, discloses the two important errors which are inherent in all aspects of the instinct theory. The first is the tendency to abstract qualities which are observed in human beings in our culture and time, and to assume that they are true for the human species as a whole. The second is the assumption that any aspect of human behavior can be explained on the basis of a single determinant such as an autochthonous instinct. In contrast to this, modern dialectical materialism asserts that human behavior is not unilaterally determined in any of its aspects but can be understood correctly only as a resultant of a complex interrelationship of forces of which the needs of the organism are but a single, often subordinate, part. Thus even so basic a biological factor as the rate of growth is never determined by genetic factors alone, but is a resultant of interaction with environmental factors. Even the basic sexual and hunger needs do not operate independently of environmental forces. The sex drive will disappear under conditions of extreme malnutrition or life-threatening danger; hunger will cease to manifest itself in the presence of overwhelming infection or certain emotional stress. This whole formulation has found recent expression in the development of the psychosomatic concept in modern medicine, which recognizes that "psyche" and "soma" in man are not separable entities but constitute a dynamic unit.

The modern materialist does not therefore expect to find an adequate explanation of the phenomenon of aggression in any such single determinant as an "instinct." He seeks instead to discover what are the forces which determine its intensity and direction. If it be charged that such an approach does away with autonomous instincts altogether, the scientist can only answer in the classic words of Laplace, who, when charged with omitting God in his theory of the evolution of the solar system, replied, "I had no need of that hypothesis" (27).

Applying this approach to the problem of aggression, we find ourselves, instead of postulating a purely hypothetical repressed aggressive instinct in cultures relatively free from manifestations of aggression, asking why it is that aggression is so prevalent in our own culture and so relatively lacking in these others. As soon as we do this it becomes apparent that the widespread hostilities in our society spring basically from the .insecurities and rivalries engendered by the individualistic competitive economic system under which we live; and different degrees or manifestations of aggression in other cultures become equally understandable in the light of their own socioeconomic organizations.*

---

*This fact is convincingly demonstrated by Kardiner, who in his psychological analyses of various cultures has made one of the major contributions in psychoanalysis towards conclusively disproving the theory of instincts. "One must believe," he writes, "that either the destructiveness must be identified in forces unleashed by external realities which confront man, or that it is unrelated to realities and determined by an autochthonous death instinct. The first view can be clinically verifiable, the second cannot. The first view can be established either by the study of comparative sociology or by a historical study of the same society. The second must remain a matter of belief. . . . In Tanala-Betsileo culture it was clearly demonstrated that both aggressive and masochistic forms of destructiveness . . . increased when there was a scarcity created in subsistence opportunities; prior to this time the compensations for

Let us consider, finally, Freud's concepts of feminine psychology. Here too the problem is not whether his *observations* were correct. There is no doubt of the widespread existence in our society of the phenomenon which Freud described as "penis envy" (although whether it is as universal even in our culture as Freud believed is open to doubt). The modern materialist's criticism of this concept springs from a questioning, not of its existence, but of Freud's interpretation of its significance. Here again Freud the biologist assumed that it sprang essentially from the anatomical difference between the sexes ("anatomy is fate") (29) and from the woman's envy of the supposed inherently superior value of the penis as compared to the vagina. Now it would be unrealistic to deny that these anatomical differences, as well as the physiological facts of menstruation, childbirth, and menopause, must and do play a role in conditioning the consciousness of women. But the organic factor is but one of many determinants, and its significance in the total pattern of forces depends on its relationship to the other elements involved. Being a woman will have one significance in an androcentric culture, a totally different significance in a gynecocentric one, and still another in a society where the sexes have complete equality of opportunity socially, economically, and culturally. To assume from the facts of our culture that "penis envy" is a basic aspect of woman's "nature" is but another example of the methodological error upon which we have already commented.

Space does not permit critical examination of all the other derivatives of the Freudian theory of instincts. They refer to clinical

---

suppression of aggression were adequate to hold this mutual aggression in check. Once these compensations were removed in the form of tangible satisfactions, the aggression broke its encapsulated bounds. This precludes the necessity for any hypothesis about autochthonous death instincts" (28). It is noteworthy, however, that Kardiner is not able to completely free himself from the influence of instinctivistic thinking even as he is engaged in refuting it! For in writing of "suppression of aggression," "holding mutual aggression in check," "aggression breaking its encapsulated bounds," he implies the very thing he is attempting to deny: namely, that aggression is an autochthonous force which must be "suppressed" and "held in check" lest it "break its encapsulated bounds." His statement about the Tanala-Betsilao would have been more accurate had he added: "Prior to this time the compensations for *cooperative relationships* were adequate to make aggression *unnecessary*."

phenomena which indubitably exist. But the theoretical assumptions underlying the classical Freudian interpretation of these phenomena reveal the fundamental errors of either mechanistic or entelechistic thinking which are implicit in the whole theory of instincts.

At the beginning of this article I indicated that psychoanalytic theory, far from being static, has been undergoing significant development and change. The evidence for this is unmistakable if one attempts even a brief survey of the psychoanalytic literature. Freud himself laid the groundwork for a significant reorientation of psychoanalytic theory when in 1926 he revised his concept of anxiety as arising from frustration of instinctual impulses, and recognized instead that it was a defense against outward dangers and a manifestation of the "ego" (30). In 1933 Wilhelm Reich took up the problem and called to the attention of psychoanalysts the importance of studying the character structure of the patient, rather than the vicissitudes of the "instincts" (31). This important turning point in psychoanalysis marked a major shift in emphasis which has characterized it ever since, a shift to "ego psychology." A period of great ferment in psychoanalytic thinking ensued in the following years. Much discussion and earnest questioning of basic psychoanalytic doctrine began to take place in a way that had never before occurred.* Ernest Jones's comment, quoted at the beginning of this

---

*A few of the leaders in this process in America were Alexander, Fromm, Horney, Kardiner, David Levy, Rado, Schilder, and Sullivan. Within the space of a few years there appeared Horney's *Neurotic Personality of Our Time* (1937) and *New Ways in Psychoanalysis* (1939), Kardiner's *The Individual and His Society* (1939) and *Traumatic Neuroses of War* (1941), Rado's *Developments in the Psychoanalytic Conception and Treatment of the Neuroses* (1939), Sullivan's *Conceptions of Modern Psychiatry* (1940), and Fromm's *Escape from Freedom* (1941), all of which made significant revisions in classical psychoanalytical theory and brought it closer to modern materialistic concepts. The publication of Alexander and French's *Psychoanalytic Therapy* (1946) stimulated a revaluation of some of the procedural techniques of psychoanalysis. In addition there have been countless articles by other analysts, too numerous to mention, which also have been adding gradually to the momentum of change in psychoanalytic thinking. It should be noted also that even among the ranks of the classical analysts there have been articles questioning one or another aspect of Freudian theory (32). The task still remains, however, for a psychoanalyst thoroughly grounded in the principles of historical and dialectical materialism to integrate all the positive contributions of psychoanalysis, in the light of these principles, into a comprehensive, definitive study of human behavior.

article, is significant of a changing viewpoint to which even Freud's oldest and most loyal followers must sooner or later begin to give cognizance.

What then are the positive concepts of the most advanced theoretical viewpoint in psychoanalysis today? In the space which remains we can only briefly indicate a few of the outstanding ones. The advanced psychoanalytic view sees the relationship between the individual and society as a dialectical one and denies that any basic conflict of interests inevitably exists between them. It affirms that the human personality is neither innately "evil" nor innately "good," and that man's potentialities in either direction depend on the incentives offered by the society in which he develops. It recognizes that human consciousness is a unique resultant of the interaction between the human organism and the social influences to which it is exposed from the moment of birth onward. It asserts that the particular medium in which this interrelationship first takes place in our society is, for most individuals, the family. In order to understand fully, therefore, how the consciousness of any individual in our society has evolved, it is important to study his relationships within his family group. In this group the influence of the parents, or parent-substitutes, is preeminent, since the parents are in most instances the "chief purveyors and reflectors to the growing child of the contradictory patterns in our culture." This does not deny the tremendous influence which school, church, the street, books, newspapers, radio, movies, etc., have upon the thought processes of every individual in our culture; and full cognizance is taken of these factors. Nor does the insistence upon the historical importance of childhood relationships in the development of personality in any way deny the potentiality of change throughout the life of the individual. Psychoanalysts affirm, however, that childhood experiences have a particular significance because it is in the formative years of childhood that basic character patterns are set down which tend to become the frame of reference in relation to later experiences. Concepts, for example, such as "I am loved (and therefore feel secure) only when I am submissive," or "I am not loved regardless of how I behave," strongly reenforced by repeated childhood experiences, acquire a dynamic importance which profoundly influences all the subsequent life relationships. Being painful in character, they tend to become repressed to protect the personality from persistent conscious conflict. Then, as unconscious "affective complexes" (Luria), they continue to exert a decisive influence upon the subsequent thought and behavior of the individual. Thus, a person who suffers from a deep conviction that he is unlovable withdraws into a defensive shell; by so doing he actually prevents people from loving him and so constantly reenforces his basic neurotic conviction through a vicious cycle.

In considering the interaction of the child with his environment, the progressive psychoanalyst does not, however, conceive of the child as a mere passive recipient or tabula rasa. He recognizes that man is born with important affirmative biological needs for food, sexual gratification, and protection from the elements, which are active factors in the dynamic interrelationship with his environment; but he insists that these biological needs "*condition* his development but do not *predetermine* it" (33). The progressive psychoanalyst therefore equally rejects any effort to explain man's behavior entelechistically in terms of autonomous instincts, or mechanistically in terms of man being simply a "product of his environment." Only out of the recognition of the active and complex interrelationship between man's biological inheritance and his social environment can a truly dialectical and materialistic conception of human nature evolve.

Which brings us to our final point. The progressive psychoanalyst of today recognizes that the forms of production and distribution in our society, and the contradictions between the prevailing Christian ethics of brotherhood and justice and an economic order which stresses rugged individualism and rewards aggression and deceit, inevitably leave their impress on the personality of every person in our culture. These influences of our society vary in their effects upon the different sociological classes, and the varying effects can be recognized in general in the members of each class. But it does not mean that the behavior of any individual can be deduced from his class relationships alone. Regardless of class similarity, there are wide variations of individual behavior within every class which are understandable only in the light of the specific life experiences of that individual. Historical materialism can explain the general character of any given society or class, but only a dynamic psychology of the individual can fully explain the specific variants in any individual within that society or class. And since circumstances are changed by men as much as men are changed by circumstances, only a combination of these two scientific methods can give us a complete understanding of both "the forest and the trees" in the social world in which we live.

REFERENCES

1. ERNEST JONES, "A Valedictory Address," *Internatl. Jour. of Psychoanal.*, Vol. 27 (1946).
2. SIGMUND FREUD, *Collected Papers* (London, 1924), 1:254.
3. *Ibid.*, p. 298.
4. *Ibid.*, pp. 297–298.
5. *Ibid.*, p. 311.
6. MILTON H. ERICKSON, "A Study of Hypnotically Induced Complexes by Means of the Luria Technique," *Journ. Genetic Psychol.*, Vol. 30 (1934); "Experimental Demonstration of the Psychopathology of Everyday Life," *Psychoan. Quart.*, Vol. 8 (1939); and numerous other papers.
7. A. R. LURIA, *The Nature of Human Conflicts* (New York, 1932), pp. 128–131, 133, 142, 155, 157, 159.
8. S. L. RUBINSTEIN, "Soviet Psychology in War Time," *Philosophy and Phenomenological Research*, 5:183 (1944).
9. JOSEPH WORTIS, "Freudianism and the Psychoanalytic Tradition," *Amer. Journ. Psychiat.*, Vol. 25 (1945); and FRANCIS BARTLETT, "Recent Trends in Psychoanalysis," *Science and Society*, Vol. 9 (1945).
10. J. MARMOR, "Theory and Practice of Psychoanalysis," *Science and Society*, Vol. 10 (1946). This article contains a more detailed exposition of modern psychoanalytic technique, for the reader who may be interested. (Chapter 8, this volume.)
11. V. J. McGILL and L. WELCH, "A Behaviorist Analysis of Emotions," *Philosophy of Science*, Vol. 13 (1946); and "Hysteria as a Conditioning Process," *Amer. Jour. of Psychotherapy*, Vol. 1 (1947).
12. V. J. McGILL, "The Mind-Body Problem in the Light of Recent Psychology," *Science and Society*, 9:342 (1945).
13. REUBEN OSBORN (i.e., Osbert), *Freud and Marx* (London, 1937); JACK RAPAPORT "Marxism and Psychoanalysis," *Science and Society*, Vol. 5 (1941); BURRILL FREEDMAN and WALTON VAN CLUTE, "Dialectical Aspects of Psychoanalysis Misunderstood," *Psychoan. Review*, Vol. 31 (1944).
14. SIGMUND FREUD, *op. cit.*, pp. 298–299.
15. SIGMUND FREUD, *New Introductory Lectures on Psychoanalysis* (New York, 1933), p. 131.
16. SIGMUND FREUD, "Psychoanalysis: Freudian School," *Encyclopaedia Britannica*, 14th ed., 18:674.
17. LUDWIG JEKELS, "Psychoanalysis and Dialectic," *Psychoan. Review*, 28:228 (1941).
18. FRANCIS H. BARTLETT, *Sigmund Freud* (London, 1938).

‌‍‌‍‍

19. HOWARD SELSAM, *What Is Philosophy?* (New York, 1938), p. 45.
20. OTTO FENICHEL, "Psychoanalytic Remarks on Fromm's Book, *Escape from Freedom,*" *Psychoan. Review*, 31:138–140 (1944).
21. *Ibid.*, p. 140.
22. KINGSLEY DAVIS, "Extreme Social Isolation of a Child," *Amer. Jour. Sociol.*, Vol. 45 (1940).
23. J. MARMOR, "The Role of Instinct in Human Behavior," *Psychiatry*, 5:515–516 (1942). (Chapter 1, this volume)
24. RUTH BENEDICT, *Patterns of Culture* (Boston, 1934); MARGARET MEAD, *From the South Seas* (New York, 1939); ABRAM KARDINER, *The Individual and His Society* (New York, 1939), and *The Psychological Frontiers of Society* (New York, 1945).
25. ABRAM KARDINER, *The Individual and His Society*, p. 111.
26. A. H. MASLOW, "A Comparative Approach to the Problem of Destructiveness," *Psychiatry*, Vol. 5 (1942).
27. Quoted by Selsam, *op. cit.*, p. 65.
28. KARDINER, *op. cit.*, pp. 402–403.
29. SIGMUND FREUD, "Some Psychological Consequences of the Anatomical Distinction Between the Sexes," *Internatl. Jour. of Psychoanal.*, Vol. 8 (1927).
30. SIGMUND FREUD, *The Problem of Anxiety* (New York, 1936).
31. WILHELM REICH, *Charakteranalyse* (Vienna, 1933); in English translation, *Character-Analysis* (New York, 1945).
32. Two examples are: LAWRENCE KUBIE, "A Critical Analysis of the Conception of a Repetition Compulsion," *Internatl. Jour. of Psychoanal.*, Vol. 20 (1939); and GREGORY ZILBOORG, "Masculine and Feminine," *Psychiatry*, Vol. 7 (1944).
33. S. L. RUBINSTEIN, "Consciousness in the Light of Dialectical Materialism," *Science and Society*, 10:260 (1946).

10

SOME CONSIDERATIONS CONCERNING
ORGASM IN THE FEMALE
(1952)

The sexual frigidity of women . . . is still a phenomenon which is insufficiently understood. Sometimes it is psychogenic, and, if so, it is accessible to influence; but in other cases one is led to assume that it is constitutionally conditioned or even partly caused by an anatomical factor.

SIGMUND FREUD—*New Introductory Lectures on Psychoanalysis*

Although much is known about both the physiology and psycho-dynamics of the male orgasm, the mechanisms underlying orgasm in the female remain shadowy and obscure. The reasons for this are both physiological and psychological. On the physiological side is the fact that the female orgasm is not accompanied by an objectively perceptible emission as is that of the male, which not only makes it difficult at times for the woman herself to recognize, but also makes it impossible for any external observer to be certain about it. On the psychological side are the taboos which so strongly surround the subject of female sexuality. The conventions of our culture are still so powerful in this respect that women themselves, who might be expected to shed the greatest light on this subject, are for the most part unable or unwilling to do so. One might speculate as to whether their very sensory perceptions of the process, having developed in the crucible of these conventions, have not been affected in such a way as to interfere with an accurate evaluation of their own sexual reactions.

143

FREUD'S CONCEPT OF GENITAL EROGENICITY

Most psychoanalytical concepts about the physiology of the female orgasm date back to Freud's classic formulation in his *Three Contributions to the Theory of Sex*. In this monograph, Freud advanced the thesis that genital erogenicity in the normal female, although first centered in the clitoris, eventually becomes transferred to the vagina; and that sexual orgasm in the mature, healthy female should be in response to vaginal rather than clitoral stimulation. "We may assume," Freud says, "that in the phallic phase of the girl, the clitoris is the dominant erotogenic zone. But it is not destined to remain so; with the change to femininity, the clitoris must give up to the vagina its sensitivity, and with it, its importance either wholly or in part" (7). Failure of such transfer to take place leads, in Freud's opinion, to sexual frigidity or "anesthesia," a condition which he believed due to "profuse sexual activities in infantile life" (8).

Horney and Lorand, among others, have suggested that vaginal sensations may be present in early childhood, but the conclusion that clitoral sensitivity must ultimately give way to vaginal sensitivity in the normal female seems never to have been seriously questioned in the psychoanalytical literature.

Freud's hypothesis was based on certain common clinical observations. It is a well-known fact that masturbation in the young female is generally centered around clitoral stimulation. It is also commonly observed that the sexually "frigid" adult female is incapable of having an orgasm through vaginal intercourse, but is often able to achieve an orgasm through direct stimulation of the clitoris. On the other hand, women who seem to have achieved the greatest degree of sexual freedom and responsiveness are able to have orgasms freely through vaginal intercourse. The intensity of the orgasm, moreover, appears to differ depending on its character. Most observers report that the "clitoral orgasm" is experienced as a localized response, while the so-called "vaginal orgasm" seems to be a more violent, intense, and generalized reaction.

Although these clinical observations seem well authenticated, recent studies of the sexual physiology of women* have thrown

---

*This article predated the research studies of Masters and Johnson. (J. M., 1973)

some doubt on their theoretical interpretation, and specifically upon the hypothesis of the transfer of erogenicity from the clitoris to the vagina. Evidence has accumulated in recent years to indicate that in the normal adult woman clitoral excitation by the penis in the process of intercourse is an important factor in the stimulation leading to orgasm. A clitoris which is located too high above the urinary meatus is believed by some investigators to reduce the capacity of the female for orgasm during intercourse. Landis measured the meatus-clitoris distance in several hundred women and concluded that individuals in whom this distance is greater than one and one-half inches are less likely to experience orgasm during intercourse than are women in whom it is less. Dickinson (3), on the other hand, questions that the location of the clitoris is the decisive factor, although he too believes that its stimulation is an essential factor in orgasm. In his opinion, the most reliable index to clitoral function is not its location so much as its susceptibility to displacement during intercourse.

Indirect corroborative evidence of this continued function of the clitoris in adult sexual life is offered by the study of the preferred sexual positions in various cultures of the world (6). Such study reveals that face-to-face coitus, which affords a greater opportunity for the woman to obtain clitoral stimulation, is the position preferred by most people in most societies. Kinsey and his collaborators found that the position which their subjects considered most conducive to orgasm in the female was that in which the man lies on his back and the woman sits or lies above him in a face-to-face position. This is a position which more than any other favors clitoral excitation during coitus. Ford and Beach found that coitus-a-tergo does not occur as a usual or preferred practice in any of more than thirty-five societies which they studied, and they conclude that this may well be due in part to the fact that stimulation of the clitoris is minimal when this position is employed.

Most significant of all, however, are histological studies in females of the sensory cells known as the genital corpuscles, which "are highly specialized end-organs for the perception of this particular sensation (i.e., orgasm) just as the retina is adapted for the sense of sight and the neuro-epithelium of the nose is adapted for the sense of smell" (10). These histological studies indicate that genital corpuscles do not occur in the vaginal mucosa and are confined predominantly to the glans clitoridis (10). Some are also found in the areas directly adjacent to the clitoris, notably the labia minora.

IMPORTANCE OF CLITORIS

The meaning of these findings is that the chief sensory area for erogenous sensation in women is localized in the glans clitoridis, just as in men it is localized in the homologous glans penis. (The shaft of the penis, like the vagina, is lacking in genital corpuscles.) This does not, of course, mean that these are the only erogenous areas. The importance of the secondary erogenous zones such as lips, breasts, and buttocks is well known. Moreover, there are kinesthetic receptors within the vaginal wall, the stimulation of which by the erect penis contributes voluptuous sensations to the normal woman. There are similar receptors in the bulbocavernosus muscles around the lower end of the vagina which contribute a sense of ejaculation during orgasm by their spasmodic pulsations. The contractions of these same muscles in the male cause actual ejaculation of semen from the penis during orgasm.

How do these observations concerning the importance of the clitoris in the sex life of the normal adult woman fit into the pattern of the previously mentioned clinical observations about "clitoral" and "vaginal" orgasms? Do they not seem to require some revision of the hypothesis concerning the shift of erogenicity from the clitoris to the vagina? If so, what hypothesis can be offered in its place?

Before considering these questions, it may be pertinent to examine, for a moment, our knowledge concerning the anatomy and physiology of orgasm in the male. It is an accepted fact that in the male there is an orgastic spinal center in the sacral segment of the spinal cord. As can be demonstrated from the evidence of neurophysiology, discharges of tension in this orgastic center can be achieved either at a reflex spinal level or by cortical stimulation. In the former instance, this discharge is achieved by simple mechanical stimulation of the genital corpuscles of the glans penis, which eventually causes a rising tension in the spinal center until reflex discharge takes place. In the latter instance, the cortical stimulation is achieved through psychological stimuli, occurring through supraspinal sensory receptors. Thus not only stimulation of secondary erogenous areas (lips, nipples, etc.) but even witnessing exciting scenes, or reading an erotic piece of literature, or merely fantasying, dreaming, or anticipating a particularly exciting or erotic experience can produce orgasm in some males in the total absence of any physical stimulation of the penis itself. In certain neurotic men it has been observed that extreme anxiety or tension of nonsexual origin may occasionally produce sexual orgasm, apparently through the medium of an overflow of cortical excitation which affects the spinal orgastic center.

In the normal masculine orgasm, however (normal from a psychodynamic standpoint), what apparently takes place is a combination of the spinal and cortical mechanisms. The male reaches a high state of sexual excitation through the combination of psychological, tactile, olfactory, and visual stimuli, even in the absence of any direct physical stimulation of the glans penis. This excitation is sufficient to produce erection but not orgasm. For orgasm to take place, a certain amount of supplementary physical stimulation of the glans penis itself, through the process of intercourse, is necessary. This physical excitation is further enhanced in the process of intercourse by the psychological stimulus from the mounting excitement of the partner. Under ideal circumstances this crescendo of excitement occurs in both partners simultaneously, and the combination of physical and psychological stimulation finally results in orgasm.

In considering the parallel mechanism of orgasm in the female, there is no reason to expect from our knowledge of anatomy and physiology that the female has two spinal orgastic centers rather than one. On the contrary, it is fair to assume that the female undoubtedly has an orgastic center located in the sacral segment of the spinal cord, exactly as the male has. From neurohistological evidence, it can be shown that the sensory receptors for this spinal orgastic center are the genital corpuscles, located predominantly in the glans clitoris, just as the homologous sensory receptors in the male are confined primarily to the glans penis. Although one might naturally assume that the tiny clitoris could hardly play as important a sensory role as the much larger penis, Dickinson points out (4, p. 42):

> The female organ is minute compared with the male organ, but the size of its nerves, and the number of nerve endings

in the glans of the clitoris compare strikingly with the same provision for the male. Indeed, Kobelt states that the glans of the clitoris is demonstrably richer in nerves than the male glans for the two stems of the dorsalis clitoridis are relatively three to four times as large as the equivalent nerves of the penis. Without dividing up, they run mostly with three branches to the edge of the glans. Here, before their entry, they are so thick one can hardly comprehend how such a volume of nerve tissue can find room between the numberless blood vessels of the tiny glans. Arrived near the surface of the glans they dispose themselves, just as in the male glans, in an intricate plexus, running also in loops in the tender membrane of the prepuce.

An indirect corroboration of the high degree of erogenicity implicit in the extremely rich nerve supply of the glans clitoridis lies in the much greater capacity of the female to have multiple orgasms as compared to the male.

ORGASTIC IMPOTENCE

Yet, in spite of all the evidence that anatomically and physiologically the female should, at the very least, be fully as able as the male to have orgastic reactions, the clinical facts are that women are much more frequently orgastically impotent than are men. Dickinson and Beam (5) in a study of one thousand married women, found that only two out of every five women experience regular orgasms during intercourse, and these figures are corroborated by other investigators.

The conclusion seems inescapable that when anatomical factors such as described by Landis (12) and Dickinson (3) are ruled out, the major difficulty must lie primarily in the psychological rather than in the physiological sphere. This does not in any way gainsay the important effect of the ovarian cycle upon the libidinal reactions of women, as demonstrated by the studies of Benedek and Rubenstein (2), but frigidity per se, as Benedek herself says, "can be related to the ovarian function only in rare cases of severe hypogonadism. In all other instances, women may have any form and degree of frigidity, and at the same time normal gonadal function" (1). Similar observations have been more recently made by Perloff.

The psychological factors involved in feminine frigidity, on the other hand, are manifold. They have been frequently and amply described in the psychoanalytical literature and do not require repetition here. The complexity of sexual maturation in women, the greater degree of sexual repression and inhibition which our culture impresses upon them, and the envy and hostility to men which stems in part at least from the position of women in an androcentric culture are only a few of the factors which interfere with the capacity of women to enter with uninhibited pleasure into a sexual relationship. Fears of being injured by the penis, fears of pregnancy and childbirth, and lack of adequate skill, tenderness, or potency on the part of the male partner are other factors which have been commonly described.

We are concerned here, however, not so much with the psychodynamics of frigidity as with the mechanisms involved in the orgastic reaction of the woman. The important consideration for our present purpose is the fact that whenever, and for whatever reason, a psychological inhibition of the capacity to enjoy sexual intercourse exists, the woman will usually be capable of responding orgastically only at a spinal level, if at all; that is to say, only through the medium of direct mechanical stimulation of the clitoris itself. On the other hand, if the woman has been able to free herself from the blanket of psychological inhibition, she will be capable of responding through the medium of enhanced cortical excitement (that is, through cortical facilitation) to vaginal intercourse.

The conclusion that such a response is the result of vaginal excitability has been due to the implicit assumption that the physical stimulation which is taking place in vaginal intercourse is primarily of the vaginal wall and mucosa. Actually, as has been pointed out, some stimulation of the clitoris almost invariably occurs in normal vaginal intercourse and is an important factor in the excitation leading to orgasm. The difference between the so-called clitoral and vaginal orgasms, therefore, is explicable not in terms of the different origin or location of the orgastic response, but in the different intensity of it and in the degree to which cortical factors are contributory. As in the male, the intensity of orgasm in the female varies with the degree of psychological excitation present. In a purely spinal reflex, due only to mechanical stimulation of either the penis or the clitoris, the orgasm is generally experienced as a localized and limited reaction. On the other hand, in both the male and female, the higher the degree of emotional and psychological participation, the greater the degree of cortical facilitation of the spinal discharge and the more general and intense is the orgastic experience. Where the cortical excitation is of a particularly high order, the orgastic reaction may be so intense and generalized as to result in convulsive twitchings which are almost like minor epileptic seizures, and which probably have a somewhat similar neurophysiological mechanism in terms of dysrhythmic cortical discharges. It would be pertinent in this regard to do electroencephalographic studies of cortical patterns during intense orgasm.

EXTRAGENITAL ORGASM

It should be noted further that there are other analogous reactions in the female which are similar to those observed in the male. For example, in women, too, orgasm is capable of taking place without any local genital stimulation at all. To quote from Dickinson and Beam's study of one thousand marriages: "The records contain instances of orgasm obtained from nipple suction, from lying beside another, from nursing a baby, from pressing (fully dressed) against another, from a shampoo at the hands of a male hairdresser, from a look, from a kiss, from touching the eye or ear, from a handclasp, and from a picture or flower which contains no figure and no likeness to any person or scene" (5). Orgasms, under most of these circumstances, represent a discharge of the spinal center which has been initiated primarily by cerebral excitation. In the normal woman, moreover, as in the normal man, the excitement of the partner, and particularly the setting off of his orgastic reaction, constitutes an intense psychological stimulus for her and often acts as a trigger for her own climactic response.

Pursuing the logic of this hypothesis, therefore, we may say that strictly speaking there is no such thing as a "vaginal" orgasm in the female, any more than we might speak of "scrotal," "anal," or "prostatic" orgasm in the male. It seems logical to assume that the actual spinal mechanism of orgasm is identical in all females, but that variations which take place in the nature of female orgasm are due to the degree to which cortical inhibition or cortical facilitation accompanies the spinal reflex. Where cortical inhibition is great, due to long-standing sexual repression or to a high degree of anxiety, hostility, ambivalence, or guilt in relationship to the sexual partner or the sexual act, the spinal mechanism may be completely inhibited, in which event we observe a total incapacity for orgasm, or so-called frigidity. Where the cortical inhibitions are not of such a high order, we observe a capacity to have orgasm only with prolonged stimulation of the clitoris. This is what is ordinarily described as a "clitoral" orgasm. However, where cortical inhibitions do not exist, where there is a freedom from psychological tension or anxiety in the sexual act, and instead there is a high degree of tender affection, love, and psychological excitement, then cortical facilitation takes place. The result is an intense orgastic response in which the intromission of the phallus into the vagina is of major importance. This is both psychodynamically and physiologically the optimum type of response, and represents what is ordinarily characterized as a "vaginal" orgasm.

CONCLUSIONS

The question may properly be asked as to what significance, if any, these considerations may have. Their importance lies in the effect which our present theories concerning female sexuality have upon the psychology of many women and upon the physicians who treat such women. Women patients are often encountered who suffer from anxiety because their subjective reactions do not fit the popular hypothesis concerning clitoral and vaginal sensitivity. Such women will often say that they enjoy sex and have orgasms regularly, but worry "because my husband has to stimulate my clitoris first," or because "most of my sensations seem to be clitoral." Obviously one cannot generalize about such reactions, and psychological disturbances are often involved even in such relatively minor limitations of orgastic function. But it may be an error to assume in advance that such reactions are necessarily of serious neurotic import. It is perfectly possible that in some instances they may be, as Freud himself suspected, "constitutionally conditioned or even partly caused by an anatomical factor."

An understanding of the function of the clitoris, moreover, is of importance to men as well as to women. Not infrequently sexual maladjustment of women can be traced to a failure of their male partners to appreciate the importance of clitoral stimulation in sexual foreplay as a factor in preparing the woman for an orgastic reaction. In addition, the woman herself all too often fears, resents, or objects to any form of clitoral manipulation for a variety of unconscious reasons—masturbatory guilt, shame about her genitals, anxiety that such manipulation is "perverse," "unnatural," or "neurotic," etc.

It seems fair to conclude, therefore, that a proper understanding of the role which the clitoris normally plays in adult female sexuality will help the physician in general as well as the psychiatrist more adequately to evaluate and treat the sexual disturbances of their patients as well as to reassure those who suffer from needless anxiety because of misapprehensions based upon faulty knowledge.

SUMMARY

Some considerations have been presented which throw doubt on the popular assumption that genital erogenicity in the female becomes normally transferred from the clitoris to the vagina. There is evidence to indicate that clitoral sensitivity is a continuing factor in adult female sexuality, and that the chief difference between so-called clitoral and vaginal orgasm is explicable not in terms of the different origin or location of the orgastic response, but in the different intensity of it and in the degree to which cortical facilitation of the spinal reaction has taken place.*

*These conclusions were, in essence, subsequently confirmed by the epochal research studies of Masters and Johnson, reported in *Human Sexual Response,* Boston, Little Brown & Co., 1966. (J. M., 1973)

REFERENCES

1. BENEDEK, T. "The functions of the sexual apparatus and their disturbances." In: ALEXANDER, F., *Psychosomatic Medicine.* New York, Norton, 1950.
2. BENEDEK, T., and RUBENSTEIN, B. B. "The Sexual Cycle in Women." *Psychosom. Med. Monog.* Washington, D.C., National Research Council, 1942, vol. 3, nos. 1 and 2.
3. DICKINSON, R. L. In: FORD, C. S., and BEACH, F. A., p. 21. (6)

4. DICKINSON, R. L. *Human Sex Anatomy.* Baltimore, Maryland, Williams & Wilkins, 1933.
5. DICKINSON, R. L., and BEAM, L. *A Thousand Marriages.* Baltimore, Maryland, Williams & Wilkins, 1931.
6. FORD, C. S., and BEACH, F. A. *Patterns of Sexual Behavior.* New York, Harper, 1951, p. 24.
7. FREUD, S. "The Psychology of Women." In: *New Introductory Lectures in Psychoanalysis.* New York, Norton, 1933, p. 161.
8. FREUD, S. "Three contributions to the theory of sex." In: *The Basic Writings of Sigmund Freud.* New York, Modern Library, 1938, p. 164.
9. HORNEY, KAREN. Denial of the vagina. *Internat. J. Psycho-Analysis 14:*57, 1933.
10. KELLY, G. L. *Sex Manual* (ed. 5). Augusta, Georgia, Southern Medical Supply Co., 1950, pp. 30 et seq.
11. KINSEY, A. C., POMEROY, W. B., and MARTIN, C. E. *Sexual Behavior in The Human Male.* Philadelphia, Saunders, 1948.
12. LANDIS, C. In: FORD, C. S., and BEACH, F. A. (6)
13. LORAND, S. Contributions to the problem of vaginal orgasm. *Internat. J. Psycho-Analysis 20:*432, 1939.
14. PERLOFF, W. H. Role of the hormones in human sexuality. *Psychosom. Med. 11:*133, 1949.

11

ORALITY IN THE HYSTERICAL
PERSONALITY
(1953)

The subject of hysteria is particularly significant for psychoanalysts, for it was in the process of the study and treatment of this condition that Freud discovered the method of psychoanalysis and developed many of its basic theories. The concepts of fixation and regression grew out of these early studies, as did the formulation that hysterics are fixated at the phallic or early genital phase of libidinal development. Over the years a psychoanalytic characterology emerged which assumed increasing clinical importance. Wilhelm Reich in his *Character-Analysis* (12) was the first to state what had become implicit in the theory and practice of psychoanalysis but had not until then been explicitly expressed—namely, that a neurotic character structure underlies every symptom neurosis, and that the optimum goal of

Among classical Freudians this is generally regarded as my best and most influential psychoanalytic article. I believe that the reason for this is that although it challenges one of the most basic tenets of orthodox psychoanalytic theory, namely the "oedipal-fixation" etiology of hysteria, it does so most tentatively and without explicitly "attacking" the existing point of view. The historical reason for this is that this was the first paper I ever presented at an Annual Meeting of the American Psychoanalytic Association. I realized that its essential thesis was an unorthodox one, and that no one had ever dared before to question the fundamental credo concerning hysteria; I therefore soft-pedaled its "revolutionary" implications in the hope that what I considered (and still consider) its essential clinical correctness would be more readily accepted. If I were rewriting this paper today, I would be far less gentle to the entire "libidinal" framework of analytic theory which I consider to be archaic in the light of our newer knowledge concerning personality development. (See Chapters 8, 9, 17, 19, and 20.)

psychoanalytic therapy must be not merely the eradication of the neurotic symptom but the changing of the neurotic character structure. It is the underlying character structure of hysteria which is the concern of this communication.

It should be emphasized at the outset that we are admittedly dealing with an abstraction. There is no pure hysterical personality any more than there is a pure compulsive personality. In personality development, residuals of earlier stages of growth can invariably be found interspersed with the characteristics of later stages. Nevertheless, broad clinical differences do exist, and there is some value in attempting to define the main patterns which are associated with these differences.

It is recognized also that there are many ways of classifying character other than that with which this communication is concerned. As Freud (6) has pointed out, it depends on which characteristics are taken as the basis of classification. It is not intended, therefore, to draw any general conclusions about human typology in this paper.

Since the early classical papers of Freud, Jones, and Abraham, the compulsive personality has been one of the most clearly delineated of all the character pictures. The hysterical personality, on the other hand, has never been as sharply clarified. One of the first descriptions of the hysterical character as such appears to have been that of Wittels (13) in 1930. The chief characteristics of the hysterical type, according to Wittels, are that it is "infantile and feminine."

> The hysteric character [he says] never frees itself from its fixation on the infantile level. Hence it cannot attain its actuality as a grown-up human being; it plays the part of a child, and also of the woman. The hysteric person has no actuality, she (or he) confuses fantasy and reality, that is to say, allows the law of the "Id" to enter into the ego.

In 1933, Wilhelm Reich (12, pp. 189 et seq.) described the hysterical character in more detailed clinical terms. The behavior of the hysterical character, he states, appears to be obviously sexualized, with disguised or undisguised coquetry in woman, and a softness and effeminacy of manner in men. "Facial expression and gait are never hard and heavy as in the compulsive character, or self-confident and arrogant as in the phallic-narcissistic character. . . . The movements are soft. . . . and sexually provocative." In both sexes there is a quality of apprehensiveness, which becomes particularly evident when the sexual behavior seems closer to attaining its goal. Other characteristics which Reich describes are: a tendency to unexpected changes of behavior, strong suggestibility, easy disappointment reactions, lack of conviction, compliance alternating with quick depreciation and groundless disparagement, imaginativeness, and pathological lying. Additional features of the hysterical character which may be noted are: a compulsive need to be loved and admired; intense feelings of inadequacy, which may be conscious or unconscious; a strong dependency on the approval of others for self-esteem; a powerful capacity for dramatization and somatic compliance; and a tendency to repress aggressive feelings or attitudes, or to act them out in concealed ways.

Wilhelm Reich explains these characteristics as being "determined by a fixation on the genital phase of infantile development, with its incestuous attachment." Any pregenital strivings which may be present, he considers to be representations of genitality.

> In the hysterical character [says Reich] mouth as well as anus, always represent the female genital while in other character forms these zones retain their original pregenital function. . . . To the extent to which other than genital mechanisms are found in the hysterical character they no longer belong specifically to this character type.

Reich explains the marked tendency of hysterics to oral regressions by the fact that the mouth, having assumed the role of the genital, absorbs much libido. Where oral fixations are relatively strong, he concludes that there will be a tendency to depressive reactions, and he believes that there are gradual transitions from pure melancholia, in which orality is predominant, to pure hysteria, in which "genitality" is predominant.

The fact that oral mechanisms and symptoms are conspicuous in hysteria has, of course, long been recognized. Globus hystericus, vomiting, anorexia, and bulemia are bywords in the symptomatology of hysteria. In "Fragment of an Analysis of a Case of Hysteria," Freud (4) takes cognizance of a number of oral symptoms presented by his patient, Dora, notably nausea, anorexia, gastric pains, and a history of prolonged thumb sucking in childhood.

The question, therefore, is not whether oral mechanisms are prominent in hysteria. That is taken for granted. The problem, rather, is whether these mechanisms may not play a more *determining* role in the dynamics of hysteria than has been generally assumed.

Edmund Bergler's idea of a basic neurosis (1) rooted in oral dependency and forming a substratum to all subsequent neurotic patterns comes to mind at this point, but this formulation seems to be an oversimplification. It is true that one can find traces of oral fixation, like leftover occupation troops, to use Freud's famous simile, not only in neurotic individuals but in everyone. It is probably inevitable, in view of the long biological dependency of the human infant and its even longer social dependency, that every person will encounter some degree of frustration of oral dependency needs, traces of which will persist in the subsequent character structure. Such traces, however, do not constitute a neurotic character, nor are they necessarily of major importance in the dynamics of the ultimate character picture. In the compulsive personality for example, one is much more impressed by the determining role of the manner in which discipline and sphincter training have been applied to the child than by the role of the oral dependency frustrations.

In the analysis of the hysterical character, on the other hand, one is struck not only by the prominence of oral mechanisms but also by their tenacity. I would like to call attention to several significant considerations in this respect.

One of the cardinal elements in the concept of fixation and regression is the clinically demonstrable fact that, generally speaking, the earlier the point of fixation, the greater is the damage to the developing ego, and the more serious the ultimate clinical picture when regression takes place. This corresponds to the popular axiom that "as the twig is bent, the tree's inclined." The younger the developing ego, the more susceptible it is to injury; and the ultimate effects of traumatic experiences in the character structure seem to be more widespread the earlier they have been sustained. An analogy to this in the biological sphere is seen in the well-known relationship between the time of injury to an embryo and the degree of defect at birth.

Thus, in psychopathology, according to present theory, as one ascends the scale of fixation points from early oral to the final genital phase, one encounters in succession certain types of schizophrenia, the manic-depressive disorders and the addictions, paranoid conditions, compulsion neuroses, hysterias and finally, "normalcy." As can be seen, there is a rough correlation between accessibility to psychoanalytic treatment (i.e., to character change) and the depth of the fixation point. On the basis of current theory, therefore, one would be inclined to conclude that of all the major functional psychiatric disorders, hysteria should be the easiest to be treated, and this indeed is the prevailing opinion in the literature.

One wonders whether this is not a clinical myth which tradition and the plasticity of hysterical symptoms have tended to perpetuate. For the fact is that although hysterical *symptoms* are indeed usually among the easiest of all clinical disturbances to resolve, the underlying hysterical *character structure* is often one of the most difficult to alter. Furthermore, although theoretically one might expect the ego-integrative capacity of the hysteric to be greater than that of the compulsive, since the depth of regression and fixation is presumably less in the hysteric, actual clinical findings do not bear this out. One is impressed by the finding that of the two types, the compulsive character seems more often to have the better contact with reality—a fact noted by Wittels (13) in his early paper—and to have the more mature ego structure.

Another notable clinical fact is that under extreme stress the hysterical character almost invariably responds with oral regression, with depressive or schizophrenic reactions, or with some form of addiction, especially alcoholism—a point which Wittels (13) also stressed. The clinical association of the hysterical personality with schizophrenic reactions, in particular, as well as the similarities in the underlying character structure of the hysteric and certain schizophrenics, is in fact a rather striking one and probably more than coincidental. The borderline between hysterical introversion and schizophrenic autism, between hysterical fantasy and schizophrenic delusion, and between hysterical materialization and schizophrenic hallucination is often a narrow one; and quantitative factors may effect the qualitative transition from one to the other (9). The fact that patients may at one time present the picture of a classical hysteria and later regress to a full-blown schizophrenia is well-known and has been frequently reported (2, 7, 10, 11, 14).

The question may be raised as to whether or not such cases were not latent or borderline psychotics in the first place and not "true hysterics"; but it appears to be a form of post hoc reasoning which the clinical facts do not justify. The prepsychotic psychodynamics and symptomatology of such cases do not differ significantly from those of other cases of hysteria which never become psychotic. Although it is recognized that hysterical symptoms (as well as obsessive-compulsive ones) may at times be defenses against psychotic regression, the fact is, as Wittels (13) points out, that the tenuous contact of the hysteric with reality is typical of him, as is his tendency at times to confuse fantasy with reality. Under extreme stress the ego of the hysteric retreats even further from reality, and the confusional states which may ensue under such circumstances probably represent transitional borderline syndromes on the road to actual psychotic regression.

> A hysterical patient, in the course of analysis, reacted with intense anxiety to a remark on the analyst's part which she considered critical. On leaving the office, she felt confused and felt as though the high buildings on either side of the street were leaning over toward her, and were about to topple over and crush her. She wandered through the streets disoriented and frightened for several hours, after which the confusion subsided and she was able to return home. This patient did not develop a psychosis, but there is little doubt that greater stress at this time could have led to a psychotic breakdown.

These clinical aspects of the hysterical character—its resistance to change, the immaturity and instability of its ego structure, and its close relationship to addictions, depressions and schizophrenia—are all, it seems to me, best explained on the basis of deep-seated oral fixations. The resistance to character change in the hysteric, no less than the responsiveness to symptom change, grows out of his oral fixations. The easy disappearance of hysterical symptoms under therapy, like the hysteric's suggestibility, is often a form of transference compliance, the unconscious formula being, "If you will love and protect me, I will be or do whatever you want of me." But this same oral dependency becomes a source of major resistance when the analysis impinges upon it directly. The patient stubbornly clings to patterns of passivity and ingratiating compliance, and the working through of these and similar character traits is often one of the most difficult of analytic tasks. Efforts to resolve the transference are met as though they represent rejection and at this time oral-aggressive manifestations as well as recurrence of old symptoms may assert themselves.

This is not in any way to deny the tremendous and unquestionable part which oedipal fixations play in the hysteric. I believe, however, that a review of the clinical material in most instances will reveal that the fixations in the oedipal phase of development are *themselves the outgrowths of preoedipal fixations, chiefly of an oral nature.* As Fenichel (3, p. 95) states: "Pregenital fixation gives the subsequent Oedipus complex an irrevocable pregenital cast." The kind of parent whose behavior keeps a child at an "oral" level is apt to be the kind of parent whose behavior favors the development of a strong Oedipus complex. The preoedipal history of most of the hysterics I have seen has revealed one of two things—either intense frustration of their oral-receptive needs as a consequence of early defection or rejection by one or both parent figures, or excessive gratification of these needs by one or both parent figures.

The following case is illustrative:

A twenty-five-year-old housewife presented a wide variety of phobic symptoms. She had fears of insects, birds and dogs; she was terrified of carousels, of high places, and of the dark; she was seized by uncontrollable panics in the dentist's chair; and she was unable to be alone in the house or to talk to anyone on the telephone. She had a number of recurrent physical symptoms, notably headaches, feelings of a lump in the throat, and transitory vomiting attacks for which no organic cause could be found. On a number of occasions in the past year she had experienced periods of total amnesia for several hours at a time, although her outward behavior during these periods was apparently normal. Since childhood, she had a need to eat excessively whenever under tension, and much of her adult life had become a struggle against a resultant tendency to obesity. In the past three years she had also acquired a pattern of excessive indulgence in alcohol.

She had weighed 11 lbs. at birth. She was an only child. The father was a chronic alcoholic who died of cirrhosis of the liver when the patient was fourteen. Her parents were separated when she was eight years old and divorced a year later. The father's work took him away from home much of the time and the patient never saw much of him. She had an idealized picture of him as a sensitive, artistic, charming man who had been driven to drink by her mother. The mother was described as a dominating, controlling and narcissistic woman who was always critical of the patient. There was great emphasis on eating throughout the patient's childhood. Whenever she complained or cried, the mother gave her much food but little affection. The mother's chief concern was that the patient be a docile and compliant child, and even minor infractions of discipline were dealt with by frequent corporal punishment. The mother never remarried. The only source of affection in her childhood that the patient could recall was a Negro maid whom the mother dismissed when the patient was about three because she felt the patient was getting too attached to her.

A factor in the mother's attitude appears to have been a pigmented nevus on the patient's cheek which had been present since birth. Throughout the patient's childhood she was made to feel as though she had a repulsive defect, and although the nevus was surgically removed when she was eight years of age, the residual scar remained for her a perpetual reminder of her original "ugliness."

The mother's attitude toward sex was strongly repressive. Sex was never spoken of in the home, and even menstruation was treated as a secret shame. The patient was brought up to believe that to wash her hair or bathe while menstruating was highly dangerous. When she was five, she was discovered in the act of masturbating by her mother. She was severely whipped and warned that if she continued this practice her brain would turn to water and God would strike her dead. The patient had no recollection of masturbating after that except for a brief, anxious period during her adolescence.

From the time she left home to go to college, the patient had led a life of sexual promiscuity, but with total frigidity. Her original pattern was "to lead men on but not have relations with them," but when one of them angrily criticized her for this, she became anxious and thereafter was almost always compliant. Intercourse meant nothing to her but she felt it was "unfriendly" to refuse a man who wanted her. During the act, she blocked off all sensation below the waist, almost to the point of anesthesia. Being kissed and fondled above the waist was the only part of sex she enjoyed, and she often wished she had "only scales below the waist, like a mermaid." Nevertheless, if she did not have intercourse for any length of time, she would become anxious, and equated it with feeling "starved."

Prior to her marriage and afterwards, she always had to have a boy friend "on the side." She described this on one occasion as "love insurance," on another as "extra food in the pantry."

Although she was a more than averagely good-looking person, she had a deep conviction that she was unattractive and that no one could love her for herself. Being loved was more important than loving. She once said: "I can't let myself love anybody unless I'm absolutely certain they love me, and I'm never certain."

She was terrified of aggressive attitudes in others, but even more so of any aggressive feelings in herself. She was so concerned with what others thought of her, and so eager to please everyone, that she had lost the sense of self and had no real identity or convictions of her own.

Her fear of talking on the telephone was ascribed to the fact that "when you talk on the telephone you can't see the reactions you're getting." For a long time in the analysis she had anxiety when lying on the couch, for the same reason. It was not until late in the analysis that she was able to feel sufficiently secure not to turn her head constantly to watch for the reaction on the analyst's face.

Responsibility of any kind frightened her, although she was both intelligent and talented. She cultivated an elaborate façade of pseudo-stupidity as a defense against having to deal responsibly with household problems, with her children or with money. The idea of growing old was frightening to her, and she clung to the pattern of the child-wife. She showed a marked tendency toward fabrication and exaggeration, which was a source of frequent friction between herself and her husband.

Her analysis was a prolonged one, extending over four and a half years. Although most of her ego-dystonic symptoms subsided during the first year of analysis, her character defenses of compliance, passivity, and apprehensiveness were far more stubborn, as were also the bulemia and the excessive indulgence in alcohol. Sex, food, and liquor were all "oral" replacements to her for inner feelings of emptiness, coldness and unlovability, and it was not until these feelings were worked through the transference relationship that she was finally able to replace her addictions with more mature behavior. Her attitude in the transference, as might be expected, alternated repetitively between one of seductive ingratiation and idealization of the analyst as a father symbol, and an apprehensive testing and retesting of him as a mother symbol who was cruel, critical and rejecting.

In the reconstruction of this case, it seems clear that the earliest and most basic fixations were oral in nature. The patient felt rejected and unloved from her earliest childhood on. Eating was the only important gratification that was freely permitted her, and oral satisfaction became the focus around which all of her affectional and security needs centered. This gave her subsequent Oedipus complex "an irrevocable pregenital cast."

The inability of hysterics to resolve the Oedipus complex and to achieve mature "genitality" is, I believe, a consequence of such earlier experiences which have resulted in preoedipal oral fixations. If this assumption is correct, and I believe that clinical evidence substantiates it, then some of the material presented by hysterical patients in analysis may require reevaluation. For example, much of the manifestly incestuous material, like the overtly expressed incestuous wishes of the schizophrenic, may conceal deeper pregenital wishes of an oral character. Thus the incestuous dream of the hysteric may conceal behind the symbolic wish to cohabit with the mother (or father) a deeper, pregenital wish to be loved and protected by her (or him) to the exclusion of the rest of the world.

In relation to the parent of the same sex, a dream or fantasy may have the manifest content of a homosexual wish or fear, while the deeper wish is to suckle at the breast as a symbol of love and protection, as in the following instance:

A young man of twenty-four, suffering from numerous phobias and hysterical conversion symptoms, reported the following dream: He was in the home of his employer, an older man; they had a sumptuous dinner together and after that the employer made sexual advances to him. The patient began to perform fellatio upon his employer, then awakened with anxiety. The manifest content of this dream was a passive homosexual one, but the deeper pregenital meaning was: "If you will feed and protect me, I shall be passively compliant to your every wish." In this instance, the dream not only had obvious transference implications in relation to the analyst, but also characterized the patient's basic way of relating to all potential parent symbols whether male or female. The phallus in the dream was in the deepest sense a breast symbol.

By the same token, many of the manifestations of the castration complex in the hysteric become more meaningful when they are understood not in terms of genital anxiety but in terms of the fear of losing love or of being cut off symbolically from the maternal breast, an interpretation of castration anxiety which Freud (5) was the first to advance in *The Problem of Anxiety*.

Similarly the wealth of oral fantasies encountered in the hysteric may deserve reevaluation. In discussing the fellatio fantasy which is so common in hysterical women, Fenichel (3, p. 229) describes it as a distorted expression for the wish to bite off and incorporate the penis and suggests four possible meanings for this wish.

It may mean [he says] (a) a displacement upward of genital wishes, (b) the idea of impregnation, (c) a revenge on the man who possesses the envied organ . . . , and (d) an incorporation of the castrated penis and an identification with the man.

While recognizing the overdetermination of such fantasies, and the fact that one or all of these meanings may be implicit in them, there is a fifth possibility which is frequently encountered in female hysterics, and that is the oral-receptive meaning of this fantasy, in which the fellatio represents a pregenital suckling at the penis as a breast-symbolic source of love and sustenance. Still another possibility is the fact that fellatio may represent for the hysterical woman a way of gaining the love of the man by gratifying him sexually without having to submit to the feared genital contact herself.

In the same way, the pseudo-sexuality of the hysteric may be interpreted too exclusively along genital lines without taking into consideration its pregenital significance. Thus the sexual coquetry of the hysterical woman is interpreted by Reich (12, p. 191) as serving "the purpose of finding out whether and from where the expected (incest) dangers will materialize"; while Fenichel (3, p. 234) attributed it to the damming up of their sexuality so that it "comes out in unsuitable places and at inconvenient times." The contradiction between the repression of sexuality in hysterics and their "sexualization" of all their relationships is, of course, more apparent than real. But there is a possible explanation for it other than those which Reich and Fenichel give. The sexuality of the hysteric is indeed a sham, but primarily *because it expresses a pregenital oral-receptive wish rather than a genital one.* The distress and surprise of the hysterical woman when her seductiveness leads to her being approached genitally is consequently understandable. She is being approached as a woman when what she really desires is to be taken as a child. Repeatedly one hears the hysterical woman say, "If only the man would just kiss me and hold me in his arms, instead of wanting sex!"

In this regard, it is of interest to consider the question of why the hysterical character is seen more commonly in women than in men. The usual explanation for this is that the course of sexual development is more complicated in women than in men, and that castration anxiety in the female tends to fixate her in the oedipal stage while in men it tends to foster the resolution of the Oedipus complex. In all likelihood, we are dealing here too with an overdetermined phenomenon, and one wonders whether there may not be still another factor operating. If oral fixations and oral receptivity play an important determining role in the etiology of the hysterical character, might it not follow in a society which tends to regard dependency, passivity and receptivity as feminine traits, acceptable in women but not in men, that the hysterical type of character structure would persist more frequently in women?

There are a number of theoretical implications which follow from the assumptions which have been advanced in this paper. The present assumption that neuroses necessarily represent later stages of fixation than psychoses ought perhaps to be reconsidered in favor of the hypothesis that an orally, anally, or phallically fixated individual may be *either* neurotic *or* psychotic, with the *qualitative* shift from neurosis to psychosis depending on *quantitative* variations in the balance between ego strength and ego stress (9).

It would appear, also, that hysterics as well as certain psychotics may show a predominance of oral fixations. The crucial point of differentiation, apart from the degree of stress at the point of breakdown, is the important question of ego development and ego strength. The psychotic, either because of still unknown constitutional reasons, or because of more severe or more prolonged damage during the crucial years of infancy, has a weaker ego-integrative capacity and consequently a lower threshold for stress.

This raises an important question concerning the usefulness of the libidinal frame of reference as a means of classifying mental disorders, unless one takes the matter of ego development into consideration. As Robert Knight (8) has aptly put it:

> The attempt to build a classification of mental disorders by linking a certain clinical condition to each level of libidinal fixation, has presented a one-sided, libidinal theory of human functioning. This psychoanalytic contribution has been of major value, but it needs to be supplemented extensively with the findings of ego-psychology which have not, as yet, been sufficiently integrated with the libido theory.

If, nevertheless, one uses the level of libidinal fixation as a frame of reference for the differentiation of neurotic character, it is suggested that a *predominance* of oral fixations favors the development of a hysterical character, a *predominance* of anal fixations a compulsive character, and a *predominance* of phallic fixations, a phallic-narcissistic character. It is of interest to note that this conception has its counterpart in one of Freud's later formulations. In his paper entitled "Libidinal Types," first published in 1931, Freud (6) suggested that in terms of the libidinal situation three main types can be distinguished, which he named the *erotic,* the *obsessional* and the *narcissistic.* As he visualized these, they represented character pictures within the boundaries of normalcy, but he recognized that "in their extreme developments, they may well approximate to clinical pictures and so help to bridge the gulf which is assumed to exist between the normal and the pathological."

The erotic type, Freud described as representing "persons whose main interest . . . is focused on love; loving, but above all, being loved, is for them the most important thing in life. They are governed by the dread of loss of love, and this makes them peculiarly dependent on those who may withhold their love from them." The obsessional type, he described as characterized by "the supremacy exercised by the superego," while in the narcissistic type "the ego has a considerable amount of aggression available, one manifestation of this being a proneness to activity; where love is in question, loving is preferred to being loved. People of this type . . . readily assume the role of leader. . . ."

Freud then goes on to discuss the various mixtures of these types which, he points out, occur more frequently than the pure types. He suggests that the ideally normal person would have elements of all three types in harmonious balance.

He concludes with a tentative suggestion that when persons of the erotic type fall ill, they will develop hysteria, and those of the obsessional type will develop obsessional neuroses. People of the narcissistic type, he felt, are peculiarly disposed to psychoses and probably to criminality.

It will be noted that this formulation of Freud's is roughly paralleled by the hypothesis presented in the present study. His erotic type closely approximates the hysterical character with its strong oral dependency, and its relationship to the clinical syndrome of hysteria was recognized by him. His other types also are analogous to present-day conceptions of the obsessional and phallic-narcissistic character types.

In conclusion, I would emphasize the following points, not as proven facts but as tentative and hypothetical suggestions toward a reevaluation of the psychodynamics of the hysterical character.

1. Oral fixations are of basic importance in the hysterical character.

2. These oral fixations give the subsequent Oedipus complex of the hysteric a strong pregenital cast.

3. There is a close psychodynamic relationship between hysteria, addiction, certain types of depression, and schizophrenia.

4. The greater frequency of hysteria in women as compared to men may be, in part at least, a cultural phenomenon due to the

fact that oral receptivity, dependency, and passivity are regarded in our society as feminine traits, and are consequently more acceptable in women than in men.

5. An orally-fixated individual may be either neurotic or psychotic, depending on the balance between ego strength and ego stress. The question of ego development is of crucial importance, not only in this respect, but also in the entire question of "choice" of mental disorder. The present correlation of diagnostic categories with the level of libidinal development needs to be integrated with the newer findings of ego psychology.

6. If, nevertheless, one uses the level of libidinal fixation as a frame of reference for the differentiation of neurotic characters, it is suggested that, although there are residuals of fixation at all levels in every neurotic character, a predominance of "oral" fixations favors the development of a hysterical character trend, a predominance of "anal" fixations a compulsive character trend, and a predominance of "phallic" fixations a phallic-narcissistic character trend.

REFERENCES

1. BERGLER, E. The Basic Neurosis. New York: Grune & Stratton, 1949.
2. CALDWELL, J. M. Schizophrenic psychoses. Am. J. Psychiat., 97:1061, 1941.
3. FENICHEL, O. The Psychoanalytic Theory of Neurosis. New York: W. W. Norton & Co., 1945.
4. FREUD, S. (1905) Fragment of an analysis of a case of hysteria. Collected Papers, 3:13–146. London: Hogarth Press, 1924.
5. FREUD, S. (1926) The Problem of Anxiety. New York: W. W. Norton & Co., 1936.
6. FREUD, S. (1931) Libidinal types. Collected Papers, 5:247–251. London: Hogarth Press, 1950.
7. JUNG, C. G. Psychogenesis of schizophrenia. J. Ment. Sci., 85:999, 1937.
8. KNIGHT, R. P. Borderline states. Bull. Menninger Clin., 17:1, 1953.
9. MARMOR, J. and PUMPIAN-MINDLIN, E. Toward an integrative conception of mental disorder. J. Nerv. & Ment. Dis., 111:19, 1950. (Chapter 2, this volume.)
10. MILLER, W. R. Relationship between early schizophrenia and the neuroses. Am. J. Psychiat., 96:889, 1940.
11. MYERSON, A. Neuroses and neuropsychoses. Am. J. Psychiat., 93:263, 1936.
12. REICH, W. Charakteranalyse. Berlin, 1933.
13. WITTELS, F. The hysterical character. Med. Rev. of Reviews, 36:186, 1930.
14. ZILBOORG, G. The deeper layers of schizophrenic psychosis. Am. J. Psychiat., 88:493, 1931.

12

THE PSYCHODYNAMICS OF
REALISTIC WORRY
(1955)

In popular scientific literature the assumption is generally made that worry is a pathological symptom from which the "normal" individual should be free. "How Not to Worry" is the major theme of countless essays which purport to promote mental health.* It is the purpose of this communication to examine the psychodynamics of worry and to offer the thesis that under certain circumstances worry performs a useful and necessary function in the service of a healthy ego.

In considering this problem, the first question with which we are confronted is that of definition of terms. Just what do we mean by "worry," and how does it differ, if at all, from such concepts as fear and anxiety? The distinction between these various terms is far from clear, and there is no general agreement concerning them in the literature. The most prevalent conception, based on Freud's distinction between realistic and neurotic anxiety (1926), identifies fear with realistic anxiety. It differentiates between fear and anxiety on the basis of fear being a reaction to a known, tangible, objective and conscious source of danger, and anxiety being a reaction to an unknown, intangible, subjective and unconscious source of danger. May (1953) has attemped to differentiate between fear and

---

*Norman Vincent Peale's *The Power of Positive Thinking,* which has occupied the best-seller lists for many months, is a classic example of this kind of approach. For an excellent popular critique of it, see William Lee Miller's "Some Negative Thinking about Norman Vincent Peale," in *The Reporter* for Jan. 13, 1955.

anxiety on a somewhat different basis. "In fear," says May, "we know what threatens us, we are energized by the situation, our perceptions are sharper, and we take steps to run or in other appropriate ways to overcome the danger. In anxiety, however, we are threatened without knowing what steps to take to meet the danger. Anxiety . . . is the feeling of being 'caught,' 'overwhelmed'; and instead of becoming sharper, our perceptions generally become blurred or vague." May seems to make a kind of quantitative as well as qualitative distinction between the two also. "Fear," he says, "is a threat to one side of the self . . . but as soon as the threat becomes great enough to involve the total self, one then has the experience of anxiety."

Rado (1950), on the other hand, is of the conviction that there is no sound basis whatever upon which to differentiate anxiety from fear, and he advocates the exclusive use of the word "fear" to denote all responses of this kind to danger.

Although I believe that Rado is basically correct in his insistence that both *physiologically* and *genetically* fear and anxiety are closely related, it seems to me, nevertheless, that *psychodynamically* it is useful to make a distinction, as Freud did, between reactions to realistic and unrealistic sources of danger. Whether one chooses to call these reactions by the terms realistic and neurotic anxiety, as did Freud, or normal and disordered fear reactions, as does Rado, is essentially a matter of semantics. In this communication I shall retain the traditional terms of *fear,* or realistic anxiety, on the one hand, and *neurotic anxiety,* on the other, to distinguish between realistic and neurotic fear reactions to danger.

Where, however, does the concept of worry enter into this picture? Is it simply a colloquial term which is completely subsumed under the concept of anxiety (as most psychoanalytic as well as popular writers have apparently assumed*), and which, therefore, has no place in a serious scientific article, or does it have a distinctive connotation which should properly be separated from anxiety?

---

*A search of the *Psychoanalytic Quarterly, Psychoanalytic Review,* and *International Journal of Psycho-Analysis* for the past twenty years fails to reveal the word "worry" in their subject indices, except for one mention in the *Psychoanalytic Quarterly* in 1938, which refers to a review of a popular book on the subject of *Worry and Its Control.*

I believe that it has. Borrowing from a suggestion of Rado's that in emergency situations the organism may respond on various levels of integration—from a crudely biological, which he calls the *hedonic*, to a somewhat higher level, which he calls the *emotional*, to the most highly organized level, which he calls the *intellectual*—I would like to advance the hypothesis that anxiety represents an *emotional* level of response to impending danger, while worry is the expression of an *intellectual* level of response to such danger. Neurotic worry in this formulation would thus bear the same relationship to realistic worry as neurotic anxiety does to realistic anxiety.

Another way of stating this formulation is that anxiety is essentially an *emotional signal* of impending danger, while worry is a form of *mental activity* which is set off by this signal. Anxiety is an alerting mechanism, worry an effort at problem-solving. In this connection I would call attention to the fact that, although fear and anxiety are readily ascribed to animals, worry appears to be a distinctively human reaction. We rarely, if ever, speak of animals as worrying (unless we are deliberately speaking of them anthropomorphically)! A related observation is the fact that we never think of infants either as worrying, although it is well recognized that infants can show fear reactions from the earliest weeks of life on. Our assumption that infants do not worry is an implicit recognition of the fact that worry represents a level of mental functioning which requires a more advanced stage of ego integration. It would be of interest to study the precise age at which the process of worry can first be observed in the young child. Such a study would, I believe, shed light on an important phase of development of the normal ego.

In Rado's system, worry might be characterized as "apprehensive thought." At this point it must be emphasized that although worry is a process distinct from anxiety, *it never exists without the latter. The mental work of worry is always set off, or triggered, by an underlying signal of anxiety.* In this context Austen Riggs's definition (1944) of worry as a "cycle of inefficient thought whirling about a pivot of fear" corresponds with the thesis which is being propounded in this paper, except that, as we shall see, the thought need not necessarily be inefficient. It is of interest here to note that worry is not merely an intransitive verb. It is also used transitively to connote the harassing of an object with the purpose of overcoming it.

Worry bears a similar relationship to anxiety as does the dream. Both represent activity of the ego—in the instance of worry, directly and consciously, in the dream, distortedly and unconsciously—to deal with something which threatens or disturbs it. Dreams might, in fact, be characterized as the worrying of the unconscious during sleep. This similarity is particularly evident, as we shall see, when we compare the dynamics of worry to those of the recurrent dream of the traumatic neurosis.

Worry over realistic matters, then, may be regarded as a defensive function of the ego, the purpose of which is either to ward off an anticipated real trauma or to deal with the painful consequences of one already experienced. The student who is concerned with his ability to pass an important pending examination would be an example of the first type of reaction; while the one concerned with the consequences of his having failed the examination would be an example of the second. In the former instance, the worry creates the anticipated threat in fantasy, and endeavors to master it. In the latter instance, the worry repetitively seeks to undo the trauma. In the first instance, the individual is concerned with "How can I deal with what is going to happen?"; in the second, with "How can I undo what has happened?" The second reaction is thus similar psychodynamically to the recurrent dream of the traumatic neurosis, which likewise represents efforts on the part of the ego to master successfully a previously unmastered traumatic experience. It is worth noting that anxiety occurs in the traumatic dream not simply through the act of re-experiencing the traumatic situation, but through the fact of failing once again to master it. When the ego is finally able to bind the stimulus cathexis provided by the experience—i.e., to integrate it within the organism—anxiety ceases to be experienced.

In this sense, realistic worry is not merely a defensive mechanism; it is also an integrative one. It represents "work" on the part of the ego, endeavoring to bind the stimulus cathexis provided by the impending danger. When successful it leads to action, i.e., to overt motor activity dealing with the danger; or else to an internalized binding of the stimulus cathexis by the integrative action of the ego, i.e., the individual "stops worrying," either by rationalizing the traumatic experience, or else by a process in which the individual detaches cathexis from the real or fantasied object of which the trauma has deprived him (e.g., the student finally "accepts" the fact that he has gotten a poor grade). If the ego fails in its integrative task, however, then decompensation takes place either in the form of ineffective or circular worrying (which is identical with what is usually clinically labeled as obsessional rumination)—or else the effort to deal with the problem at an *intellectual* level is given up entirely, and regression takes place to the *emotional* level, in which anxiety, bound or unbound, is the dominant feature. The clinical picture may then be that of an anxiety state, a phobia, or a conversion hysteria.

If these neurotic defenses fail to cope with the stress situation, even further regression may then take place to a psychotic (affective or schizophrenic) level of response (Marmor & Pumpian-Mindlin, 1950).

There is, of course, still another type of reaction to anxiety which totally "short-circuits" the worry respone, and that is the well-known mechanism of "denial." Although the mechanism of denial is widely employed, even among "normal" individuals, psychodynamically I would consider it to be a less healthy response than that of realistic worry, since it indicates a lesser ego capacity to deal effectively with a stress situation.*

The "work" of worry may be further likened to the work of mourning. Actually worry, as we have indicated above, like mourning, is often related to a lost "object." The object may be a tangible and real one—as when a person worries about the possibility of losing his job—or it may be a relatively intangible one, such as

---

*Almost a year after this paper was written and presented, I received a copy of a research study by Irving L. Janis of the Dept. of Psychology of Yale University, which arrives independently at similar conclusions. In his study (see pp. 119–154) Janis demonstrates that "surgical patients who develop an illusion of invulnerability based on a *total denial* of the impending threat (e.g., 'there will be nothing at all to this operation') are more likely to be traumatized or to show acute emotional disturbances afterwards than those who rely on a more limited sense of invulnerability that takes account of realistic anticipations . . . A central postulate suggested by the case studies and the correlational findings is that there is a 'work of worry' which . . . enables the person to cope more effectively in the long run with a painful reality situation . . ."

prestige, success, or self-esteem. The person who worries about the possibility of doing poorly in a contest or debate would be an example of the latter kind of object loss. The work of worry differs from that of mourning, however, in that it is an intellectual process, while mourning is an affective one. In mourning the preoccupation of the ego is with emotionally missing the loved object; in worry, it is with the problem of "What am I going to do now?" It will be recalled that in his classic paper on "Mourning and Melancholia," Freud (1917) explained the work of mourning as a struggle on the part of the ego to withdraw libido from its attachment to the object. Every one of the memories and hopes which bound the libido to the object is brought up and hypercathected, thus detaching the libido bit by bit. Freud has likened melancholia to an open wound drawing to itself cathectic energy from all sides. This is equally true of worry, in which the ego in its work draws unto itself cathectic energy from all sides (Freud called this "anticathexis"), so that a person who is extremely worried can consequently think of nothing else, and often has neither desire nor interest in anything else. Sleep also often becomes impossible because the cathectic demands of the work of worry do not permit the general withdrawal of cathexis which is necessary for sleep.

Examples demonstrating this mechanism are numerous. The worried mother, who cannot sleep or eat during the critical illness of a loved child; the wage earner who has been laid off from the job upon which his family depends for sustenance, and who spends a restless, tossing night trying to figure out what to do next; the adolescent with the lead in the high-school play who has no appetite before opening night, and who keeps going over the lines which he fears he may forget; these are common illustrations from everyday life. In clinical practice, on the other hand, the obsessional and hypochondriacal patients whose symptoms of "worry" are associated with insomnia, anorexia, and loss of libido are all too familiar to require elaboration.

This explanation, in terms of mental economics, of the work involved in the process of worrying also serves to explain why individuals who find themselves suddenly or unexpectedly relieved of worry often react with a period of great jubilation or high spirits. This is precisely what Freud (1917) was describing in "Mourning and Melancholia" when he wrote, "All states such as joy, triumph, exultation, which form the normal counterparts of mania, are economically conditioned in the same way. First there is always a long, sustained condition of great mental expenditure . . . upon which at last some influence supervenes, making it superfluous so that a volume of energy becomes available for . . . discharge—for example, when some poor devil, by winning a large sum of money, is suddenly relieved from perpetual anxiety about his daily bread, when any long and arduous struggle is finally crowned with success, when a man finds himself in a position to throw off at one blow some heavy burden or false position he has endured" (pp. 164–165). In all such situations, Freud points out, the freeing of the ego from its heavy task permits the whole amount of anticathexis to become suddenly available, thus giving the ego a sense of great exultation, energy and power.

The economic explanation may also clarify why realistic worry often neutralizes neurotic anxiety while the worry lasts. The cathectic demands of the ego in coping with the realistic threat may be so great that no libidinal energy is available for the neurotic conflict during such periods. Thus a severe obsessional neurotic, who for months had been preoccupied with fears of cancer and insanity, was totally free of these symptoms during a two-week interval in which he was in serious danger of being dropped from his job under cirumstances which would have been not only humiliating, but seriously damaging to his entire future. Interestingly enough, when he successfully combatted and overcame this threat, he experienced an interval of several days in which he felt jubilant, strong and healthy—after which his neurotic symptoms recurred.

It is possible that similar economic mechanisms are involved in the well-known temporary return to reality of psychotic patients under circumstances which constitute a life threat.

A few additional questions require clarification at this point. What about the patient who utilizes what appears to be a realistic worry as a resistance against dealing with his inner psychological conflicts? The answer, I believe, is that the worry in such instances is clearly not a real worry, but a sham one, a defense against concealed and repressed sources of anxiety. Realistic worry always rests on a foundation of realistic anxiety, and the ego threat in such instances is an objective and conscious one.

Another question which may be raised with regard to the problem of worry is its relationship to time. A formulation which suggests itself is that worry is a process which deals with future dangers, in contrast with anxiety which deals with present ones, and grief which is concerned with past ones. Although there is a certain persuasiveness to this thesis on first glance, more careful reflection has led me to discard it for several reasons. First, this formulation ignores what I believe to be the essential differentiating feature between worry on the one hand, and anxiety or grief on the other, namely, the fact that worry is an intellectual or thinking process, while anxiety and grief are affective ones. Second, although it is true that worry most often seems to be concerned with impending or future dangers, this is not invariably so. A person can be worried about a present danger, such as the fact that he is unemployed, or ill, or about a past one, as in the instance of the student who has failed an examination. Third, neither anxiety nor grief can on closer inspection be rigidly limited to time sequences. Grief can deal with present as well as past loss, while anxiety can be related to impending threats as well as present ones. In spite of these facts, however, I believe there may be a special relationship between worry and the future in the sense that even when worry deals with present or past traumata, its goal is invariably to achieve a more effective mastery in the future. The formula "What am I going to do now?" carries this implication.

In concluding, the question may properly be asked: what, if any, is the significance of a concept of realistic worry, such as has been outlined in this paper? To answer this, I would turn for a moment to the problem of fear. In the past twenty years, psychiatrists have come to an awareness of the fact that fear, under realistic conditions of danger, is a normal reaction of the healthy ego. This realization was of enormous help in strengthening the morale of World War II soldiers, who by learning to accept their fear as normal were relieved of the additional burdens of guilt and self-condemnation which characterized their predecessors in World War I. I believe it is equally important for psychiatrists to recognize the normalcy of realistic worry, and I am of the opinion that the mental hygiene value of such recognition, just as in the case of fear, can be extremely valuable for the public at large. One is impressed by how many people operate upon the assumption that to worry about anything is ipso facto "neurotic," and that the "normal" person should never worry.* Most people apparently seem to be unaware of the rather obvious fact that to be unworried in the face of a distressing or threatening reality situation may sometimes be a symptom of a serious mental disorder rather than a sign of mental health. As in the case of fear, the problem with which we must be concerned in worry is not the fact that it exists, but rather the question of whether or not *it has a realistic basis, and whether it leads ultimately to some action or thought which liberates the ego cathexes or anticathexes and restores the mobility of the ego.* Similar considerations are involved in the distinction between healthy and neurotic fantasy, and between normal grief and depression (Jacobson, 1957).

The entire area of the psychodynamics of normal mental processes is one which has been relatively neglected by psychoanalysis but which deserves more attention (Liddell, 1953; Shakow, 1953). All too often patients have the illusion that mental health and happiness are synonymous, and that when they are "cured" they will "live happily ever after." One gets the impression that occasionally even an analyst or psychotherapist, seduced by the omnipotent expectations of his patients, may set for himself this same kind of illusory therapeutic goal. Obviously even the most successful analysis cannot guarantee happiness for anyone. The world in which we live presents us with a continuous procession of real problems and difficulties. The difference between "normalcy" and neurosis lies not in the absence of problems but in the ego resources which the individual is able to bring to bear upon them—not in the absence of anxieties and worries but in their effectiveness in mobilizing contructive ego activity. The capacity of the individual to move in a healthy direction, in every instance, is dependent upon the balance of forces between the severity of the stresses to which the ego is being subjected,

---

*Contrast this with the moving statement of Warren Weaver of the Rockefeller Foundation in the December 11, 1954 issue of the *Saturday Review of Literature:* "Are you satisfied with the state of the world? Are you content with the behavior of modern men? Have you reached the point where soporific relaxation is the real goal, where more than anything you want rest and quiet and protection from stimulation? . . . I want no sluggish languor, no bovine complacency. A phenobarbital philosophy does not appeal to me. I want to be concerned, stimulated, stirred, worried."

on the one hand, and the integrative ability of the ego ("ego strength"), on the other. The task of mental hygiene, therefore, is always a twofold one—to reduce the stresses, and to strengthen the ego. It is hoped that a better understanding of the psychodynamics of worry may contribute to this goal.

REFERENCES

FREUD, S. (1917), Mourning and Melancholia. *Collected Papers*, 4:152–170. London: Hogarth Press, 1925.

———— (1926), *The Problem of Anxiety*. New York: Norton, 1936.

JACOBSON, E. (1957), On Normal and Pathological Moods. *The Psychoanalytic Study of the Child*, 12:73–113. New York: International Universities Press.

LIDDELL, H. S. (1953), The Biology of Wishes and Worries. *Mid-Century Psychiatry*, ed. R. R. Grinker, Springfield, Ill.: Charles C. Thomas, pp. 104–112.

MARMOR, J. & PUMPIAN-MINDLIN, E. (1950), Toward an Integrative Conception of Mental Disorder. *J. Nerv. & Ment. Dis.* (Chapter 2, this volume.)

MAY, R. (1953), *Man's Search for Himself*. New York: Norton, pp. 38 f.

RADO, S. (1950), Emergency Behavior. *Anxiety*, ed. P. Hoch & J. Zubin. New York: Grune & Stratton, pp. 150–175.

RIGGS, A. (1944), Quoted in D. B. Klein, *Mental Hygiene*. New York: Henry Holt, p. 367.

SHAKOW, D. (1953), Some Aspects of Mid-Century Psychiatry. *Mid-Century Psychiatry*, ed. R. R. Grinker. Springfield, Ill.: Charles C. Thomas, pp. 104–112.

A SPECIAL NOTE

This paper, like "Orality in the Hysterical Personality" (Chapter 11), was presented at a meeting of the American Psychoanalytic Association, and was couched in terminology designed to facilitate communication with my listeners. Although I feel its essential thesis about the function of worry is a correct one, I would no longer use some of the theoretical concepts that I employed at that time. The constructs of "libidinal cathexis and anticathexis," for example, although metaphorically descriptive, can no longer be considered scientifically tenable; there is no justifiable basis in the light of current neurophysiological knowledge for operating within a "psychic energy" frame of reference (cf. Young, J. Z. *A Model of the Brain*, London: Oxford University Press, 1966). If one conceives of the brain as a problem-solving, model-building, living kind of computer, one can understand the function of worry in terms of efforts of the organism to revise its overall "working model" (for the achievement of security, gratification or mastery) in the light of an experienced or expected trauma that has upset or seems likely to upset, the previous working model. Following Miller, Galanter, and Pribram (ref. Miller, G. A., Galanter, E. and Pribram, K. H. *Plans and the Structure of Behavior,* New York: Holt, Rinehart & Winston, 1960) we can postulate that human beings, consciously or unconsciously, usually operate with a hierarchy of plans some of which are concerned with long-term goals, others with short-term goals. When a major change in the environment or within the organism occurs that disrupts one of these set goals, central nervous system activity is triggered to alter or modify the impaired plan. When this can be done easily we experience little or no anxiety. When the solution is less clear, we experience more anxiety, and the "work" of replanning is experienced as worry. Also, the relief one feels when a new solution is achieved is quite understandable simply in terms of the pleasure at regaining a sense of mastery or security without necessitating the employment of concepts of shifting energy patterns or cathexes. (J. M., 1973)

13

SOME COMMENTS ON EGO
PSYCHOLOGY
(1957)

The term "ego psychology" is often used in different ways. My own use of it in this discussion will be within the framework of the id-ego-superego constructs of Freudian psychology, to designate the action system of that portion of the personality which is concerned with the perceptual, integrative and executive functions of the personality. I am not, in other words, using the term "ego" as synonymous with "total personality." Let me emphasize, however, that this does not indicate an unawareness of the basic fact that the human organism, like any other biological organism, functions holistically, and that an "ego psychology" is as much of an abstraction as an "id psychology." In the final integrative synthesis of human behavior theory, there can be only a psychology of the total organism, the resultant of the dynamic interaction of biological, psychological and sociological factors. Once we accept this fact, however, we can, I believe, usefully employ the constructs of id, ego and superego to designate symbolically some of the vectors in this interaction, without losing sight of the fact that they are not independent entities.

It is customary to speak of early psychoanalytic theory as being primarily an id-oriented psychology, and this was, of course, true. Although originally Freud was only rarely preoccupied with the dynamics of the ego, in later years he gradually began to give it more attention, culminating in his study on *The Ego and the Id* in 1923 (2); but it was not until 1926, when he revised his concept of anxiety and reformulated it as an ego signal rather than as a

180

consequence of repressed libido (3), that Freudian ego psychology really received a major impetus forward. Two subsequent important landmarks in this area were Wilhelm Reich's *Character-Analysis* in 1933 (6), and Anna Freud's significant study on *The Ego and the Mechanisms of Defense* in 1936 (1).

All of these earlier classical writings on ego psychology, however, discussed it primarily in terms of the ego's defensive role in mediating the conflicting demands of id, superego and outer world. This led to the justified criticism by many observers that in Freudian theory there was no adequate conception of the *nondefensive* aspects of ego function. Moreover, in these earlier writings, the ego was not regarded as having any original identity of its own—it was conceived of merely as the outer crust of the id, formed by contact with the outer world, with all of its energies being ultimately "borrowed" from the id.

Then in 1939, Hartmann, taking cognizance of the fact that "conflicts are not the only sources of ego development," formulated his theory of the "conflict-free ego sphere" embracing such functions as "perception, intention, object-comprehension, thinking, language, recall phenomena, productivity, motor-development, grasping, crawling, walking . . . and the maturation and learning process implicit in all these and many other [activities]" (4).

Although there has been the usual lag in the understanding and dissemination of Hartmann's significant contribution in the psycho-analytic literature, it seems to me that its implications for modification of classical libido theory are quite considerable and that it presents an important bridge of rapprochement to other variations of psycho-analytic ego psychology.

For one thing, Hartmann's modification changes what has hitherto been a cornerstone of Freudian theory, namely that all pleasure strivings are ontogenetically related and are part of a unitary libido. By recognizing that there are primary ego strivings for mastery which are pleasurable in themselves (although they may and generally do become *secondarily* cathected with libidinal affects), Hartmann goes a long way toward meeting one of the major criticisms of classical Freudian theory. These primary ego drives in Hartmann's system are not too dissimilar, I believe, to the "autonomous strivings toward growth and self-realization" in Horney's system, and to some of the "dynamisms" concerned with "the feeling of ability or power" in Sullivan's system.

In general there are two major aspects to human ego development—that which proceeds from intrinsic biologic growth or maturation, and that which proceeds from learning. In actuality, of course, there is constant interplay and interaction between these two vectors, and neither of them proceeds independently of the other. In fact the biological aspects of man gradually become so interpenetrated with social influences that as time goes on the biological as such is no longer, in my opinion, isolable in human behavior and thought. This dialectical fusion has its anatomical and physiological basis in the development of the language and association centers of the cerebral cortex, which goes on concomitantly with the maturation and socialization of the child. I would agree with Sullivan, therefore, that what is *human* in the human personality grows out of man's social relationships and cannot be separated therefrom.

To return to the factors involved in ego development, it has always seemed to me that most psychoanalytic theories, rooted as they have been in psychopathology rather than in normal development, have laid excessive stress upon frustration and anxiety as prime factors in ego development. Now one cannot, of course, question the universality of some frustration and anxiety in the life history of any child in our culture, and probably in any culture. What I am questioning is the excessive degree of importance placed on them in most theories of ego development. Very recently, on the program of the American Psychoanalytic Association, Gerhart Piers (5) pointed out that there are generally three main ways in which learning takes place: (1) by *trial and error,* which falls into the class of reward and punishment learning, or frustration and reward learning. This is the kind of learning which most psychoanalytic theories have emphasized. But in addition, Piers reminded us, learning can also take place through (2) sudden awareness of a *gestalt* (which would be akin to what we often describe as sudden insight, and which Karl Bühler described as an "a-ha" awareness), and (3) through a process of *identification.* These latter two forms of learning, and particularly the third, have been relatively neglected in psychoanalytic theories of ego development.

I would like to advance the suggestion that in addition to the intrinsic maturational forces whose existence we can take for granted, and in addition to the developmental consequences of anxiety and frustration which have been so well studied in psychoanalysis, human ego development also takes place *optimally* through a process of identification with loved objects. You will note that I am using the concept of identification differently here than in the sense where it is used to designate a mechanism of *defense*. While I recognize that identification can be utilized as a defense, I believe it to be an intrinsic ego dynamism which grows out of the primitive tendency of the young infant toward *imitation* (or *fascination*, to use Bernfeld's term). Such conflict-free learning processes as are involved in walking, for example, are acquired primarily, I believe, through this mechanism of positive identification. Most other aspects of human acculturation are more involved with parental value systems (i.e., cultural value systems), which in turn lead to much greater admixtures of frustration and anxiety for the child in the learning process, which may account for why these other functions more often become entwined with psychopathological processes. I suspect that when such aspects of acculturation as talking, weaning, sphincter-training, and eating are allowed to be learned "naturally," so to speak, through positive identification—as they can be—rather than through premature disciplinary training involving frustration or punishment, the child is more likely to grow up not only free from conflicts in these areas, but also with the kind of flexible adaptability which stems from feelings of trust toward others, as well as that trust in self which we call self-confidence. I believe that we need much more study in psychoanalysis of this kind of ego development, which takes place through gratification rather than through frustration, and its implications for child rearing and education would be very great.

The implications of ego psychology for psychoanalytic practice have been tremendous. I think it is fair to say that regardless of how dedicated a psychoanalyst is to the libido theory, in practice he must always deal with the ego psychology of the patient. Any other approach is not only therapeutically ineffective, it is therapeutically meaningless. One still occasionally—fortunately less and less often, I believe—encounters the attitude in some analytic circles that analysis focused on the ego rather than on the id is somehow or other superficial and not really psychoanalysis. Anna Freud (1) criticized this attitude as far back as 1936: "The view held," she wrote, "was that the term *psychoanalysis* should be reserved for . . . discoveries relating to the unconscious psychic life, i.e., the study of repressed instinctual impulses, affects and fantasies. With problems such as that of the adjustment of children or adults to the outside world, with concepts of value such as those of health and disease, virtue or vice, psychoanalysis was not properly concerned" (pp. 3–4). Anna Freud then went on to point out that the ego is and must be the focus of psychoanalytic therapy, since it is only through the medium of the ego that the unconscious needs of man are observable.

Obviously, then, ego psychology is neither superficial nor deviant in modern psychoanalytic therapy. It is the only proper theoretical tool which can be practically employed, and failure to understand this usually leads to "wild" analysis.

I am convinced that many of the differences in approach among the different schools in analysis today can be resolved through better communication among them. One of the difficulties involved is semantic; and if we can ultimately agree on a common terminology, it will facilitate the resolution of these differences. Another practical difficulty is the fact that the raw clinical data which we all observe are in themselves products of the transactional relationship between patient and analyst. It is not surprising, therefore, that the patients in each school of analysis tend to produce the kind of memory material, symbols, dreams and fantasies which tend to confirm the frame of reference in which they are working. This is an aspect of psychoanalytic practice, I believe, which requires much additional study and research. A group of investigators with whom I am working at present is engaged in an intensive study of the nature of the therapeutic process, and one of the things which we are hoping for is that we will ultimately be able to extract and identify precisely those factors which are common to the therapeutic process in all of the various schools of psychoanalysis.

I am certain of only one thing. Ours is still a very young science. Only by preserving an attitude of genuine open-mindedness to new ideas, from whatever avenue they come, can we hope to make progress in it. We have much to learn, not only from one another, but from other areas also, areas such as field theory, communications theory, cybernetics and general systems theory, to mention a few of the most outstanding. Alfred North Whitehead (7) once wrote, "Nothing is more curious than the self-satisfied dogmatism with which mankind at each period of its history cherishes the delusion of the finality of its existing modes of knowledge." As long as the proponents of any psychoanalytic theory can remain free of that delusion, we shall continue to advance the frontiers of our knowledge.

REFERENCES

1. FREUD, A.: *The Ego and the Mechanisms of Defense* (1936). New York: International Universities Press, 1946.
2. FREUD, S.: *The Ego and the Id* (1923). London: Hogarth Press, 1927.
3. FREUD, S.: *The Problem of Anxiety* (1926). New York: Norton, 1936.
4. HARTMANN, H.: Ego Psychology and the Problem of Adaptation (1939). In: *Organization and Pathology of Thought,* ed. D. Rapaport. New York: Columbia University Press, 1951.
5. PIERS, G. & M.: Learning Theories and the Analytic Process. Presented at the Annual Meeting of the American Psychoanalytic Association, May, 1957.
6. REICH, W.: *Character-Analysis.* New York: Orgone Institute Press, 1945.
7. WHITEHEAD, A. N.: Collapse of Certitude. In: *The Dialogues of Alfred North Whitehead,* ed. L. Price. Boston: Little Brown, 1954.

14

PSYCHOANALYSIS AND PSYCHIATRIC
PRACTICE
(1961)

Psychoanalysis did not, as many people seem to think, spring full-blown and de novo out of Freud's head, like Athena out of Zeus's. Freud's earliest formulations were significantly rooted in the concepts and techniques of the psychiatric practice of his time, particularly those of hypnosis and suggestion. That psychoanalysis subsequently became alienated from the main body of psychiatry was in a sense an historical accident, deriving from the intense opposition and hostility which its theories initially aroused in official medical circles. The relative isolation of Freud and his small group of followers that ensued led to the formation of psychoanalytic societies, journals and training institutes, which for many years remained outside the mainstream of organized psychiatry.*

Over the past 50 years, however, the influence of psychoanalysis upon psychiatric thought, particularly in America, has steadily increased, so that it may now fairly be said that there is no field of American psychiatry today that has not been deeply influenced by the impact of psychoanalytic concepts. Psychoanalysts in America, from the time Freud delivered his famous introductory lectures at Clark University in 1909 down to the present, have affirmatively sought to disseminate its doctrines and expand its influence among

---

*A secondary outgrowth of this was Freud's welcoming of nonmedical allies into psychoanalysis and his defense of their right to treat psychiatric patients, a not insignificant historical factor in the challenges which have increasingly arisen in recent years to the medical profession's claim to exclusive prerogatives in the field of psychotherapy.

the psychiatric profession at large. The names of James Putnam, Ernest Jones, Abraham Brill, William Alanson White and Smith Ely Jelliffe stand out particularly as early pioneers in this effort.

Today almost all of the major medical schools in America accept psychoanalytically oriented psychodynamics as the basis of their psychiatric teaching both to medical students and to psychiatric residents. Indeed, in a number of medical schools postgraduate psychoanalytic institutes have already been established. There is an increasing trend in this direction, and it is not inconceivable that in another 25 years the independent psychoanalytic institutes will be outnumbered and perhaps even replaced by such university training centers. When one recalls Sigmund Freud's deep sense of personal frustration at being denied official recognition by the University of Vienna one can appreciate to what an extent psychoanalysis has completed a full circle in the rich academic acceptance that it now enjoys!

The psychiatric resident of 25 years ago generally worked in a state hospital and was exposed almost exclusively to diagnostic Kraepelinian psychiatry. If he wanted training in dynamic psychotherapy he had practically no alternative but to seek psychoanalytic training in the independent psychoanalytic institutes. In contrast, the average psychiatric resident of today gets a great deal of exposure, not only to the theories of psychoanalysis but also to the principles of psychoanalytic psychotherapy, from instructors, a large proportion of whom are psychoanalysts or psychoanalytically oriented psychiatrists. As a result, the young psychiatrist entering upon clinical practice today, after his residency, is much more psychodynamically sophisticated than were his predecessors 25 years ago (1).

The effect of this profound interaction of American psychoanalysts with other areas of clinical psychiatry has not been only in one direction, however. Just as psychoanalysis has importantly influenced the entire spectrum of clinical psychiatry, so it has itself been significantly affected by its closer contacts with other currents of thought. The result of all of this has been a blurring of the sharp line of demarcation which originally existed between psychoanalysis and other forms of clinical psychotherapy, and a wide borderland has developed in which it has become increasingly difficult to differentiate definitively between "true" psychoanalysis and "psychoanalytically oriented psychotherapy." So true has this become that efforts on the part of a special committee of the American Psychoanalytic Association, which was charged in 1948 with the task of clearly defining the differences between psychoanalysis and psychotherapy, resulted, after four years of study, in a frank admission that no agreement could be found for such a differentiation. As Robert Knight (2) has said, there is gradually evolving only one psychotherapy which "must rest on a basic science of dynamic psychotherapy."

If there is any fundamental dichotomy in the broad field of psychotherapy today it is not between "psychoanalysts" and "psychotherapists," but rather between those psychiatrists who are primarily psychologically oriented and those who are primarily physiologically oriented, though even in this respect there is considerable overlapping. Hollingshead and Redlich (3) have suggested the designation of A-P (analytic-psychological) and D-O (directive-organic) to these two groupings. They describe the A-P group as essentially non-directive in its psychotherapeutic approach and as utilizing a psychodynamic orientation. Among this group, the basic psychoanalytic concepts of unconscious mental activity, conflict, repression and transference are widely accepted and utilized. The D-O group, on the other hand, is described as biologically oriented, tends to be largely directive and authoritarian in its psychotherapeutic approach, and for the most part is outspokenly antagonistic to psychoanalytic teaching. Yet even this latter group is much more deeply influenced by psychoanalytic ideas than it realizes. Moriarity (4), who consciously deprecated psychoanalysis in a recent article, nevertheless described one aspect of his therapeutic work as "working through . . . emotionally charged matters of 'unfinished business,' " of making a "direct attack on resistances . . . with emphasis on broadening of the 'ego boundaries,' " and of "direct uncovering of unconscious needs and wishes, carried over from infancy and childhood." Indeed, many such psychiatrists, even in their utilization of biological techniques such as drug injections, CO_2 therapy, electrotherapy, and more recently, LSD therapy, often seek to justify their techniques with reasons derived from psychoanalytic theory, e.g., that their techniques assist in bringing repressed conflictual material into consciousness, or in aiding emotional abreactions, in facilitating regression and the development of transference reactions, etc.

What are some of the modifications in theory and technique which have been taking place in psychoanalysis and have been bringing it into closer integration with general psychotherapeutic practice? Perhaps the most fundamental shift in the emphasis of modern psychoanalysis began with Freud's revision of his theory of anxiety in 1926. The reformulation of the concept of anxiety as an ego-signal rather than as the consequence of repressed libido opened the door to the further development of psychoanalytic theory as an ego psychology* and diverted it from its previous almost exclusive preoccupation with the id. Wilhelm Reich's *Character-Analysis* in 1933, Anna Freud's *The Ego and the Mechanisms of Defense* in 1936, and Heinz Hartmann's *Ego Psychology and the Problem of Adaptation* in 1939 were important landmarks in this development.

With the shift in psychoanalysis from an id- to an ego-orientation, the path was cleared for other modifications in ego psychology. There was, in fact, an enormous fermentation of ideas in psychoanalysis in the thirties, which reflected this shift. An early leader in these changes was Sandor Rado, one of the pioneers in the early psychoanalytic movement, who, influenced by the classic work of Walter Cannon on bodily changes in pain, hunger, fear and rage, introduced into psychoanalysis concepts based on adaptational psychodynamics.

Around the same time, as a consequence of increasing interaction with sociologists and anthropologists, a number of other psychoanalysts began to emphasize the interrelationship between personality and culture. Leaders in this area, albeit with different approaches, were Karen Horney, Erich Fromm and Abram Kardiner. Within the same broad framework, Harry Stack Sullivan developed a theory of personality development with special emphasis on the central importance of interpersonal relationships. The field theory concept,

---

*Although Alfred Adler had anticipated many of the subsequent developments of ego psychology in his writings, his emphasis upon the fallacious concept of organ-inferiority, as well as his awkward style of communication, limited his early influence among psychiatrists. In recent decades the value of some of his contributions has been receiving increasing recognition.

developed by the eminent social psychologist, Kurt Lewin, also lent ideological support to the personality and culture group.

In still another area, the researches of psychoanalysts in psychosomatic medicine were greatly enriching the understanding of psychiatrists dealing with problems in this field. The names of Flanders Dunbar, Franz Alexander, Thomas French, Roy Grinker, Arthur Mirsky, Sidney Margolin, and George Engel are but a few of those who have been prominent in bringing psychoanalytic concepts to bear on the large realm of psychophysiological disorders. More recently, James Miller and his Institute for Behavioral Research at Ann Arbor, Michigan, and Roy Grinker in Chicago have been active in the attempt to integrate psychoanalytic theory with the significant contributions which have been made in other areas of behavioral science, notably the open-systems theory of von Bertalanfy, the information-communications theory of Shannon and Weaver, and the cybernetics of Norbert Wiener.

In recent years there has been a considerable revival of interest in the theory and practice of hypnotherapy, a revival in which psychoanalytic concepts such as suggestion, repression, resistance, regression, introjection, displacement, substitution and transference have played an important part. Among the psychoanalysts and psychoanalytically oriented psychiatrists who have made notable contributions in this area the names of Schilder, Wolberg, Kubie, Erickson, Gill, and Rosen come to mind.

There have been many other influences also which have contributed to modifications and broadening of psychoanalytic theory and practice. The research with infants and children of Margaret Ribble, Rene Spitz and David Levy; the animal experimentation of Jules Masserman, Howard Liddell, and others; the work on war neuroses of Kardiner, Grinker, Spiegel and others, and the widening interdisciplinary relationships with clinical psychologists, social workers, sociologists and anthropologists, have all left their own imprint on psychoanalytic thinking.

Meanwhile, psychoanalytic techniques have also been undergoing significant modifications which have been diminishing the gap that has hitherto existed between psychoanalysis and dynamically-oriented psychotherapy. Analysts have been coming more and more to the realization that their therapeutic techniques must be adapted to the needs of the patient. The modifications which have grown out of the application of psychoanalytic principles to the therapy of psychotics and of children have played a particularly important part in this awareness. Prominent among the changes which have been taking place has been a gradual lessening of emphasis on some of the more ritualistic aspects of psychoanalytic technique. As early as 1938 Frieda Fromm-Reichmann challenged the concept that a patient must lie on a couch for "true" psychoanalysis to take place. This dogma, which grew historically out of the fact that it was associated with the hypnotic techniques of Freud's time, also had a practical basis in the fact that it was subjectively very difficult in Freud's day to discuss freely sexual and other intimate topics face to face with another person. In mid-twentieth century America, however, largely, in fact, because of the liberating influence of Freud's revolutionary doctrines, it is much less embarrassing to do so. As to the hardship on the analyst to be looked at for eight hours daily, which Freud had commented on as an additional reason for this rule, Fromm-Reichmann pointed out that this inevitably followed from Freud's technical requirement that the analyst not react outwardly in any way to what the patient might say. If, however, the psychoanalyst permits himself to interact with the patient as a "participant observer" (to use Sullivan's phrase), being looked at becomes considerably less of a strain. In any event, the fact that the use of the couch may make the therapist feel more comfortable, does not necessarily mean that this technique is optimal for the patient. Fromm-Reichmann's challenge of this dogma, which grew out of her adaptation of psychoanalytic techniques to the therapy of schizophrenics, led to a more flexible understanding of the use of the couch as a technical tool. We have come to understand that the fundamental issue, after all, is how we can best facilitate the communicative process, both verbal and nonverbal, between patient and therapist. To the extent that the couch does accomplish this for many people it is indeed a valuable technical adjunct to therapy. For dependent compliant personalities, for example, who guide their every word by anxiously watching the expression on the analyst's face for approval or disapproval, the partial separation from the analyst offered by the couch is of unquestionable help. On the other hand, for the emotionally detached patient who tends to avoid intimate human relationships, the couch tends to facilitate further emotional withdrawal, and for such patients it may be of the utmost importance therapeutically to work in a more direct face-to-face manner.

Another technical dogma which has gradually been undergoing change is the rigid insistence on a five-times-a-week frequency of visits. One of the leaders in the trend toward modification of this rule has been Franz Alexander, who, with a number of his colleagues at the Chicago Institute for Psychoanalysis, began in the late thirties to experiment with altering the frequency of visits. What has become clearer over the years is that the five-times-a-week rule, which, like the use of the couch, grew historically out of the special circumstances of Freud's pattern of practice, need not necessarily be adhered to rigidly for the achievement of the goals of psychoanalytic therapy. The advantage of frequent visits is that they make it easier for both patient and therapist to maintain the thread of continuity between visits, and to work more intensively and in great detail with the day-to-day material of the patient. On the other hand, in some instances, daily visits may tend to intensify the dependency patterns of the patient and to cause his life to become too strongly centered upon the analysis, in a manner that is unfavorable to his therapeutic interests. A large proportion of American analysts now see many of their patients only three times a week, and there is a widespread tendency, even when they have begun with a higher frequency, to reduce the frequency as the patient makes progress. The fact that in addition many analysts see patients for "psychotherapy" once or twice a week has further served to obliterate the demarcation line between psychoanalysis and psychotherapy.

Perhaps the most important of the technical changes which have been taking place in psychoanalysis is the changing conception of the therapist's role. The original dictum that the analyst must be a shadowy, neutral, impersonal and value-free figure is coming to be recognized not only as a practical impossibility, but even as being, in some instances at least, of questionable therapeutic value. We are beginning to realize that in the transactional relationship between patient and therapist there is no such thing as a "neutral" position on the part of the therapist. The very effort to be neutral, passive, or impersonal constitutes an attitude which must *actively* affect the patient either positively or negatively. To some patients, silence and passivity on the part of the therapist may be perceived as a kind of comforting reassurance, absence of pressure and freedom from moral judgment, but to others the identical behavior may mean coldness, lack of empathy, or even critical rejection.

The corollary assumption that the psychoanalyst in his therapeutic role can be value-free, or can refrain from reflecting his values to the patient, is another traditional dictum of psychoanalytic theory which has been gradually undergoing modification. Psychoanalysts, like all psychotherapists, are inevitable purveyors to their patients of some of the fundamental mores and values of their time and milieu. What the analyst chooses or does not choose to comment upon, what he regards as healthy or neurotic, are all inextricably involved in value-judgment. The psychoanalytic goal of "genital love," for example, involves a particular kind of interpersonal and sexual relationship which is by no means universal, but reflects the values of Western culture. This is equally true of others of our basic concepts such as masculinity, femininity, emotional maturity, and "healthy aggression." This is not to deny that the psychoanalyst's approach to these concepts is often a broader and less rigid one than those of conventional society, and that this *relatively* more tolerant attitude has genuine therapeutic merit for the patient. It is, of course, in this fact that the kernel of truth in the classical dictum of the "non-evaluative" analyst lies.

What this all points to is an increasing recognition among psychoanalysts that the psychoanalytic process is a dynamic two-way interaction between the therapist and the patient—an interaction which Grinker and Spiegel, borrowing a term from Dewey and Bentley, have called the transactional process. In this process the therapist's personality, his value system, and his techniques of interaction, nonverbal as well as verbal, are being recognized as at least as important, and in many instances even more important, than the uncovering of repressed content which has been the cornerstone of the traditional model of the psychoanalytic process. The increasing awareness of this among psychoanalysts has been reflected in recent years in the growing literature on the subject of "countertrans-ference" attitudes in the analyst and their effect upon the analytic process.

In summary, then, psychoanalysis shows evidence with every passing year of increasing integration into the mainstream of Ameri-can psychiatry. In child psychiatry, in psychosomatic medicine, in the neuroses of war, in the psychotherapy of psychoses, in social casework, in group therapy, and in research and education, its theories and its techniques are being adapted and integrated to a point where the previously sharply delimited borders between psychoanalytic and psychiatric practice no longer exist. Although this development seems to be an inevitable one, and one that in the long run must benefit and broaden the purviews both of psychoanalysis and psychiatry, one must not overlook the fact that the early isolation of psychoanalysis was by no means without value. The detachment and the freedom from conventional ways of thinking in psychiatry which it entailed was of tremendous importance in the generation and fermentation of fresh and original ideas and insights into human behavior. That this isolation finally reached a point of diminishing returns should not cause us to forget our enormous indebtedness to the heroic pioneers of the psychoanalytic movement. Without their dedicated devotion to their unpopular ideas, and their willingness to withstand the abuse, the ridicule, the ostracism, and the economic privation which their nonconformity entailed, psychiatry would be immeasurably poorer today.

REFERENCES

1. The Psychiatrist—His Training and Development. Washington, D.C.: Ameri-can Psychiatric Association, 1953.
2. KNIGHT, R. P.: Bull., N.Y. Acad. Med., No. 25, 1949, p. 101.
3. HOLLINGSHEAD, A. B., and REDLICH, F. C.: Social Class and Mental Illness. New York: John Wiley and Sons, Inc. 1958.
4. MORIARITY, J. D.: J. Neuropsychiat. 1:116, 1959.

15

PSYCHOANALYTIC THERAPY AS AN EDUCATIONAL PROCESS

Common Denominators in the Therapeutic Approaches of

Different Psychoanalytic "Schools"

(1962)

Thus psychoanalytic treatment acts as a second education of the adult, as a correction to his education as a child.

> Sigmund Freud: "Psychoanalysis,"
> Encyclopaedia Britannica (14th ed.)

It was little more than sixty-five years ago that the genius of Sigmund Freud gave birth to the theory of personality and the system of psychological therapy that now goes by the name of psychoanalysis. The remarkable saga of the survival and expanding influence of his ideas in spite of the resistance which they first encountered is now a matter of history.

Within the psychoanalytic movement itself, however, significant rifts have developed which even today are sources of intense polemic among their respective adherents. The initial defection of Alfred Adler in 1911 was followed a year later by that of Carl Jung. Some thirteen years later Otto Rank went his own way, embittered by the hostile reception which the publication of his *Trauma of Birth* had encountered from Freud's followers. Less than a decade later, in the early thirties, the rise of ego psychology initiated a rich fermentation of new ideas which terminated in a number of disputes and splits within the psychoanalytic movement from which it is still reverberating. Some of the theorists in the forefront of this ideological ferment were Sullivan, Horney, Fromm, Kardiner, and Rado. Followers of the former three ultimately set up separate schools of psychoanalysis outside of the American Psychoanalytic Association, while the latter two initiated the formation of the first so-called "Neo-Freudian" institute within the framework of the American Psychoanalytic Association.

It is not the intention of this paper to examine the various theories espoused by these different schools of thought or to compare their merits. This has been done by others at great length (17, 18, 23). I wish, however, to emphasize a conviction advanced by Ernest Jones in his valedictory address to the British Psychoanalytic Society in 1946 (12). In commenting upon the fact that in the early history of psychoanalysis there had been a strong tendency to insist on a high degree of conformity both in theory and practice among all who professed themselves to be psychoanalysts, Jones stated:

> The impossibility of this ideal is being recognized and it is being replaced by the more practicable, though difficult enough, endeavor to distinguish between what constitute the essential characteristics of psychoanalysis and what are super-imposed and more varying features. Here we cannot do better than follow Freud's own definition. Psychoanalysis is simply the study of mental processes of which we are unaware, of what for the sake of brevity we call the unconscious. The psychoanalytic method of carrying out this study is that characterized by the free association technique of analyzing the observable phenomena of transference and resistance. As Freud himself said, anyone following this path is practicing psychoanalysis even if he comes to conclusions different from Freud's . . . and it is plain that we should be forsaking the sphere of science for that of theology were we to regard these conclusions . . . as being sacrosanct and eternal.

In the light of this statement I would affirm that the various schools of thought to which I have made reference are all practicing psychoanalysis despite their theoretical differences. What I hope to demonstrate in this paper is that in spite of these *theoretical* differences the *therapeutic* approaches of these psychoanalytic schools have certain basic factors in common which, so far as therapy is concerned, *are more significant than their theoretical differences.*

My initial premise is that all of the major psychoanalytic schools have essentially similar therapeutic objectives, although they may attach different names to these objectives. Whether they are subsumed under the concept of "genitality" as in libido theory; or under "active creative will" as in Rankian theory; or under the concept of "social interest" as in Adlerian theory; or in terms of "full development of the self" as in Jungian theory; or in the "integrated self" of Sullivan; or the "self realization" of Horney; or the "productive personality" of Fromm—all are concerned with basically similar goals of helping the neurotic individual to achieve greater emotional maturity, to love unselfishly, to have meaningful and satisfying sexual relationships, to work effectively, and to be a socially responsible and productive human being within the limits of his capacity. In other words, although there is disagreement about the sources of neurosis and about how to conceptualize personality development, there is fundamental agreement about what constitutes mental health. These therapeutic goals, incidentally, are not unique to psychoanalysis. Insofar as they represent a normative ideal which is widespread in our culture, they are common to many other educational, therapeutic, or spiritual orientations. What is unique to psychoanalysis is not its goals but its *method* of bringing unconscious mental processes into the awareness of the patient, and its deliberate utilization of the subtleties of the interpersonal relationship between the analyst and the patient as a means of bringing about a therapeutic result.

My second premise is that mature and experienced therapists in all of these varying psychoanalytic schools of thought, by and large, achieve comparable therapeutic results with their patients. Although reliable statistical results are admittedly unavailable on this point, I know of no evidence to the contrary. In twenty-five years of psychiatric and psychoanalytic practice, I have had the good fortune to work closely over long periods of time with a good many psychoanalysts of diverse theoretical orientations—classical Freudians, Neo-Freudians, Horneyites, and Fromm-Sullivanians, as well as some who defied any classifications but borrowed what they considered useful from all groups. My experience strongly confirms the findings of Fiedler (4) and Heine (11) that favorable therapeutic results are less dependent upon the theoretical inclination of the analyst than they are upon his personal characteristics, experience and empathic capacity. As Fiedler has pointed out, the more expert therapists from different schools of thought are more apt to agree with each other as to what constitute optimal therapeutic relationships than they are to agree with less experienced therapists within their own schools. Apparently a capable therapist would be a capable one within any of these theoretical frameworks, and a poor therapist would be a poor one regardless of his theoretical point of view.

But how is this possible? How can therapeutic approaches based on radically divergent theories be equally efficacious for the patient? To answer this question it is necessary to examine the crucial problem of the nature of the psychoanalytic therapeutic process.

In general, there have been two principal viewpoints about this. The first of these has assumed that the analytic process depends fundamentally upon giving the patient correct insight into the nature of his unconscious conflicts. If the proper interpretations, properly timed, are made, presumably the patient's "insight" gradually or suddenly increases and, ipso facto, he becomes healthier. As Freud eloquently stated: "In the early days of analytic technique . . . we regarded the matter intellectually and set a high value on the patient's knowledge of . . . the forgotten traumas of childhood . . . in the certain expectation of bringing the neurosis and the treatment to a rapid end by this means" (6). Later, Freud placed major emphasis on the insights involved in the "working through" of the patient's resistances, stating that this was "the part of the work that effects the greatest changes in the patient and that distinguishes analytic treatment from every kind of suggestive treatment" (7).

But what is insight? To a Freudian it means one thing, to a Jungian another, and to a Rankian, a Horneyite, an Adlerian or a Sullivanian, still another. Each school gives its own particular brand of insight. Whose are the correct insights? The fact is that patients treated by analysts of all these schools may not only respond favorably, but also believe strongly in the insights which they have been given. Even admittedly "inexact" interpretations have been noted to be of therapeutic value (9)! Moreover, the problem is even more complicated than this; for, depending upon the point of view of the analyst, the patients of each school seem to bring up precisely the kind of phenomenological data which confirm the theories and interpretations of their analysts! Thus each theory tends to be self-validating. Freudians elicit material about the Oedipus complex and castration anxiety, Adlerians about masculine strivings and feelings of inferiority, Horneyites about idealized images, Sullivanians about disturbed interpersonal relationships, etc. The fact is that in so complex a transaction as the psychoanalytic therapeutic process, the impact of patient and therapist upon each other, and particularly of the latter upon the former, is an unusually profound one. What the analyst shows interest in, the kinds of questions he asks, the kind of data he chooses to react to or to ignore, and the interpretations he makes, all exert a subtle but significant suggestive impact upon the patient to bring forth certain kinds of data in preference to others. I shall elaborate upon this important point a little later. Just now, I should like to suggest that *what we call insight is essentially the conceptual framework by means of which a therapist establishes, or attempts to establish, a logical relationship between events, feelings, or experiences that seem unrelated in the mind of the patient.* In terms of the analyst's objectives, insights constitute the *rationale* by which the patient is persuaded to accept the model of more "mature" or "healthy" behavior which analysts of all schools, *implicitly* or *explicitly,* hold out to him. Now, since interpretations that put the patient's material within one frame of reference seem to be just as effective for the patient as interpretations that put it within another frame of reference, it is logical to conclude that the specific insight given *cannot* be the only or exclusive basis for the therapeutic reaction.

The second major theory about the therapeutic process, in contrast to the rationalistic emphasis upon insight, has stressed the importance of liberating repressed emotions and/or repressed traumatic memories. This has led to emphasis on techniques designed to facilitate either emotional abreaction or the release of repressed memories, on the assumption that such abreaction is productive of therapeutic effects. Unfortunately, with the possible exception of certain traumatic hysterias, where such abreaction may cause the disappearance of the traumatic *symptom,* this assumption simply is not borne out by clinical experience. The dramatic evocation of anger or tears or a repressed memory in a patient may, it is true, leave him feeling transitorily calmer, or more relaxed, but I have never seen it, in and of itself, produce the lasting personality changes which are the therapeutic objectives of the psychoanalytic process. Moreover, as Alexander demonstrated as long ago as 1930 (2), the recovery of repressed memories is often the *result* of therapeutic progress rather than its cause.

I would like to suggest that the truth about the nature of the therapeutic process lies somewhere in between the rationalistic overemphasis upon the acquisition of insight and the emotionalistic overemphasis upon abreaction, and that the process of achieving the characterological growth and emotional maturation which are the goals of psychoanalytic therapy is essentially a learning process. This is by no means a new idea, but it has not had wide acceptance among psychoanalysts. Freud himself seemed to recognize it when he wrote in the *Encyclopaedia Britannica* that "psychoanalytic treatment acts as a second education of the adult, as a correction to his education as a child," but in later writings he argued against the analyst's being an educator, stating: "However much the analyst may be tempted to act as a teacher, model, and ideal to other people . . . this is not his task in the analytic relationship . . ." (8) Psychologists, however, have for some time suspected that psychotherapy in general, as well as psychoanalysis in particular, involved a learning process. Notably Shoben in 1949 (20) and more recently Strupp (22) have made valuable contributions to this conception.

My own conviction is that whether or not the analyst is *consciously* "tempted to act as a teacher, model, and ideal" to his patients, he *inevitably* does so to a greater or lesser extent; and this is a central aspect of the psychoanalytic process. In one of his last writings, Freud himself advanced the idea that the analyst becomes a "new superego" who "corrects blunders" made by the patient's parents (8). Strachey in 1934, writing on the nature of the therapeutic action in psychoanalysis, stated the matter even more explicitly:

> The principal effective alteration consists in a profound qualitative modification of the patient's superego . . . This modification . . . is brought about in a series of innumerable small steps by the agency of mutative interpretations, which are effected by the analyst in virtue of his position as object of the patient's id impulses and as auxiliary superego. The dosed introjection

of good objects is regarded as one of the most important factors in the therapeutic process. (21)

The fact that the analyst generally does not explicitly hold himself forth as a model for his patient does not negate the fact that in the presence of a positive transference he invariably tends to become a model which the patient consciously or unconsciously attempts to emulate (i.e., "introjects"). As the therapist's implicit values and behavioral characteristics are gradually communicated, overtly or subtly, to the patient, they become part of a learning process in which the patient is involved. The process of identification with the analyst, which has often been described, is an aspect of this learning process. This too is not unique to psychoanalysis. Identification with a loved or admired person is one of the earliest and most basic techniques of learning in human beings. Walking, talking and many of our most characteristic mannerisms are acquired chiefly by this route.

It is probable that relatively few psychoanalysts today, of any school, would still insist that the analyst is or must be a "mirror-like" figure who does not interact with the patient but merely reflects the latter's own feelings and thoughts back to him. It has become increasingly clear that such "neutrality" is actually a fiction; that in the transactional relationship that exists between patient and therapist, the very effort to be impersonal or "neutral" is an *active* attitude which must affect the patient either positively or negatively, depending on his needs. Thus, Mandler and Kaplan (16) have demonstrated in an interesting experimental study that the same "mm-hmm" on the part of a therapist may be interpreted as approval by some patients and disapproval by others, thus influencing some positively, others negatively. By the same token, the myth that the psychoanalyst is free from moral values in his relationship to the patient seems also finally to be disappearing. Although psychoanalysts as a group are undoubtedly less conventional in their value-systems than society at large, there can be little doubt that our psychoanalytic concepts of mature love, emotional maturity, masculinity, femininity, "healthy" aggression, etc., are not universals, but generally reflect certain of the outstanding values of contemporary Western culture. These become inevitably communicated to our patients in what we choose or do not choose to interpret, in the kinds of questions we ask, in what we implicitly approve of as "healthy" or focus upon as "unhealthy" and even in our nonverbal mannerisms.* In face-to-face transactions the expression on the therapist's face, a questioning glance, a lift of the eyebrows, a barely perceptible shake of the head or shrug of the shoulder all act as significant cues to the patient. But even *behind* the couch, our "uh-huhs" as well as our silences, the interest or the disinterest reflected in our tone of voice or our shifting postures all act like subtle radio signals influencing the patient's responses, reinforcing some responses and discouraging others. That this influence actually occurs has been confirmed experimentally by numerous observers (14, 19). Krasner (15) has recently prepared a comprehensive and impressive review of the evidence in this area.

An important contributory factor which heightens the patient's responsiveness to the analyst's implicit attitudes, of course, is the tendency towards the development of a positive transference reaction. This is a point which Frank (5) has emphasized in terms of the patient's faith and expectancy. The analyst's social role as a person who is endowed by the help-seeking patient with knowledge, prestige, authority, and help-giving potential, as well as the therapist's own confidence in his method and his ability to help the patient, are potent factors in the development of such transference reactions, but one should not ignore the real attributes of the analyst either. To the extent that the analyst is a person of intelligence, objectivity, integrity, empathy, and humanistic values, the patient's tendency towards a positive transference is further facilitated. Thus the patient begins to seek the analyst's love and acceptance; and the analyst's attitudes of approval or disapproval, in whatever way they manifest themselves—through questions, confrontations, interpretations, or

---

*In the four-year study of the therapeutic process which Dr. Franz Alexander and co-workers (this author included) have been conducting at the Mount Sinai Hospital, Los Angeles, under a grant from the Ford Foundation, we have been particularly impressed by the significance of the nonverbal communication which goes on between therapist and patient.

through the myriads of subtle nonverbal cues—thus come to function as a kind of reward-punishment system to the patient.

What part does insight play in all of this? Insight in the therapeutic process might be roughly compared to the understanding which a golf pro or a tennis pro gives his pupil when he tells him what is wrong with his swing as well as what is right with it.* It is an important factor in the pupil's being able to improve, but in itself does not *make* the pupil improve. Before this can take place, countless hours of practice must intervene. The tendency of the student is almost always to fall back upon the old, habitual, faulty patterns. This is analogous to the "resistance" of the psychoanalytic patient. It requires repeated "interventions" on the part of the pro, confronting the pupil with his "resistances." *All of this, however, should occur in a climate of empathic emotional support and mutual confidence if the pupil is to persist in the difficult learning process despite frequent feelings of discouragement and resistance.*** This is particularly true if the pupil, like the neurotic patient, has little self-confidence. It is for analogous reasons that the psychoanalytic process, like any difficult learning procedure, of necessity takes considerable time. The acquisition of insight is only a small part of the process. The "working through" process is what takes by far the longer time. Insight consists, in effect, of saying to the patient, "Look what you are doing"; working through consists of countless repetitions of "There you go again!" Ultimately the patient is able to anticipate the awareness himself: "There *I* go again"; and finally to short-circuit the old, habitual faulty reactions into the more constructive, more effective, and more mature patterns of adaptation, which are *implicitly* or *explicitly* being held up to him by the therapist. The basic

---

*Parenthetically, anyone who has taken such lessons will realize that golf and tennis pros, no less than psychoanalysts, belong to different "schools," and that the "insights" which are given to the pupil may vary considerably from school to school.

**On the other hand, one must recognize that there are pupils who, for reasons inherent in their personality structure, may respond more favorably to overt or covert disapproval. These would be analogous to patients who respond therapeutically to a frustrating or nongratifying kind of relationship with the therapist, as is implied in the classical psychoanalytic doctor-patient model.

significance of making what is unconscious conscious lies not in any magical change which is spontaneously forthcoming as a result, but in the fact that only by becoming aware of what is disturbing his functioning does it become possible for the patient to bring it under the conscious integrative control of his ego.

I realize, of course, that all that goes on in the analytic process is by no means as logical, rational, or intellectual as the above paragraph might imply. The subtle interplay of transference and countertransference reactions, and particularly the very important role which transference-interpretations and dream-interpretations play in psychoanalytic procedures are unique aspects of the psychoanalytic educational process which are not present, at least to the same degree, in other learning experiences. Nor is all learning in psychotherapy as gradual or trial-and-errorish as my crude golfing analogy might suggest. One must also include in this model the more sudden "flashes" of "insight" and more rapid changes of behavior which often occur in the analytic process. Such sudden "insights" and changes, however, are in my opinion simply varieties of "gestalt" learning, and do not invalidate the basic learning model which I have been describing as the essence of the psychoanalytic therapeutic process.

It may be asked at this point whether defining psychoanalysis as an educational process tends to minimize the importance of the interpersonal relationship between the analyst and patient as one of the fundamental ingredients of the analytic therapeutic process. My reply to this would be strongly in the negative. There is nothing mystical about the interpersonal relationship. It is the fundamental matrix in which the educational process takes place, and the quality of this relationship, like that of any teacher to his pupil, is of prime importance either in facilitating or hindering the patient's learning. For such learning to take place optimally, or in some cases, even at all, a favorable emotional climate between the patient and therapist is essential. This involves not only a basic confidence and trust in the analyst, but also a feeling on the part of the patient that the analyst understands him, is genuinely interested in his welfare, and believes in his fundamental worth as a human being. However, the way in which the analyst interacts with the patient is not only a matrix. It is also a basic part of the patient's learning experience. Since the perceptual and affective distortions which are involved in the patient's neurotic difficulties have largely grown out of disturbed interpersonal relationships with significant persons in his past, it is usually important that the patient experience a "corrective" relationship (1) with the analyst. This need not, however, involve any artificial or feigned "role-playing" on the part of the analyst. Rather, to the extent that the analyst in his professional role is consistently encouraging and empathic, yet firm and objective, he *inevitably* presents a corrective emotional relationship to the patient in contrast to the ones the patient has experienced with the significant figures in his past. The effect of this is to facilitate teaching the patient in a here-and-now situation that his previously learned attitudes and expectations in relation to authority figures are erroneous.

A more fundamental question now suggests itself. Does not this conception of the psychoanalytic process imply that the patient is being guided or pressed into a mold of the analyst's making, with no opportunity for free or spontaneous growth or choice on his part? I do not think so. While it is true that the analyst sets a goal of more mature behavior, we must not forget that this is, more often than not, the patient's conscious goal also. But more importantly, to the extent that good analytic therapy is nonauthoritarian, as it should be, it implies a respect for the patient's right to seek his own paths to the achievement of such maturity. Moreover, the concept of the dissolution of the transference carries with it the implicit assumption that one of the basic goals of analytic therapy is the enabling of the patient to achieve autonomy and self-determination, and to free him of childhood dependencies on and overevaluations of all authority figures *including* the analyst.

At this point it may be appropriate to ask whether the concept of psychotherapy as an educational process applies to nonpsychoanalytic types of psychotherapy also. I believe it does. In nondirective therapy of the Rogerian type, the values and goals of the therapist are also conveyed to the patient, but almost entirely implicitly. Despite the fact that the Rogerian therapist makes few or no actual interpretations, he, too, by the kinds of material he chooses to reflect back to the patient as contrasted to those which he does not choose to reflect, by the tone of his voice, and by the quality of his personality, communicates his implicit therapeutic objectives, presents himself to the patient as a model for identification, and influences the patient's productions. I believe, in short, that the assumption that the Rogerian therapeutic relationship enables the patient to spontaneously cure himself tends to overlook the subtle transactional processes that are going on even in this technique. Nevertheless it is true that psychoanalysts in general have paid insufficient attention to the circumstances and types of disorders in which self-correcting mechanisms in the patient may be expected to play an important role in the therapeutic interaction. That such mechanisms exist can hardly be denied. Cures and significant alterations of personality do not occur only in the offices of psychiatrists. In psychoanalysis, however, in contrast to counseling, therapists are generally dealing with the more severe types of neurotic disorders, in which self-correcting mechanisms are less operative. In the more directive psychotherapies an educational process is also taking place, of course, but there is an important difference in their underlying philosophy of education as compared to that of the nondirective approaches. As Klein has suggested, the differences between directive and nondirective therapists are comparable to those between progressive and traditional teachers. The nondirective therapist, like the progressive teacher,

> permits the student to set his own goals, encourages independent and spontaneous expression, shows respect for the pupil's worth and promise, prefers a democratic to an authoritarian learning atmosphere, and abhors techniques of domination and coercion. (13)

This philosophical difference is of fundamental importance in the outcome of therapy. If the goal of the therapy is emotional maturity, this implies the capacity for autonomy and self-determination. Directive psychotherapy which perpetuates the interpersonal climate of an authoritarian parent-child relationship, by its very nature makes the achievement of such a goal for the patient more difficult.

In summary, then, I have advanced the thesis that in successful psychoanalytic therapy, in all psychoanalytic schools, what actually goes on is a unique kind of educational process in which the analyst employs his particular theoretical frame of reference as a rational basis for explaining the patient's past and present difficulties and, by nonverbal as well as verbal cues, uses the instrument of a warm, empathic and meaningful human relationship as a means of helping the patient to persist in the difficult task of combatting his anxieties, overcoming his resistances and learning more mature patterns of adaptation. Such differences in technique as may exist—e.g., with regard to frequency of visit or use of the couch—are, I believe, of secondary importance in comparison to the above described common denominators. It may be argued that these technical differences are important in that they either help or hinder the learning process—and this is undoubtedly true—but if agreement can be reached on the essential nature of the therapeutic process, I believe that these other differences can be resolved. I suspect that ultimately the question that will be asked will not be—is it better for the patient to come three times a week or five times a week, or is it better to have the patient use the couch or sit up—but rather—*under what circumstances and with what kinds of patients* is this or that technical device preferable.

One final question remains to be discussed. If the assumption is correct that different theoretical frames of reference may be equally efficacious as a basis for psychoanalytic therapy, does it follow that the basic truth or error of a theory is of no practical consequence? In order to answer this question it is necessary to examine the problem of what constitutes "scientific truth."

Even in more exact areas, such as physics and chemistry, scientists do not assume that they are dealing with ultimate truth. Science is concerned with the amassing, testing, coordinating and systematizing of data. A scientific hypothesis is considered better or "truer" than another to the extent that it fulfills three criteria more effectively than the other. These criteria are:

1. Does it explain all the available data with the least degree of complexity? This is the so-called "rule of parsimony."
2. To what extent does it lend itself to experimentation and validation? What, in other words, is its heuristic value?
3. To what extent does it make it possible to predict future events? What, in short, is its predictive value?

Only that theory which meets all of these criteria most satisfactorily can truly lay claim to being the most "correct" one scientifically.

The theory of predestination, for example, is an extremely simple one which explains all human behavior quite logically and consistently. However, since it does not lend itself to testing or validation, and has no predictive value whatever, it is outside the realm of what is considered scientific. When, however, current psychoanalytic theories are compared with one another, such a clear-cut differentiation is not always possible. All of them represent honest efforts to systematize in a scientific way the known data about human behavior. None of them is strikingly more simple than the others, all of them lend themselves to some degree of testing and validation, and none of them is dramatically superior to all of the others in predictive capacity—largely because our ability to predict individual human behavior is still at a relatively crude and primitive level as compared with the predictive capacity of the physical sciences.

This should not be taken as implying that all the current theories in psychoanalysis are equally "true." It does mean, however, that the relative merits of any scientific theory cannot be proved in abstract debate but only by vigorous and meticulous experimentation and research. Clearly the challenge that faces us all is to find a theoretical framework, a "unified theory of human behavior" (10) which will not only synthesize and integrate those "truths" which are inherent in the various current psychoanalytic schools of thought, but will also lend itself more effectively to objective validation and research. To accomplish this, it may well be that psychoanalysts of all schools will ultimately have to find a common frame of reference by bringing their theories into accordance with basic concepts of adaptation and with theories of learning. This communication represents an effort to do this with regard to the nature of the therapeutic process.

REFERENCES

1. ALEXANDER, F.: The principle of corrective emotional experience. In: Psychoanalytic Therapy. New York, Ronald Press, 1946, pp. 66–70.
2. _____: Ibid., p. 20.
3. BANDURA, A.: Psychotherapy as a learning process. Psych. Bull. 58:143–159, 1961.
4. FIEDLER, F. E.: A comparison of therapeutic relationships in psychoanalytic, nondirective and Adlerian therapy. J. Consult. Psychol. 14:436–445, 1950.
5. FRANK, J. D.: The dynamics of the psychotherapeutic relationship. Psychiatry 22:17–39, 1959.

6. FREUD, S.: Further recommendations in the technique of psychoanalysis. In his: Collected Papers. London, Hogarth Press, 2:342–365, 1933.
7. _____: *Ibid.*, pp. 366–376.
8. _____: An Outline of Psychoanalysis, New York, Norton, 1949, p. 67.
9. GLOVER, E.: The therapeutic effect of inexact interpretation. Internat. J. Psychoanal. *12*:397–411, 1931.
10. GRINKER, R. R., ED.: Toward a Unified Theory of Human Behavior. New York, Basic Books, Inc., 1956.
11. HEINE, R. W.: A comparison of patients' reports on psychotherapeutic experience with psychoanalytic, nondirective and Adlerian therapists. Am. J. Psychother. *7*:16–23, 1953.
12. JONES, E.: A valedictory address. Internat. J. Psychoanal. *27*:7–12, 1946.
13. KLEIN, D. B.: Abnormal Psychology. New York, Henry Holt & Co., 1951, p. 521.
14. KRASNER, L.: Studies of the Conditioning of Verbal Behavior, Psychol. Bull. *55*:148–170, 1958.
15. _____: The therapist as a social reinforcement machine. *Paper presented at* Second Conference on Research in Psychotherapy. University of North Carolina, Chapel Hill, May 17–20, 1961.
16. MANDLER, G., AND KAPLAN, W. K.: Subjective evaluation and reinforcing effect of a verbal stimulus. Science *124*:582–583, 1956.
17. MULLAHY, P.: Oedipus Myth and Complex. New York, Hermitage Press, 1948.
18. MUNROE, R. L.: Schools of Psychoanalytic Thought. New York, The Dryden Press, 1955.
19. SALZINGER, K.: Experimental manipulation of verbal behavior: a review. J. Gen. Psychol. *61*:65–94, 1959.
20. SHOBEN, E. J., JR.: Psychotherapy as a problem in learning theory. Psychol. Bull. *46*:366–392, 1949.
21. STRACHEY, J.: The nature of the therapeutic action of psychoanalysis. Internat. J. Psychoanal. *15*:127–159, 1934.
22. STRUPP, H. H.: Toward an analysis of the therapist's contribution to the treatment process. Psychiatry *22*:349–362, 1959.
23. THOMPSON, C.: Psychoanalysis: Evolution and Development. New York, Hermitage House, 1950.

16

PSYCHOANALYTIC THERAPY AND
THEORIES OF LEARNING
(1964)

In a previous communication (14) I advanced the suggestion that psychoanalytic therapy is a learning procedure and that its underlying modus operandi is essentially the same in the various "schools" of psychoanalysis despite their ideological differences. Now I wish to look more closely at some contributions of learning theory which have relevance to psychoanalytic therapy, and to consider more thoroughly some of the inherent problems.

Learning has been defined by Hilgard (8) as "the process by which an activity originates or is changed through reacting to an encountered situation, provided that the characteristics of the change in activity cannot be explained on the basis of native response tendencies, maturation, or temporary (physiological) states of the organism." It should be noted that in human beings such a definition encompasses all behavior which cannot be attributed to the exclusive effects of biological drives (i.e., instincts), growth and maturation, or transitory states caused by drugs, fatigue, infections, etc. Clearly, all neurotic and deviant behavior which is not entirely physiologically determined falls within the scope of this definition; it is "learned" through experiential vicissitudes with parents, siblings, peers, and all of the other people, objects and relationships which are encountered by an individual in the course of his development. Together these constitute the infinite variety of unconditioned and conditioned stimuli which subtly shape his adaptive responses from the moment of birth on.

Over the past half-century an enormous body of experimental

work has accumulated, representing the efforts of behavior scientists to elucidate the nature of this learning process, and although there are at least as many schools of learning theory as there are of psychoanalysis, certain basic points of agreement have gradually emerged which ought not to be disregarded in our efforts to refine the core of our own psychoanalytic theories and practices.

As Hilgard (9) points out, learning theories fall into two major families: *stimulus-response* theories—represented by those of Thorndike, Guthrie, Skinner and Hull—and *cognitive* theories—exemplified by those of Tolman, Kurt Lewin, and the gestalt psychologists. The former tend to regard most learned behavior as a process of gradual accretion acquired through conditioning and trial-and-error sequences in which responses are reinforced by reward or success, or inhibited by punishment or failure. The cognitive group, on the other hand, tends to emphasize the greater importance in learning of more rapid perceptual "insights" or understanding.

The eclectic learning theorist recognizes that both types of learning take place in life. Trial-and-error learning is more apt to take place when the essence of the adaptive problem is beyond the immediate cognitive grasp of the learner and where imitation is not possible; even here, however, one has to make a distinction between random fumbling and an intelligent search for solutions. On the other hand, where cognitive solutions are possible, human beings tend to learn by insight and, in social situations, to a considerable extent by imitation (17). Freud's concept of the reality-principle clearly refers to patterns of thought and behavior which are learned partly through cognitive insights and partly through trial-and-error—all influenced by experienced rewards and punishments.

With regard to personality development in general, early psychoanalytic theory tended to emphasize "libidinal" pleasure-strivings and *defenses* against anxiety as the primary shaping forces. It has been only in the past 25 years that more adequate recognition has been given in psychoanalytic theory to the "nonlibidinal," "nondefensive," *adaptive* and maturational strivings of the organism, as well as to indirect effects of the social and cultural environment. Over the same quarter-century, psychologists too, particularly Skinner and Hull, have laid increasing stress upon "reinforcing" stimuli in the environment, and particularly upon positive or rewarding reinforcers, as primary motivating factors in the acquisition of new behavior patterns.

In general it can be said that psychoanalytic theory has tended to focus more strongly on the *internal* motivational aspects of personality development, while learning theories have tended to focus their attention more strongly on the nature of the *external* conditions which facilitated or retarded the acquisition of new behavioral patterns. In this respect the effect of each has been to enhance and deepen the understanding of the total learning situation in humans.

The fundamental problem with which we are faced in psychoanalytic therapy is that of how we can enable or cause the patient to give up certain acquired patterns of thought, feeling, or behavior in favor of others which are considered more "mature," "adaptive," "productive" or "self-realizing." The learning theorist, if he is a member of the stimulus-response school, structures this as an effort to teach the patient new habit patterns; or, if he belongs to the cognitive school, as an effort to teach the patient new patterns of perception and new cognitive "insights."

Psychoanalytic theories have generally favored the latter conception as the essential model for what happens in therapy. In his earlier papers, Freud assumed that the insights involved were related to repressed memories of childhood traumata (6) and that the mere recovery of these memories would ipso facto result in altered patterns of behavior very rapidly. Subsequently (7), Freud modified these expectations and placed emphasis instead upon the more arduous and prolonged task of the "working through" of the patient's "resistances."

It is clear that an important difference between the analytic situation and any de novo learning situation is that in the treatment of personality disorders the task is complicated by the fact that the previously learned behavior—the neurotic pattern—is particularly resistant to change. Learning theorists have suggested various reasons for this "resistance" that differ from the usual psychoanalytic explanation of repression. One of the major explanations offered is that the neurotic behavioral pattern had adaptive value originally or still does. On the basis of the original adaptive value, it is thought that the neurotic habit-patterns tended to become "overlearned," as a result of which they have become more resistant to extinction.

In terms of their current adaptive value the learning theorist suggests that there are conflicting environmental stimuli in which the pain or discomfort of some aspects of the neurotic behavior is constantly being offset by the positive reinforcement of its benefits to the patient. This corresponds to what analysts call the "secondary gain" of the neurosis.

In any event, there is little doubt that the problem of overcoming the resistance to change in the neurotic patient—in whatever conceptual framework this resistance is seen—remains the basic challenge of the psychoanalytic and psychotherapeutic process. Let us consider the contributions of learning theories to two major aspects of this problem: (1) the role of cognitive insights; (2) the role of the patient-therapist interaction.

In the aforementioned communication, I suggested (14) that since the insight given by therapists from differing psychoanalytic schools differed in content and yet their patients were all capable of showing favorable therapeutic responses, the specific insight given could not logically be the only or exclusive basis for the therapeutic response. I would like, however, to elaborate upon this problem.

A rather important distinction needs to be made first, it seems to me, between the "insight" *given* by the analyst and the "insight" which is *perceived* by the patient. I have suggested that insight, as given by a therapist, "is essentially the conceptual framework by means of which a therapist establishes, or attempts to establish, a logical relationship between events, feelings, or experiences that seem unrelated in the mind of the patient," and that "in terms of the analyst's objectives, insights constitute the *rationale* by which the patient is persuaded to accept the model of more 'mature' or 'healthy' behavior which analysts of all schools, implicitly or explicitly, hold out to him" (14). In looking back upon this formulation, however, it occurs to me that it is subject to the misinterpretation that insights given by analysts of different schools may be capriciously different, and that they do not necessarily have any relationship to the actual realities of the patient's life and behavior. Such an interpretation would be misleading. *The insights given by psychoanalysts of different schools all bear a definite relationship to clinical reality* and all fit the observable facts reasonably well, although the proponents of each theory, of course, believe theirs to be the most valid and fruitful way of organizing these facts.

Consider a specific clinical example. A young man, descriptively, is passively dependent in his interpersonal relationships. A Freudian might organize the observable data of the patient's life around the fact that he was either excessively indulged or excessively frustrated in the early years of childhood, that he is consequently fixated at an "oral-receptive" level of libidinal development, with an unresolved Oedipus complex, etc. An Adlerian might organize the same data around the patient's having developed expectations of being taken care of, with a consequent "life-style" of passivity and helplessness as a way of achieving this objective. A member of the Horney school might interpret the same material in terms of a neurotic need for affection and a basic pattern of "moving towards" people. A Rankian might derive his interpretations from the basic problem of separation-anxiety and defenses against it. A Jungian might bring in the concept of the archetypal Mother and the patient's deep strivings for reunion with her. A follower of Erich Fromm might think in terms of "receptive-orientation," "symbiotic relationships," and "non-productivity," in dealing with the same data. A Sullivanian might theorize in terms of "oral-dynamisms" and emphasize the patient's "interpersonal relationships" in his interpretations; while a student of Rado might speak of "emergency controls" and "adaptational mechanisms." *The critical point, however, is that fundamentally they are all dealing with the same data, and that there is a central core of common reality underlying all of these "insights"*—they all refer to observed or inferred patterns of passivity, dependency, and immaturity in the patient, and the implicit or explicit message which is inherent in the various interpretations is essentially the same— namely, that the patient's behavior ought to become more mature, self-assertive, and autonomous.*

----

*Subsequently, patients of each school, as a result of the suggestive impact of their analyst's interpretations, inevitably tend to bring out data in their dreams and "free-associations" which appear to confirm the theoretical frame of reference of their analysts. This is why each theory seems to be self-validating and this is what makes the "dialogue" between members of differing schools so difficult. For this reason, too, the relative validity of the various psychoanalytic theories can never be established from their respective analytic data, but must be sought for in phenomena and experimental findings which can be reproduced and objectively verified by members of all schools, as well as by nonanalysts.

What I have sketchily set forth with passive dependency, can be done equally with any other specific clinical pattern of behavior, whether it be aggressiveness, competitiveness, fearfulness, withdrawal, compulsiveness, etc. In each instance proponents of different schools may explain these phenomena with theoretical constructs which represent different ways of organizing the same data but which are fundamentally saying the same thing to the patient. The relative merit of each theory, then, is not a matter of which is more "true" but rather a matter of which is more parsimonious, and which has the greater heuristic and predictive value. One should not even rule out the possibility that for certain kinds of data one theoretical approach seems more meaningful while for other kinds, another might be. This would correspond to Bohr's theory of "complementarity" in the field of physics.

But what about "insight" on the part of the patient? Is it the same thing? Unfortunately the term "insight," as applied to what goes on in the patient, is used very ambiguously in psychoanalysis. Occasionally it refers merely to a cognitive awareness of the analyst's interpretation. It is then usually described as "intellectual insight." If, on the other hand, the cognitive awareness is accompanied by a simultaneous display or "release" of emotion, the insight is believed to be "deeper" and is then referred to as "emotional insight." The latter is considered to be more efficacious than the former in changing neurotic behavior, yet every analyst knows that frequently even emotional insight does not result in alterations of the neurotic pattern. Under such circumstances, the analyst who is convinced that insight is the key to therapeutic change, will sometimes argue that the insight is still not sufficiently deep or thorough, and that resistance to a full awareness still has to be overcome. This is implicitly utilizing a behavioral criterion for insight without making it explicit. Presumably, when the patient *really* understands, he will behave differently; which is merely another way of saying that when he begins to behave adaptively, it will then be assumed that his insight is genuine!*

It is of interest in the context to consider what the Gestalt theorists,

---

*e.g. Zilboorg: "Insight is a state of personality or ego functioning as much as a neurosis is a special state of ego functioning. It should be considered the ultimate and crowning point of integration of ego functioning." (21)

who more than any other school of learning theory concerned
themselves with the problem of insight, had to say about it. Hilgard
(10), in summarizing the experimental work of the Gestaltists,
describes three distinctive criteria of insight in an experimental
subject: (1) A period of survey, inspection and attention which is
then followed by the critical solution. (2) The ready repetition of
the solution after a single critical solution. (3) The ability to generalize
the insight to new situations that require mediation by common
principles or awareness of common relationships. Exemplifying these
criteria, once Kohler's or Yerkes' apes grasped the gestalt of the
experimental problem, they were able, immediately and thereafter,
not only to solve the problem, but also to generalize the insight
to new problems based on similar principles (20).

It is worth noting that by these criteria, the definition of insight
is linked to the ability of the subject to solve a previously unsolved
problem. Such a sequence of events can and occasionally *does* take
place following a psychoanalytic interpretation or confrontation. The
patient may have what Karl Bühler has called an "a-ha" experience
(4) and from that point on no longer reacts with the neurotic pattern,
the maladaptive nature of which has now become clear to him.

More often, however, the mere acquisition of intellectual or even
emotional insight does not result in any immediate alteration of
the neurotic patterns. There still remains the arduous and time-consuming task of (1) overcoming the patient's tendency to cling
tenaciously to his previously learned patterns of perception and
behavior, and (2) enabling him to generalize the acquired "insights"
to all situations in which similar principles are operative. These
two tasks are essentially what is involved in the concept of "working
through."

It is with regard to the nature of this "working-through" process
that proponents of the Skinner and Hull schools of learning theory
in recent years have come up with some particularly interesting
findings. A host of experimental studies (2,11,12,18) seem to indicate
that the nonverbal as well as the verbal reactions of the therapist
act as positive and negative reinforcing stimuli to the patient,
encouraging certain kinds of responses and discouraging others.
According to these investigators, what seems to be going on in the
working-through process is a kind of conditioned-learning, in which

the therapist's overt or covert approval and disapproval—expressed in his nonverbal reactions as well as in his verbal confrontations, and in what he interprets as neurotic or healthy—act as reward-punishment cues or conditioning stimuli.* The analyst's implicit or explicit approval acts as a positive reinforcer to the more "mature" patterns of reacting, while his implicit or explicit disapproval tends to inhibit the less "mature" patterns. As with experimental studies in animals, this process requires frequent repetition before the previous overlearned conditioned-responses become extinguished, and the new conditioned-responses ("habit patterns") become firmly established.**

Interestingly enough, experimental studies have demonstrated that intermittent and irregular reinforcements are more effective than frequent or regular ones in changing patterns of behavior or maintaining desired ones (19). This would appear to bear out Franz Alexander's claim (1) that variations in the frequency of analytic visits as well as intermittent vacations from analysis appear to have a beneficial effect on the course of therapy. This is a fruitful area for further research, not only with regard to the question of frequency and regularity of visits but also with regard to the question of the length of therapeutic sessions. There is no reason to assume a priori that the traditional 50-minute hour, which is a historical carry-over from what Freud found personally convenient, necessarily represents an optimum time-arrangement for all patients.

Some interesting findings on the relative value of positive (rewarding) reinforcers and negative (punitive) ones in effecting behavioral changes also have a bearing on certain problems of analytic and psychotherapeutic technique. Kurt Lewin (13) was the first to point

---

*As I have pointed out elsewhere (15), the so-called neutrality of the analyst is a fiction, and constitutes an attitude which invariably affects the patient either positively or negatively, depending on his needs.

**It is of interest to note that in the course of this therapeutic transaction, the therapist, as well as the patient, undergoes a learning experience. By the end of an analysis it can usually be observed that the analyst's perceptions of and relationship to his patient are quite different from what they were originally. The patterns of *mutual* trust and understanding that develop between therapist and patient are important ingredients in the therapeutic process. One must also recognize that self-correcting mechanisms within the patient himself, as well as fortuitous events in his life outside of the analyst's office, also enter into the complex of forces which produce change in the patient.

out the differences in the field-situation that exist between reward techniques and punishment techniques. If a subject is kept at an intrinsically disliked task by the threat of punishment, he is being forced to choose between two disagreeable alternatives, and his impulse then will be to "leave the field" altogether, to avoid both alternatives. To prevent him from leaving, usually some kind of policing, authoritarian measures become necessary. In this connection one is reminded of the classical psychoanalytic assumption that an atmosphere of frustration favors the analytic process—thus the patient may be forbidden to smoke, his questions may go unanswered, the analyst maintains an aloof attitude, etc. Now it is true that moderate anxiety often increases a learner's motivation, but it is also true that too much anxiety disrupts the learning process. The usual consequence of too frustrating a technique in psychoanalysis is either that the patient leaves the field altogether—i.e., breaks off the treatment—or else that he regresses into more primitive patterns of behavior. Although this so-called reactivation of the "infantile neurosis" is considered to be an essential aspect of classical analysis and an important desideratum, it is by no means proved that this is either the only or the best route to the eventual establishment of more mature patterns of behavior.

Another example of the rule of frustration is the common assumption that the patient must make a sacrifice—generally a financial one—if he is really to benefit from therapy. The implicit rationale here is that the pain of having to give up substantial portions of his security will help to overcome his inner resistances to change. As Lewin's work indicates, however, if both of these alternatives are sufficiently disagreeable, the more likely outcome is that the patient will quit the therapeutic field altogether. As I have stated elsewhere (16), the patient's motivation in therapy depends "on how much the suffering from his illness outweighs any secondary gains which he obtains from it. While the amount of money he is willing to pay to get rid of his illness may *reflect* the degree of his motivation, it is not the *source* of it. . . . There is by now a vast body of experience which indicates that patients in free and low-cost psychoanalytic clinics can respond to therapy just as well as patients in private offices."

In contrast to a punitive situation, the attractiveness of a reward-situation tends to keep the learner in the field rather than drive him out of it. Lewin's work indicates, however, that the reward must be obtainable only by the performance of the desired task—otherwise the learner will simply short-circuit the feared or disliked activity and fail to change. Assuming the immediate rewards which the patient seeks in the transference situation is the therapist's "love" and approval, then Lewin's findings suggest that the common psychological assumption that "love should be unconditional," if it is interpreted to mean an unconditional positive reaction to anything the patient says or does, may be neither good psychology nor good therapy. The approach which is most likely to effect changes in behavior, according to him, would be to give approval when the desired behavior takes place, but to withhold it when it does not take place. Furthermore, as indicated previously, intermittent approval is more effective than constant approval, even when the desired behavior is forthcoming.*

Lewin also makes a significant distinction between reward and success, particularly when the desired goals are intrinsic, as they are in the analytic situation. The reward of approval enables a patient to make progress towards his goals, but only the achieving of a goal constitutes a success experience. Success leads to the development of a sense of mastery which is one of the chief objectives of the therapeutic process. This underlines the importance for both the therapist and the patient of setting realistic and attainable goals.

Estes, a follower of Skinner, did a number of experiments on the effects of punishment on learning which also have a bearing on psychotherapeutic techniques (5). Estes' experiments demonstrated that a response cannot be eliminated from an organism's repertory by the action of punishment alone—i.e., punishment alone suppressed the response, but the tendency towards the response continued to exist.** Moreover, he found, punishment not only did not hasten the elimination of a response, but actually retarded its

---

*This should not be misunderstood as negating the paramount importance in the therapeutic transaction of the therapist's genuine interest in the patient's welfare and belief in his fundamental worth as a human being. It may be useful, however, to make a distinction between such basic *acceptance* of the patient and *approval* of his behavior.

**This is a validation of the psychoanalytic concept that if an impulse is repressed it will nevertheless continue to exist in the unconscious.

elimination. Permanent weakening of a response came about only when it failed to elicit any reinforcement at all, positive or negative, and this weakening process was prevented if the punishment did not permit the response to occur at all! To put this in a familiar clinical context, a child's tantrums are more likely to stop occurring if they elicit no response at all than if they incur punishment. Within the therapeutic situation this implies that apart from the positive reinforcing value of approval, the simple withholding of approval may be a more potent therapeutic instrument for changing the patient than the direct expression of disapproval. This, it seems to me, confirms the value of the traditional psychoanalytic technique of avoiding attitudes of moral condemnation towards socially-dystonic behavior in the patient. To carry over this "neutrality," however, to avoiding a show of approval towards desirable behavior patterns may not be equally therapeutic.

Still another experimental finding was that punishment tends to suppress other responses in addition to the one punished. In analytic parlance we would say that it leads to ego-restriction, while reward tends to lead towards expansion of ego-function.

One of the consequences of the increased awareness of psychotherapy as a learning process is the emergence of a school of therapists which lays stress on techniques of modifying the *behavior* of the patient without reference to his subjective cognitive or emotional processes and without recourse to interview psychotherapy. This school utilizes theoretical constructs of learning theory and stresses principles of counterconditioning, extinction, discrimination, operant conditioning, reciprocal inhibition, and social limitation. Significantly, most of the clinical examples dealt with in their case reports are phobias and circumscribed symptom-complexes, rather than personality disorders.

Bandura, in a recent book entitled *Behavioristic Psychotherapy* (3), attacks the prevailing theories of psychopathology as essentially an amalgam of "medical and demonology models, which have in common the belief that the underlying pathology and not the symptomatic manifestations must be treated." "Consequently," he says, "therapeutic attention is generally focused not on the deviant behavior itself, but on the presumably influential internal processes." He argues further that what is called a symptom is merely a learned reaction which is regarded as deviant, and that "when the actual social learning history of maladaptive behavior is known, 'psycho-dynamic' explanations become superfluous." Moreover, he contends, once the maladaptive *behavior* is altered by the application of appropriate social learning procedures it is unnecessary to modify or remove "an underlying pathology," and symptom substitution will not occur. He emphasizes that concepts such as ego strength, or emotional maturity or mental health are hypothetical constructs which in the final analysis can be inferred only from observable behavior. He regards behavior as the only modifiable reality available to the psychotherapist.

I have quoted Bandura's views in some detail not only because they are representative of this new movement in psychotherapy, but also because they reflect a basic blind spot which is characteristic of this school of therapists. Although my central thesis in this paper has been to stress the value of an understanding of learning theory for psychoanalytic therapy, and although I am in agreement with some of the criticisms leveled by the members of this school against certain aspects of psychoanalytic theory and practice, I believe that people like Bandura, Wolpe and Eysenck are making the serious error of throwing the baby out with the bath water, and of returning to a kind of oversimplified behaviorism which cognitive learning theorists, no less than Freud, have demonstrated long ago to be inadequate. To assume that what goes on subjectively within the patient is irrelevant and that all that matters is how he behaves is to discard a half-century of psychodynamic insights. We know that two people may behave in externally identical ways for entirely different internal reasons. A socially adjusted schizophrenic whose outward behavior is apparently normal is nevertheless a considerably different individual from one with identical outward behavior but without the inner delusional system. Moreover, symptoms are obviously not always behavioral, and the."free-floating" panic reactions of a person with an anxiety state may have no objective stimulus precipitating them against which the patient can be countercondi-tioned. In addition, certain behavioral symptoms, like those in conversion hysteria, are clearly only symbolic expressions of an underlying psychological conflict, and the mere removal of the symptom, which is often a simple matter, does not touch the underlying conflict at all. This is a clinical fact which decades of clinical experience have repeatedly verified. It is precisely the vast and complex area *between* stimulus and response that constitutes the major concern of modern dynamic psychiatry. It is what *cannot* be objectively seen or measured that is our chief challenge and preoccupation. It was Freud's genius, regardless of whatever limitations some of his theoretical assumptions have turned out to have, that he was the first to present us with a technique and a key to a rational understanding of this vast subjective, symbolic, and largely unconscious realm which exerts so profound an influence upon both our perceptions and our actions.

Bandura quotes with obvious approval the case of a fetishist with an impulse to smear mucus on ladies' handbags, who was treated by the counterconditioning technique of the paired presentation of a collection of handbags with the onset of nausea produced by injections of apomorphine; and claims that an 18-month follow-up study revealed not only that the fetish had been successfully eliminated but that the patient showed a "vast improvement" in his social, legal, vocational and sexual relationships. I have no way of evaluating the validity of this particular case report, but certainly there have been many years of experience with similar counterconditioning therapies in cases of alcoholism; and the ineffectiveness of such an approach, when used exclusively, in modifying the inner psychodynamic problems of the alcoholic is a matter of common knowledge. When Bandura asserts that no symptom substitution occurs in such cases he seems to be assuming that symptoms must be behaviorally manifested since the persistence of tension and anxiety states in alcoholics treated by counterconditioning therapy is a matter of common observation and is the basis for the general recommendation that any such therapy, if utilized, must be combined with psychotherapy aimed at the patient's underlying inner conflicts.

Moreover, the evidence of learning theory itself reveals that neurotic disorders are not the simple product of an exposure to a painful conditioned stimulus. The work of Pavlov, Liddell, Masserman and others has clearly demonstrated that neurotic symptoms ensue when an animal is faced with incompatible choices eliciting simultaneous approach and avoidance reactions, or with confusing conditioned stimuli which it is unable clearly to differentiate. This corresponds to the psychoanalytic concept of conflict which is at the root of the vast majority of neurotic disorders in humans. Once such a neurotic conflict is set up, the secondary elaborations, defensive adaptations and symbolic distortions become extensively involved in every aspect of the individual's thought and behavioral processes.

I am not attempting to deny the potential usefulness of counter-conditioning techniques as a part of our total psychotherapeutic armamentarium. I believe that the proponents of these views have a contribution to make and that there may well be types of behavioral disorders, particularly those which have been induced by a single traumatic experience or series of such experiences, in which such forms of therapy have a great deal to offer. It should not surprise us that certain techniques work better than others with different patients and different problems. Just as there is no single best way of teaching all people and all subjects, there is no single best way of treating all patients. To assume, however, that behavioral disorders and personality distortions which have been subtly inculcated by 5, 10 or 20 years of daily disturbances in interpersonal experience, by an entire climate of faulty relationships, confused communications, inconsistent disciplinary cues, etc., can be totally eradicated by the application of a dozen or two counterconditioning sessions aimed at some specific behavioral symptom, is to simply misjudge the complexity of the problems that are being dealt with.

For such problems I believe there is still no satisfactory substitute for the time-consuming process of patiently reeducating the patient concerning the nature of his perceptual, emotional, symbolic and behavioral distortions and of enabling him, by the working-through process, to generalize and apply his increased understanding to many different life-situations. The therapeutic techniques of all the current psychoanalytic "schools," regardless of their conceptual differences, operate upon this basis, either explicitly or implicitly. In this process cognitive learning, imitation (identification with the analyst) and a subtle conditioning procedure all usually take place, in varying degrees.* Precisely because this is a learning process we as analysts have much to gain by a better acquaintance with the contributions of the various theories of learning to see what applica-

---

*That therapeutic change *can* take place with hardly any cognitive insight is a matter of common experience. Not infrequently, successfully analyzed patients report that their feelings and functioning have improved enormously, but that they have no idea of what it was that made them better! In such instances unconscious identification processes, subtle conditioning and corrective emotional experiences have probably been the chief sources of the therapeutic modifications.

tion we can make of their findings in our own work. I shall not pretend that I have made more than a bare beginning in this direction with this paper; I have not even touched, for example, on the possible applications of communications theory, cybernetics, game theory, and general systems theory to psychoanalytic theory and practice. I would hope, however, that this effort may encourage others to explore these fruitful areas.

References

1. ALEXANDER, F.: The principle of flexibility, In F. Alexander and T. M. French, Psychoanalytic Therapy. New York, Ronald Press, 1946, Ch. 3.
2. BANDURA, A.: Psychotherapy as a learning process. Psychol. Bull. 58:143, 1961.
3. _____: Behavioristic Psychotherapy. New York, Holt, Rinehart and Winston, 1963.
4. BÜHLER, K.: Die Krise der Psychologie, 2nd Ed., Jena, Gustav Fischer, 1929, p. 136.
5. ESTES, W. K.: An experimental study of punishment. Psychol. Monogr. 57, No. 263, 1944.
6. FREUD, S.: Collected Papers, London, Hogarth Press, 1933, Vol. 2, p. 362.
7. _____: Ibid., p. 376.
8. HILGARD, E. R.: Theories of Learning, 2nd Ed. New York, Appleton-Century-Crofts, Inc., 1956.
9. _____: Ibid., p. 8.
10. _____: Ibid, p. 238.
11. KRASNER, L.: Studies of the conditioning of verbal behavior. Psychol. Bull. 55:148, 1958.
12. _____: The therapist as a social reinforcement machine. In H. H. Strupp and L. Luborsky, (Eds.) Research in Psychotherapy. Am. Psychol. Assoc., Washington, D.C., 1963.
13. LEWIN, K.: Field theory and learning. In The Psychology of Learning. Nat. Soc. Stud. Educ., 41st Yearbook, 1942, Ch. 4.
14. MARMOR, J.: Psychoanalytic Therapy as an Educational Process. In Psychoanalytic Education, J. H. Masserman, Ed. New York, Grune & Stratton, 1962, p. 286. (Chapter 15, this volume.)
15. _____: A reevaluation of certain aspects of psychoanalytic theory and practice. In Modern Concepts of Psychoanalysis, L. Salzman and J. H. Masserman, Eds. New York, Philosophical Library, Inc., 1962, p. 191.
16. _____: Ibid., p. 203.
17. MILLER, N. E. and DOLLARD, J. C.: Social Learning and Imitation. New Haven, Yale Univ. Press, 1941.
18. SHOBEN, E. J., JR.: Psychotherapy as a problem in learning theory. Psychol. Bull. 46:366, 1949.
19. SKINNER, B. F.: The Behavior of Organisms: an Experimental Analysis. New York, Appleton-Century-Crofts, 1938.

20. YERKES, R. M.: The mind of a gorilla. Genetic Psychol. Monogr. 1927, p. 156.
21. ZILBOORG, A.: The emotional problem and the therapeutic role of insight. Psa. Quart. 21:1, 1952.

17

PSYCHOANALYSIS AT THE CROSSROADS
(1966)

About six months ago (in December, 1965) I gave up a psychoanalytically oriented private practice of almost 30 years duration to take a full-time position as director of the department of psychiatry in a general hospital.* Perhaps it is no accident, therefore, that at this junction in my own career I find myself concerned with the crossroad at which psychoanalysis currently finds itself. I come, however, neither to bury psychoanalysis nor to sing its praises—neither as a hostile iconoclast nor as a devout worshipper—but rather as one who has toiled, affectionately but, I hope, with some degree of objectivity, in its vineyards for most of his working life, and who now pauses to take a backward look at the professional route he has traveled, as well as to survey the road that lies ahead.

In May 1965, in discussing Roy Grinker's paper on "Fields, Fences and Riders" at the joint session of the American Psychoanalytic Association and the Section on Psychoanalysis of the American Psychiatric Association, I said in part, "Whether we like it or not, those of us who have dedicated most of our professional lives to the study and practice of psychoanalysis must face the fact that our specialty has reached a critical crossroad. The direction we choose will determine whether the psychoanalytic community will continue to exert a paramount influence upon the mainstream of modern psychiatric thought, or will gradually recede into an unimportant sidestream by virtue of its failure to keep abreast of modern developments in the behavioral sciences. The handwriting is on

---

*At the Cedars-Sinai Medical Center, Los Angeles, Calif.

the wall for all to see. Already many of the brightest young minds in psychiatry, who for the past 20 years have flocked to the psychoanalytic institutes for training, are turning their eyes in other directions. The frontiers of research and creativity in psychiatric theory and practice—once the proud domain of psychoanalysis—have now shifted to other areas, and psychoanalysis is in serious danger of becoming a tight little island of devoted technicians plying a fading trade in the gathering twilight of its senescence."

In looking backward over the history of our field, it is fair to ask why it is that psychoanalysis finds itself in this critical situation. There is no need, for this audience, to recapitulate the early history of the psychoanalytic movement, and the heroic struggle of its early pioneers against the hostility of the professional establishment of their times. I want to point out, however, that even in the thirties, when I first entered upon psychoanalytic training, there was still a sense of excitement about what we, as candidates, were doing and learning, a sense that we were in the vanguard of psychiatric theory, where the most sophisticated thinking in our field was taking place. Indeed, the independent psychoanalytic institutes of the thirties were the only places where a young psychiatrist could get the kind of psychodynamic training and experience that would enable him to understand the hidden motivations and conflicts that lay behind his patients' symptoms and behavioral patterns.

But over the years, fresh theory has ossified into rigid dogma and the revolutionaries of the past have become conservatives. Although this has often been the history of revolutionary movements, certain of the factors involved in this shift in the psychoanalytic movement are unique to it and worth touching upon.

First, at least historically, was Freud's own attitude. Although it has often been said, and correctly, that Freud was less Freudian than most of his followers, it is nevertheless true that the hostility of his contemporaries and the professional isolation that this imposed upon him pushed him into an attitude of dedicated militancy toward his discoveries that subsequently, as the Freud-Bleuler correspondence (1) demonstrated so beautifully, drove him to equate theoretical disagreement on the part of others with personal hostility or disloyalty.

More important over the long run, however, has been the nature of psychoanalytic training as it has evolved historically. The isolated psychoanalytic institutes, independent of university interdisciplinary connections, which grew out of the enforced isolation of the early psychoanalytic movement, have tended, for the most part, to become perpetuators of a tradition rather than centers for the exploration of new frontiers in our field. The rigid hierarchy of relationships within these institutes, from lowly candidates to exalted training analysts; the ambiguous and indeed contradictory role of the training analyst as both therapist and judge, with his almost unlimited power to affect his candidate's professional life; the tendency within many of these institutes to characterize scientific doubts in a student as "resistance" and even to drop him from training if his doubts persisted or were openly expressed; the tendency of most classical psycho-analytic institutes to teach psychodynamics as a talmudic history of Freud's writings rather than as a living, changing theory of human behavior—all of these factors in psychoanalytic training have tended to harden psychoanalytic theory and practice into dogma and ritual instead of keeping it open to the new currents of scientific thought that were sweeping around it.

One of the results of all this is that the majority, but fortunately not all, of psychoanalysts today, even when they pay lip service to ego theory, still tend to think in terms of libido theory concepts, of stages of libido development, of shifting libidinal cathexes, of closed energy systems, etc. Moreover, they do so often with a degree of emotional fervor that belongs more within the confines of a religious organization than in the halls of science. Part of this fervor, as I have just suggested, undoubtedly derives from the very nature of psychoanalytic training and indoctrination. As Alexander has pointed out, part of it also stems, at least for older analysts, from the difficulty of giving up the "great inner gratification derived from [having been] a militant member of a new spiritual movement" (2). But I believe that there is also another fundamental source of the anxiety and emotion and anger that is stirred up in so many analysts when their theoretical convictions are challenged. To explore this, however, it will be necessary for me to digress in another direction.

It has become traditional to say of psychoanalysis that it is not one thing but three things: (1) a technique of psychological investigation; (2) a theory of human personality; and (3) a technique of therapy. I should like to submit to you that in this linking together of three really very disparate things (which most of us, myself included, have accepted unquestioningly for many years) lie the roots of some of the most serious institutional problems of the psychoanalytic movement.

There is no doubt, in my judgment, of the unique value of the psychoanalytic method as an *investigative tool.* No other approach that I know of has been able to explore the deepest realms of man's unconscious motivations, feelings, and fantasy life as thoroughly and meaningfully as it has. In some distant future, when the final page of the history of psychiatry is written, I am convinced that the psychoanalytic method of exploring the human unconscious will remain the brightest jewel in Freud's crown of monumental contributions. I cannot conceive that the subjective data of the nature and the quality of the symbolic abstractions that guide man's inner mental and emotional life, and that are most effectively obtained by the psychoanalytic method, will ever be less relevant to the understanding of man than the so-called hard and quantifiable data concerning his external behavior.

On the other hand, the unhappy fact is that classical psychoanalysis as a *body of theory* has failed to meet the challenge of modern scientific scrutiny in recent years. What began as a revolutionary breakthrough in the understanding of human personality development and psychopathology, has unfortunately become increasingly esoteric and dated by its stubborn ignoring of the contributions of modern biological, behavioral, and social sciences. The criticisms to which it has been subjected can no longer be lightly charged to ignorance, bias, or unconscious resistance in its critics as they were in Freud's day. The concepts of repression, unconscious motivation and conflict that stirred up our nineteenth century forbears are no longer matters of serious debate. Thanks to the tenacious courage of Freud and his early followers, they are now accepted as givens in most modern psychodynamic theories. The points that are now at issue are much more complex and sophisticated. For example, is the entire tortuous maze of Freudian metapsychology—particularly its topographic and economic aspects—the best framework for a modern theory of human behavior, or are there other theories that are equally effective, more parsimonious, and more open to scientific testing and validation? Is libido theory still tenable in the light of modern developments in ego psychology? Do the laudable efforts of sophisticated theoreticians like Hartmann, Rapaport, and Erickson to fuse the findings of ego psychology with libido theory represent the optimum and most economical approach to a theory of human behavior, or is it possible to arrive at a unified theory of human behavior that makes such a fusion unnecessary? Has not the classical nineteenth century closed-system concept of shifting libido cathexes been thoroughly outmoded by the new open-system theories concerning living organisms, and if so, is it not long past due for the disappearance of the closed-system models in psychoanalytic thinking and teaching? These are the kinds of questions that behavioral scientists both within and outside of our psychoanalytic profession have been asking with increasing insistence in recent years. Clearly, passionate personal conviction in this area is not a substitute for controlled scientific experimentation. Unfortunately, psychoanalysts, who were the first to make the world aware of the significance of the phenomenon of resistance, have themselves in large measure become its most striking exemplars. Not too long ago, one of the most prominent leaders of the American and International Psychoanalytic Associations (3) insisted that Freud's psychoanalytic paradigm was a cohesive whole and that no part of it could be discarded without destroying its unity, ignoring the fact that Freud himself had been constantly revising and disavowing parts of it throughout his life. Genius that he was, Sigmund Freud would not and could not have ignored modern developments in field theory, communications and information theory, or the exciting integrative potential of general systems theory. It will no longer suffice in today's scientific world to argue that psychoanalytic inferences need only be confirmed within the framework of the psychoanalytic method. If these inferences are correct, they must, like any other scientific inferences, lend themselves to validation by alternative techniques and methods and by independent observers. Otherwise they simply do not qualify as scientific hypotheses. There is little doubt that the alienation of formal psychoanalytic education from the main body of psychiatric training has now outlived its original usefulness and has been contributing to psychoanalytic sectarianism. Surely at this moment in history, when psychoanalysis still enjoys considerable medical prestige, and when psychoanalytically trained psychiatrists still play an important role in medical schools and psychiatric residency programs throughout the United States, the time has arrived for psychoanalytic institutes to make every effort to abandon their heroic isolation and to return psychoanalytic training to an academic setting where it can be stimulated and enriched by interdisciplinary cooperation and challenge. In such academic settings the hypotheses of psychoanalysis can be subjected to the kind of probing, testing, and research that is a necessary catalytic force in the healthy growth and progress of any science. Ultimately, and hopefully, the various current approaches to psychiatric thought and practice will be integrated into one fundamental science of dynamic psychiatry encompassing all the relevant findings of the biological, psychological, and social sciences.

Psychoanalysis has been justly compared to microscopy or to microscopic analysis. No other approach to the psychology of man concerns itself so thoroughly with the basic minutiae of his inner life. But one can no more build a comprehensive theory of human behavior out of data derived only from man's intrapsychic life than one could build an adequate theory of brain function only out of the intimate analysis of single neurones. A comprehensive modern theory of human behavior must encompass not only man's intrapsychic mechanisms and his interpersonal relationships but also our newer knowledge of relevant brain chemistry and neurophysiology, and must see all of these within the context of man's total field situation—the time, the place, and the culture within which and in relationship to which these biological, intrapsychic, and interpersonal mechanisms are operating.

As we stand here at the crossroads we must face the additional fact, however reluctantly, that as a rigidly defined *technique of therapy* classical psychoanalysis has also had serious limitations. It is cumbersome, expensive, and time-consuming, and under what conditions, if any, it deserves to be employed in preference to all other modifications of psychotherapeutic technique, still remains to be convincingly demonstrated. Freud himself, in later life, had many doubts about the therapeutic efficacy of his method; and its applicability, at best, has always been restricted to a relatively small segment of the total neurotic population. It is only in recent years that the nature of the psychotherapeutic process has begun to be subjected to rigorous scientific studies, and already many of the dogmatic assumptions of classical psychoanalytic technique, such as those concerning the behavior of the analyst, the role of insight and abreaction, the importance of the recovery of early memories, the value of induced transference-regression, the length and frequency of interviews, the importance of the fee, and the use of the couch, have begun to be seriously questioned. *Unfortunately, by tying their identities as professionals to this narrowly defined and cumbersome technique of therapy, many psychoanalysts have developed such an enormous emotional investment in proclaiming its superiority over all other techniques, that they have stopped being scientific students of the psychotherapeutic process and have become instead a guild of craft unionists defending the value of their particular craft above all others.* I believe that it is this self-created threat to their sense of professional identity and adequacy that accounts for much of the intense emotional reaction of many classical analysts when any of their doctrinaire assumptions are questioned. (Indeed, as an analyst, one may be excused for wondering whether in part this extreme defensiveness does not stem also from an unconscious awareness of the vulnerability of their position.) One of the ultimate absurdities of this emotional commitment has been the formulation in recent years that psychoanalysis was not a branch of psychiatry at all, but an entirely separate specialty—a formulation that has wrought serious and unjust income tax hardships upon hundreds of young psychiatrists undergoing psychoanalytic training.

Another significant aspect of this approach to the problem is the light that it sheds upon the whole matter of lay analysis which has plagued psychoanalysis almost from its inception. If psycho-analysis as a methodology is indeed at the same time a self-encom-passing theory of human behavior and a uniquely superior technique of psychotherapy, then it follows with absolute logic that there is no reason whatever for a competent psychoanalyst to have any medical training. Indeed, one could argue with equal cogency that it does not really require even a college degree—it is something that any reasonably intelligent and perceptive layman could be taught as a totally separate profession. On the other hand, if, as I think the facts of the past half-century have clearly demonstrated, psychoanalysis is inadequate in itself as a comprehensive theory of human behavior, and too narrowly based to be an adequate form of therapy for most psychiatric problems, *then it follows inescapably that the chief value of psychoanalysis is as a methodological tool within the context of a total psychiatric armamentarium for which medical training is indeed essential.* In saying this, I am not attempting to imply that psychotherapeutic techniques, in properly selected cases, *cannot* be performed by nonmedical personnel. On the contrary, in the years to come I think we can expect to see various forms of psychotherapy being performed more and more often by such personnel, although hopefully most of it will be in community mental health centers under qualified medical guidance and supervision. What I *am* saying, however, is that the ability to practice modern comprehensive psychiatry *does* require medical training and that psychoanalytic training per se no more qualifies a person to be a psychiatrist than biochemical training would qualify one to be a physician.

Indeed, many of the shortcomings of classical psychoanalysis as a therapeutic technique stem precisely from its exclusive preoccupation with intrapsychic dynamics. This has led classical analysts to insist on a purely dyadic therapeutic relationship, with an exclusion not only of contacts with, but even of information from, other significant figures in the patient's life, as well as to a minimization of other relevant biological, social, economic, and cultural factors. Those psychoanalysts who early made pleas for greater flexibility of therapeutic approaches with regard to such factors as frequency of visits, length of sessions, or use of the couch, or for exploration of other therapeutic parameters such as family therapy, group therapy, or the conjoint use of drugs with psychoanalytic therapy, were generally viewed with suspicion and hostility, and indeed often attacked as "not being psychoanalysts at all!" And yet, in all of these therapeutic parameters as well as in many others, psychoanalytically trained psychiatrists have made significant and basic contributions, contributions dependent on the unique insights derived from psychoanalysis.

Let us not make the mistake, therefore, of throwing the baby out with the bath as we face up honestly to some of the shortcomings of our specialized area of interest. The psychoanalytic method *is* an exceptional tool for the investigation and understanding of individual psychodynamics, and when it is not employed exclusively or with compulsive rigidity, it is an invaluable addition to our armamentarium. If we recognize and use it as just such a tool, we will find that it enriches every aspect of our clinical work, whether it be individual psychotherapy, psychopharmacotherapy, family therapy, group therapy, or social and community psychiatry.

There are still important frontiers in psychoanalysis, but they are no longer the traditional ones of uncovering the psychodynamic mysteries behind individual neurosis. That ground has been pretty thoroughly explored. The new frontiers are in other areas. A few of these (and I shall mention only a few) are: the new parameters of dream research; studies into the nature of the psychotherapeutic process, both dyadic and in groups; the relationship between biochemistry, brain function, and certain patterns of behavior; the interrelationship between individual and family psychodynamics and various social, economic, and political parameters; and the never-ending challenge to utilize all of our skills and knowledge in the quest for more effective and efficient techniques of ameliorating psychic distress and of facilitating emotional maturity.

In the search for a unifying theory of human behavior, we who are students of depth psychology have much to contribute; the subjective data of man's inner experiences cannot be ignored in any comprehensive evaluation of the human animal. If we wish to be taken seriously by our colleagues, however, the *inferences* that we draw from our data will have to be subjected to the same kind of rigorous evaluation and testing that is applied in any other field of scientific endeavor. In science nothing is sacred except the *method* of science, and to modify John Dewey's paraphrase from the Book of Job, although this method challenge our most cherished beliefs, yet we must be prepared to trust it!

REFERENCES

1. ALEXANDER, F., and SELESNICK, S.: Freud-Bleuler correspondence. Arch. Gen. Psychiat. 12: 1–9, 1965.
2. _____: The Scope of Psychoanalysis, New York. Basic Books, 1961, p. 539.
3. GITELSON, M.: On the identity crisis in American psychoanalysis. J. Amer. Psychoanal. Ass. 12: 451–476, 1964.

18

CHANGING PATTERNS OF FEMININITY: PSYCHOANALYTIC IMPLICATIONS (1968)

There is probably no area in Freud's writings more fraught with theoretical and clinical contradictions than his pronouncements concerning feminine psychophysiology. In what follows, I shall examine these pronouncements in the light of certain developments and changes in the behavioral patterns of twentieth-century women, with some consideration to the impact of these changes on the institution of Western marriage.

The exact nature of the relationship of primitive man and woman is shrouded in conjecture (the popular fantasy pictures a masterful caveman dragging his willing and passively inert mate along the ground by her hair). We know, however, that since recorded history there has been no fixed pattern to this relationship. There is evidence to suggest that in most primitive, nomadic, communal societies family descent was reckoned through the mothers (probably for the obvious reason that maternity, in contrast to paternity, could not be doubted), and clans were consequently organized along matrilineal lines. With the evolution of agriculture, and the gradual development of private property, the transfer of property from father to son became a paramount socioeconomic factor, and families began to be organized along patrilineal lines. The risk of false paternity was protected against by the development of the institution of wifely chastity, and gradually woman began to occupy a more and more subordinate role as a sexual chattel of man.

However, there has not been a straight line of social evolutionary development in the relationship between the sexes. The social status of woman has changed at various times both within the same society and in different societies. Thus, in ancient Greece up to the reign of Cecrops, families were matrilineal; women enjoyed considerable status and voted with men in the popular assembly. Yet subsequently, in the Platonic era, the position of the woman in the family became a degraded and depreciated one, and she was strictly confined to the home, without political or economic rights. There were important social and economic factors involved in these shifting vicissitudes, but they are beyond the purview of this chapter.

THE EMANCIPATION OF MODERN WOMAN

What concerns us more directly here is that in American and European history, up to the end of the eighteenth century, woman's position, for the most part, was distinctly subordinate to that of man. She was totally dependent upon him economically, had no vote and relatively few legal rights, and was denied access to formal education. Early in the nineteenth century, however, in the wake of the egalitarian spirit set into motion by the American and French revolutions and of the sociological changes engendered by the Industrial Revolution, women in England and America began, for the first time in modern history, to assert their prerogatives in relationship to men. Nevertheless, it was almost a hundred years before they obtained the right to vote and began to move toward fuller equality before the law. Even now, in the second half of the twentieth century, there are many states of the Union in which such equivalence does not exist; and the constitutional amendment on equal rights for men and women has repeatedly failed to pass Congress. Despite this, the decades since 1920 have seen remarkable changes in the status of women throughout the world. They are able to vote in most countries where voting franchises exist, to enter many professions previously reserved for men, and to move out of the confines of the home into the broader arena of social, cultural, and political life.

However, even within our lifetime there has been a discernible ebb and flow to this pattern. The "feminine revolt" that was so manifest in the twenties through the forties seems to have given way to the "feminine mystique" of the fifties. Where after World

War I women were struggling to get out of the home, the current trend seems to be back to the home. A smaller percentage of college graduates today are women than were thirty years ago, and American women constitute a smaller proportion of the professional world today than they did then. (By contrast, women in some Eastern European countries have more than doubled their representation in professional occupations.)

The reasons for this apparent recession in the revolutionary upsurge of women in America are complex. Some classical Freudians would argue that the entire feminine revolution was essentially a neurotic outbreak of "penis envy" and that what we are now witnessing is a healthy return to "normal" patterns of femininity. Such a statement, however, merely attaches value-laden labels to the phenomenon without really explaining it. Indeed, there are those who claim (1) that the post-World War II popularity of Freudian theory in America has been in itself a potent factor in "pushing" American women back toward a more subordinate and passive role. While this view may have some validity, it seems more likely that certain broad socioeconomic factors have been involved, notably the gradual increase of automation and the pressure from men to push women out of the shrinking labor market except in those areas traditionally reserved for them (domestic work, secretarial and teaching positions, retail selling, and so forth). Friedan suggests that an additional factor may have been the increased awareness of American business and merchandising executives that "women will buy more things if they are kept in the under-used, nameless-yearning, energy-to-get-rid-of state of being housewives" (2).

Nonetheless, the increased emancipation of women that began in the twenties has left an important imprint on the relationship between the sexes that deserves our further consideration.

CHANGING MALE-FEMALE RELATIONSHIPS

What are some of the changes that have taken place?* By and large there has been a considerable relaxation of the social

---

*The comments that follow refer to broad trends and are not intended as universal generalizations; obviously there are many individuals who do not fit into these patterns. The existence of these trends, however, regardless of their extent, is sufficient to document the points I shall be making.

and sexual restrictions placed upon female children born after World War I. Little girls are now allowed to play more vigorously and competitively, with resultant greater muscular strength and athletic capability. During the preadolescent and adolescent years, contacts between the sexes have become freer, and adolescent as well as preadolescent petting occurs with much greater frequency than in previous decades. This increased freedom, both socially and sexually, has led to a higher degree of sophistication and self-confidence in young girls. This, combined with the earlier physiological matura- tion curves of most girls, tends to give them a considerable degree of relative dominance and mastery over boys of similar age levels, particularly during the adolescent years. Post-World War I mores have also accorded women greater freedom in taking the initiative in reaching out to men both socially and sexually, and, as a result, much feminine assertiveness that would have been dampened or totally inhibited by the convention of earlier eras has been enabled to flourish. Many other time-hallowed conventions have also changed. For example, it is no longer considered "unfeminine" for women to wear slacks, wear short hair, or smoke cigarettes.* Indeed, we are beginning to see evidences that before too long women will also be smoking cigars and pipes without loss of feminine status.

These changing conventions have been reflected in current pat- terns of marital relationships also. Women have tended to become more dominant in the home, in an interpersonal sense. Discipline, once the exclusive domain of the father, has been increasingly delegated to the mother. Indeed, in many homes it is now father rather than mother to whom the children turn for redress from discipline or as the "soft touch." Similarly, women are playing a more important role in family decision-making. The popular joke that wives make all the minor decisions (those concerning the family), while husbands make all the major ones (those concerning interna- tional relations), is a reflection of this shift in family dominance.

Another important indication of this shift in marital equilibrium has been the increasing emphasis upon female orgasm. In the

---

*An amusing sidelight on these changing patterns was afforded some years ago by a resolution passed by a Midwestern college fraternity forbidding cigarette smoking by any of its members on the grounds that it was too effeminate!

Victorian era, "it was considered unfeminine for a woman to acknowledge or display sexual feelings of any kind, even in the conjugal relationship" (3). Now a significant proportion of women express their sexual desires quite openly and engage in the sexual act not as passive recipients but as active participants, indeed often taking the initiative in arousing the man. Sexual intercourse now is expected to culminate in orgasm for the woman no less than for the man, and failure to achieve orgasm is generally as disappointing to the woman as it would be to the man.

The changing status of women has had noteworthy reverberations outside the home also. The percentage of women in the American labor force (excluding the actual war years) has slowly but steadily increased in the past forty years. According to Bureau of Labor statistics for 1962, 24 million, or just over one-third of all working people for that year, were women (4).

Thirty-six percent of all women were working women. Of these 24 million working women, moreover, less than 25 percent were single, and slightly over 20 percent were widowed, divorced, or separated. The remaining 56 percent, or 13-1/2 million working women, were married and living with their husbands. These figures indicate that American women are assuming an increasingly important economic role in the family, not merely as the primary spenders of the family income, but also as wage earners. An additional factor in this growing economic importance is the fact that many women outlive their husbands and end up controlling their estates.

Because it is generally easier for Negro women to obtain work than it is for their husbands, the Negro woman in America is often the *only* wage earner in the family, and the Negro family therefore tends to be matriarchal, with the father occupying a depreciated status position. Although these effects are easily recognized in the Negro family, the corresponding, more subtle consequences in the white American family as a result of the economic factors described above are less easily recognizable but no less real.

Women who are not in the labor force also occupy a different psychological position than do men. The man who does not work in our society is apt to be left with a loss of identity and severe impairment of his morale; he generally becomes either depressed or apathetic, or aggressively antisocial.* The nonworking wife, however, still retains a meaningful identity as a wife and mother. She is thus able to use her leisure time more constructively. Increasing numbers of middle-class wives attend adult-education classes, read books, and participate in various artistic and creative activities. The result is that while many working husbands become progressively narrower in their areas of interest and knowledge, their wives become the chief purveyors of cultural and aesthetic interests in and outside the home. These factors tend also to increase the relative importance of the mother in the family vis-à-vis the father, and their effects upon the identifications formed by children in the family can be of great significance. It is possible, for example, that they play a part in the increasing incidence of homosexuality in modern society; a common thread in the histories of many homosexuals is the identification with the "more cultured and aesthetically oriented mother."

The progressive technological development of society in the coming decades can be expected to have continuing important effects on the relations between the sexes. Not only does the increase in automation mean that women will become more and more able to do "men's jobs," but also the sharp decline in total jobs available is bound to mean an enormous increment in leisure time for both sexes, with profound changes in family relationships.

PSYCHOANALYTIC IMPLICATIONS

The classical psychoanalytic position on women as outlined by Freud (5) is too well known to require detailing here. Its salient features, however, can be outlined briefly as follows:

1. *Anatomy is fate.* The basic nature of woman is determined by her anatomy; most importantly by her discovery that she does not possess a penis.

---

*This fact may change in coming decades as increasing automation creates larger numbers of unemployed men. The traditional Puritan ethos associating personal identity with work identity may in time have to give way to a new ethos in which identities are based on other factors, such as specific cultural interests, or skills, and so forth.

2. *Penis envy.* All female children naturally envy males for having penises, and the desire for a penis is a universal fact of normal feminine psychology, only partially compensated for by giving birth to a male child. Helene Deutsch (6) asserts that penis envy is a natural consequence of the fact that the clitoris actually is "an inferior organ" in terms of its capacity to provide libidinal gratification, as well as for its lack of "the forward thrusting, penetrating qualities of the penis."*

3. *Masochism and passivity.* These are outgrowths of normal feminine development and are natural and essential components of healthy femininity.

4. *Faulty superego development.* Due to the fact that the feminine castration-complex (precipitated by the little girl's discovery that she has no penis) pushes the little girl *away* from her mother *into* an oedipal attachment for her father, the little girl has greater difficulty than the boy in resolving the oedipal complex. Consequently, she tends to develop a defective superego (because the latter presumably comes into being only as the "heir" of the repressed oedipal complex). The result in women, according to Freud, is an inadequate sense of justice, a predisposition to envy, weaker social interests, and a lesser capacity for sublimation.

Let us now consider these formulations in the light of contemporary knowledge.

1. *"Anatomy is fate."* That the anatomical differences between the sexes must inevitably be reflected in some personality differences, regardless of variations in cultural patterns, would seem to be almost axiomatic. Differences in body image, in the experience of menstruation at puberty, in the subsequent monthly cyclical variations of endocrine function, and in the experiences of sexual intercourse, pregnancy, childbirth, and menopause are all aspects of bodily sensation and function that are uniquely different for the woman as compared to the man; and in the biological-environmental interac-

---

*Freud believed also that genital erogenicity in the normal female, although first centered in the clitoris, eventually becomes transferred to the vagina, and that sexual orgasm in the mature, healthy female should be in response to vaginal rather than clitoral stimulation. I have discussed the reasons for questioning this theory in Chapter 10.

tion that leads to personality formation, these *must* result in significant personality variances between the sexes. To deny this, and to argue, as some strongly-oriented feminists have done, that personality differences between the sexes have *nothing* to do with biological differences but are *totally* a reflection of cultural factors is to miss the mark no less than do those who have overemphasized the importance of the biological factor.* The fact is that only by taking into consideration *both* the biological differences between the sexes *and* the variations in cultural reactions to these differences—that is, the *field situation*—can the personality similarities and dissimilarities between men and women, at any given time and place, be fully understood.

Even as sophisticated an observer as Erik Erikson tends to fall into the error of trying to derive some of woman's psychological characteristics *solely* from her anatomical structure. In his recent, beautifully written "Inner and Outer Space: Reflections on Womanhood" (7), he advances the thesis that women are prone to be more concerned with "inner-space" as compared to men's greater preoccupation with "outer-space," and that this is somehow due to "the existence of a *productive inner-bodily space* safely set in the center of female form and carriage" (8). He presents as evidence for this conclusion the fact that in a study of 150 boys and 150 girls, aged ten to twelve, in which they were asked to construct a "scene" with toys on a table, two-thirds of the girls constructed *peaceful interior* scenes, while two-thirds of the boys constructed *aggressive exterior* scenes, or else structures with protruding walls. One need not question the accuracy of Erikson's observations to raise serious doubts concerning his conclusions that these differences derive somehow only from the anatomical differences between the sexes. What about the enormous multitude of acculturation factors— the toys, the games, the adult expectations, and so forth—that have played a part in shaping the fantasies, the perceptions, and the activities of these ten- to twelve-year-old children? Erikson himself notes that in almost one-third of the subjects the girls constructed "male" configurations and the boys constructed "female" configu-

---

*The reaction of feminists to the latter point of view, however, is understandable since the emphasis on innate differences has almost always been used to prove man's "inherent superiority."

rations. Obviously these were the results of experiential, not anatomical, variations. The point, simply, is that to attempt to derive such differences solely from anatomical or physiological considerations inevitably results in oversimplifications. One must always take into consideration the interaction between these factors and the experiences they encounter in the environment—in time, place, family, and culture.

2. "*Penis envy.*" It is, for example, a massive oversimplification to assume, as Freud did, that the lack of a penis must inevitably be considered as a defect by the female child, in all times and cultures. Clara Thompson (9) and others have quite correctly pointed out that the phenomenon of "penis envy" that Freud observed and described in his women patients was not a universal feminine occurrence but was related to the "culturally underprivileged" position that these women occupied. That this is so is confirmed by what has been happening to this phenomenon as the position of Western women has changed in the past four decades. Not only is it manifesting itself with much lesser intensity than it used to, but more and more psychoanalysts report that they do not even always find evidences of it. Meanwhile, another manifestation has begun to make its appearance with increasing frequency, a phenomenon in men which has been variously described as breast envy, womb envy, and woman envy, and which is derived from men's supposed jealousy of women's ability to bear and suckle children. In the past, when such a reaction was encountered in men, it was assumed to be deeply neurotic,* but now it is beginning to be described as a more "universal" phenomenon. But how is it possible that a clinical genius like Freud would have failed to recognize such a common aspect of male psychology? The answer, of course, is that it was *not* a frequent occurrence in his time, and has become so only as a consequence of the shifting equilibrium between the sexes. The fact is that womb envy, like penis envy, can only be understood by taking into consideration the total field situation in which it appears. The presence or absence of a penis may be regarded by the developing child as an asset *or* a deficit

---

*As might have been expected in an androcentric culture, however, women's envy of men was always assumed to be normal and "natural"!

depending on the nature of the cues that he or she is getting from the environment. When a society places greater value on the birth of a son than on that of a daughter, children in the family become aware of this in a myriad subtle ways; the same is true when little boys are accorded greater freedom of movement and play, and when fathers are accorded greater respect and deference than mothers. In such a society little girls, and later women, will inevitably manifest many indications of penis envy, while indications of woman envy in men will be relatively rare. On the other hand, when these conditions no longer hold true, or become reversed (as has begun to happen in Western society in recent decades), *then we can expect to find that unconscious manifestations of penis envy will begin to diminish, and those of woman envy will begin to increase.*

A male patient of mine—not a homosexual—grew up as the only boy and youngest child in a family of three children. The father was a relatively weak and incompetent person in contrast to the mother, who was a warm, competent, and dominant individual. The two older sisters were also extremely effective and assertive children. Little wonder that my patient recalled as a child strongly wishing he were a girl, and fantasying that the front of his body was smooth and penis-less just like his sisters'! *For his milieu,* his envy-reaction was no less "normal" than the penis envy of the little girl who grows up in a male-centered environment.

In this connection, Helene Deutsch's dismissal of the clitoris as "an inferior organ" in terms of its capability to provide libidinal gratification is a remarkable example of culturally-influenced amblyopia, coming as it does from a woman. The actual fact, as Dickinson (10) has pointed out, is that although "the female organ is minute compared with the male organ . . . the size of its nerves . . . and nerve endings . . . compare strikingly with the same provision for the male. Indeed . . . the glans of the clitoris is demonstrably richer in nerves than the male glans, for the two stems of the dorsalis clitoridis are relatively three to four times as large as the equivalent nerves of the penis . . ." Little wonder that this "inferior organ" enables the orgastically potent female often to have multiple orgasms to every single orgasm of the male!

More recently, in the most definitive article to date on female sexuality in the psychoanalytic literature, Sherfey (11), leaning heavily on the unprecedented and significant research findings of Masters and Johnson,* puts the finishing touch to the myth of clitoral inferiority. Not only is clitoral stimulation capable of producing multiple orgasms to an extent unknown in men (as many as twenty to fifty consecutive orgasms have been recorded within the span of an hour!), but also the average orgastic response in women in generally more prolonged than that of men and just as intense in terms of their muscular capacities.

3. *"Masochism and passivity."* The assumption that normal men are naturally dominant and aggressive, while normal women are naturally submissive and masochistic, is another myth that the changing patterns of relationship between the sexes has begun to dispel. Even the biological evidence has never justified these conclusions. It is well known that among lower animals the female of the species can be fully as vicious and aggressive as the male, while dominance per se, as biologists have long recognized, is not a simple sex-linked trait but depends on a number of variables, including relative size and strength, motivation, previous experiences, social setting, and so forth.**

A variant of this, the effort to justify this myth on the basis of the differences in roles in sexual intercourse, similarly fails to stand up under careful analysis. The common argument advanced here is that in the sexual act it is the male who must be the penetrator, while the woman is merely the recipient, and that the aggressivity of the male and the passivity of the female naturally follow from this.† The error here lies in confusing a *behavioral* phenomenon with a *motivational* one. A male can be a passive and submissive

---

*The researches of Masters and Johnson also explode with finality the fiction of the exitence of a vaginal orgasm distinct from clitoral orgasm. Their studies reveal beyond a doubt that the nature of orgasm in the female is the same regardless of the stimulus that produces it, and consists of rhythmic contractions of extravaginal musculature against the greatly distended circumvaginal venous plexi and vestibular bulbs surround the lower third of the vagina (12).

**According to Harlow (personal communication, 1965), in primates, *all other things being equal,* males tend to be dominant to females. If the female is larger and heavier, however, she may be dominant. In human beings, the significant variables in dominance behavior are much more complex and include social and psychological parameters as well as physical ones.

†Even Erich Fromm, despite his strong cultural orientation, succumbed to this fallacy in his essay on "Sex and Character," *Psychiatry,* VI (1943), 21–32.

penetrator, while a female can be an aggressive and dominant recipient, in the sexual act. Indeed, recent researches (13) indicate that the female genital apparatus during orgasm is extremely active. Receptivity and passivity are not synonymous. It is a striking commentary on the power of a cultural prejudice that both male and female classical Freudians have always assumed that the vagina, as a hollow organ, *had* to be a passive receptacle, although they came to no such conclusions about either the mouth or the anus. "Oral" and "anal" aggression were readily recognized, but the same theoreticians, caught in the meshes of an unconscious common prejudice, were unable to see that, under certain conditions, the vagina, too, could be an aggressively seeking, grasping, holding, or expulsive organ. The analogy between the mouth and the vagina has, of course, been recognized unconsciously by many males in the symbolism of the "dentate vagina," but most psychoanalysts have tended merely to dismiss this as a neurotic construction, without recognizing the important kernel of truth that it contains.

An additional refutation of the myth of "normal feminine masochism" is that women who are passive and submissive in relation to men are *less* apt to be orgastically potent than those who are more assertive, self-confident, and dominant (14).

It may be argued by some that one cannot ignore the impact of fantasy on character formation and that the sexual fantasies of men and women are inevitably different: the male adolescent's fantasies deal with penetration; the female's with presumably anxious fears of being penetrated, and deflorated. The experience of periodic menstruation with its bleeding also is supposed to contribute in some way to an inevitable masochistic inclination in women as compared to men. Perhaps. But here, too, I must caution that the psychological impact of what appear to be simple biological events in men cannot ever be divorced from their sociocultural context. Fantasies of being penetrated *may or may not* be associated with anxiety or masochistic implications. The little girl, relatively early in her life, under conflict-free circumstances, experiences the insertion of objects (or her finger) into her vagina as a pleasurable, not a painful experience. It is man, not woman, who assumes that to experience such penetration is painful and therefore masochistic.

The fact that so many women in our culture are indeed apprehensive about their first sexual experience is not a biological inevitability but the result of a puritanical culture which, in its effort to maintain a completely artificial sexual morality, fills little children, and particularly little girls, with fears of sex as something dirty, sinful, and even dangerous. Even the bleeding of menstruation need not necessarily be anxiety-provoking. I have known a number of adolescent girls—and I am sure there are many—who welcomed their first menstrual period with tremendous elation and excitement and could not wait to tell their parents and friends that at last they had achieved the visible evidence of maturity. The fantasies and self-images of men and women are indeed different—and inevitably so, for both biological and cultural reasons—but these differences do not necessarily lead to sex-linked patterns of masochism or sadism.

4. *"Faulty superego development."* Nowhere does the cultural bias inherent in Freud's views about the nature of women become more apparent than in his bland assumption that women have less adequate superegos than men. (One is reminded of Professor Higgins's plaintive cry in *My Fair Lady:* "Why can't a woman be like a man?") Certainly no objective mid-twentieth-century American behavioral scientist would seriously argue any longer that women inherently have a lesser sense of justice, a greater disposition to envy, weaker social interests, or a lesser capacity for sublimation than men. The record of women in England and America in the past four decades on behalf of social justice and human brotherhood compares more than favorably with that of men.

It is important to note, however, that Freud's views on women were not merely an outgrowth of his position as a nineteenth-century middle European male; they flowed quite logically from his theory about superego development. If they were in error, as they obviously were, his theory of superego development must also be fallacious. It simply cannot be that the development of the superego results only from the resolution of the Oedipus complex, as classical psychoanalytic theory has long held. This is not the place to enter into a detailed dissertation on how the personality phenomenon that Freud designated as superego comes into being, but suffice it to say that it is obviously an acculturation phenomenon that develops from the child's gradual incorporation of the do's and dont's from its environment—beginning from the time the child is first able to comprehend the significance of such interdictions. The impact of this acculturation process is felt by girls as fully and as early as it is by boys. Indeed, the evidence is that since, culturally, little girls are expected to be better behaved than little boys, the pressure of this process is *greater* upon girls than upon boys. As a result, as might be anticipated, females in our culture, at least in their early years, are apt to show evidence of *better* superego development than do males—the very reverse of Freud's theoretical assumption.

THE PROBLEM OF GENDER ROLE

Actually, much of what we have been talking about in this essay revolves around the problem of what modern social psychologists would call "gender role"—that is, what is considered "masculine" or "feminine" behavior. The fact is that gender-role patterns have varied widely in different times and in different cultures. As Opler (15) has put it:

> A Navajo Indian may be a he-man, a gambler, and a philanderer while dressing in bright blouses adorned with jeweled belts, necklaces, and bracelets. French courtiers in the retinues of effete monarchs were equally philanderers, though rouged, powdered, and bedecked with fine lace. The Andaman Islanders like to have the man sit on his wife's lap in fond greetings, and friends and relatives, of the same or opposite sex, greet one another in the same manner after absences, crying in the affected manner of the mid-Victorian woman. Like the Ute, they value premarital sexual experimentation and sexual prowess and technique in any later life period. Obviously, the style of social and sexual behavior is something of an amalgam and is culturally influenced.

Gender role and gender identity, although generally related to the biological sex of a child, actually are not shaped by biological factors but by cultural ones. Once the child's biological ascription is settled, a myriad of culturally defined cues begin to be presented to the developing infant which are designed to shape its gender identity to its assigned sex. Little girls are handled more gently than little boys, are given different toys to play with,* are expected to be quieter and cleaner, are spoken to in different tones, and are addressed in different terms. The little girl who wheedles is spoken of fondly as a "charmer" and a "coquette"; the little boy is told to stop being a baby and to act like a man. The little girl's clothes and hairdos are noticed, complimented, and fussed over. Not so the little boy's; he is more apt to be praised for his agility and courage. The girl is expected to help with "inside" chores (cleaning up, doing dishes); the boy, with "outside" ones (shoveling snow, mowing the lawn). So powerful are these acculturation processes that, as the Hampsons (17) have demonstrated, in certain cases of pseudo-hermaphroditism in which the child's biological sex is mistaken for that of the opposite sex the incorrect gender identity becomes so powerfully established by the age of two or three that it becomes psychologically destructive to the child to try to change it.

What is important to our present thesis, however, is not that this acculturation occurs, but that, as we have seen, its *content* can and does change. What we have been observing in recent decades is a gradual change in certain female gender-role patterns that have previously been traditional in Western culture.

The implications of these changing patterns extend beyond psychoanalytic theory to psychoanalytic therapy. Erich Fromm once observed that a psychoanalyst's value-system would profoundly affect how he would treat a female patient who presented the problem of Nora in Ibsen's *A Doll's House*. If he held to classical psychoanalytical views concerning femininity, he would focus his interpretations upon her "penis envy" and her rejection of the "normal" feminine goals of wifehood and motherhood. On the other hand, if he were a feminist, he would, instead, focus upon her "healthy" rebellion against her husband's infantilization of her and would encourage her to move out of the home as a laudable effort at self-realization. Still another alternative to these two extremes exists, however. One need not assume that motherhood and a fulfilling life in the outside world are incompatible, any more than fatherhood and such a life.

---

*The assumption that all girls "naturally" prefer dolls to boys' toys is not borne out by objective studies (16).

In contrast to men, however, who are *expected* to combine these two aspects of life, women have alternatives now; they may or may not choose to combine them, and the choice is theirs. The task of the analyst is to help them make this choice, freely, without guilt, and in relationship to the realities of their specific life situations.

REFERENCES

1. BETTY FRIEDAN, *The Feminine Mystique* (New York: W. W. Norton, 1963).
2. *Ibid.*, p. 207.
3. MAY ROMM, "Sexuality and Homosexuality in Women," in J. Marmor, ed., *Sexual Inversion: The Multiple Roots of Homosexuality* (New York: Basic Books, 1965), p. 282.
4. ESTHER PETERSON, "Working Women," *Daedalus*, Spring 1964, p. 672.
5. SIGMUND FREUD, "The Psychology of Women," in *New Introductory Lectures on Psycho-analysis* (New York: W. W. Norton, 1933), pp. 153–185.
6. HELENE DEUTSCH, *The Psychology of Women*, Vol. I (New York: Grune & Stratton, 1944), pp. 228 ff.
7. ERIK ERIKSON, "Inner and Outer Space: Reflections on Womanhood," *Daedalus*, Spring 1964, pp. 582–607.
8. *Ibid.*, p. 587.
9. CLARA THOMPSON, "Penis Envy in Women," *Psychiatry*, VI (1943), 123–125.
10. R. L. DICKINSON, *Human Sex Anatomy*, 2nd ed. (Baltimore: Williams & Wilkins, 1949), p. 42.
11. MARY JANE SHERFEY, "The Evolution and Nature of Female Sexuality in Relation to Psychoanalytic Theory," *Journal of the American Psychoanalytic Association*, XIV (1966), 28–128.
12. W. H. MASTERS and VIRGINIA JOHNSON, *Human Sexual Response* (Boston: Little, Brown & Co., 1966).
13. MASTERS and JOHNSON, *op. cit.*
14. A. H. MASLOW, "Self-Esteem (Dominance-Feeling) and Sexuality in Women," *Journal of Social Psychology*, XVI (1942), 259–294.
15. M. OPLER, "Anthropological and Cross-Cultural Aspects of Homosexuality," in Marmor, ed., *Sexual Inversion*, p. 116.
16. MIRRA KOMAROVSKY, *Women in the Modern World* (Boston: Little, Brown & Co., 1953).
17. J. L. HAMPSON and JOAN G. HAMPSON, "The Ontogenesis of Sexual Behavior in Man," in W. C. Young, ed., *Sex and Internal Secretions*, 3rd ed., Vol. II (Baltimore: Williams & Wilkins, 1961), pp. 1401–1432.

19

NEW DIRECTIONS IN PSYCHOANALYTIC THEORY AND THERAPY

(1968)

The panorama of psychiatric thought in the modern era can be divided into three successive major trends. The earliest of these encompassed the somatically-centered theories of the nineteenth century, in which man was conceptualized essentially as a *biological* machine. If disturbances occurred in the behavior of this machine, they were presumed due either to faulty manufacture—a hereditary defect or constitutional weakness—or to some external noxious agent—an injury, germ, or toxin.

Although many psychologists and psychiatrists had begun to question various aspects of this formulation, the major shift away from it, and the beginning of the second trend, occurred with the emergence of Freud's theoretical system at the turn of the century. Freud, without negating the importance of the organism (indeed he placed great stress on its unfolding evolutionary patterns), was the first to lay significant emphasis on the early environmental experiences of the infant and child. His focus, however, was on the intrapsychic reverberations of these experiences and his module was the *individual as a developmental unit*.

Finally, the revolutionary change that has been taking place in psychodynamic thought in the latter half of the twentieth century has been, not the gradual evolution of the Freudian model from a libido-oriented one to an ego-oriented one—although that has been important—but rather a shift from the closed system of the

251

individual model to an *open-system module in which the individual's functioning is always examined in the context of his group or field situation.* Thus, while Freud's conceptual framework was psychodynamic but individual-centered, the emerging newer patterns of psychiatric thinking may be described as psychodynamic but system-centered. In advanced psychoanalytic circles today the focus of psychopathology is no longer being sought—at least to the same degree as formerly—within the individual's psyche, but rather in his system of relationships, his family, his small groups, his community, his society. This does not mean, however, that the valuable understanding acquired during half a century of interest and research in the dynamics of intrapsychic functioning needs to be discarded. It is my conviction that these insights continue to be relevant even as we move on to concern with various other modules of human interaction.

There are no ultimates in science. It is the exciting challenge and eternal frustration of the scientific method that the truth it pursues is an ephemeral will-o'-the-wisp which the pursuer can only approach but never totally grasp. Indeed, even in fields such as physics or chemistry, in which the variables are infinitely more controllable than those of behavioral science can ever hope to be, scientists do not assume that they are ever dealing with ultimate truths. Science is concerned with the amassing, testing, coordinating, and systematizing of data. A scientific hypothesis is considered better or "truer" than another if it fulfills three criteria more effectively than the other. (1) Does it explain all the available data with the least degree of complexity? (Parsimony.) (2) To what extent does it lend itself to experimentation and validation? (Heuristic value.) (3) To what extent does it make it possible to predict future events? (Predictive value.)

Some contemporary approaches to psychodynamic theory satisfy these criteria more adequately than Freud's unwieldy classical metapsychology. Of equal importance is the fact that the constructs which they are beginning to use have dispensed, for the most part, with the highly specialized jargon of cathexes, countercathexes, fused and defused instincts, repetition compulsions, and the like, that have for so long separated psychoanalysis from the rest of the behavioral sciences. The constructs of adaptation, learning, information processing, communication, and systems theory, which modern psychoanalysts are beginning to use, are bringing psychodynamic thinking back into the mainstream of modern psychobiological thought. Some readers might well ask, "That is all very well, but is it *psychoanalysis?*" I am tempted to reply irreverently that the question is an irrelevant one since what really matters is whether or not these approaches, regardless of what names or labels are attached to them, fulfill the criteria of science more effectively than previous ones. In science nothing is sacred except the method of science, and although this method challenges our most cherished beliefs, we must be prepared to trust it. Nevertheless, my response to this emotionally-laden question is that modern psychoanalysts do accept what I believe to be the essence of Freud's great contribution—the recognition that human behavior is motivated; that the nature of this motivation is often largely concealed from awareness; that our personalities are shaped not only by our biological potentials, but also by experiential vicissitudes; that functional disturbances in human cognition, affect, and behavior are the result of contradictory and conflictual inputs or feedbacks; and that early developmental experiences are of particular significance in shaping subsequent perceptions and reactions in adolescence and adulthood. If the corollary question of whether or not they do sufficient honor to Freud were a meaningful one—and basically, as far as science is concerned, it is not—I would argue that they do him greater homage by standing on his giant shoulders and trying to extend his vision than by worshipping blindly at his feet.

Psychoanalysis traditionally has been considered to be three things: a *method* of investigation of thoughts and feelings of which the subject is unaware ("the unconscious"), a *theory* of human personality, and a *technique* of therapy. At this point in history, roughly three-quarters of a century after Freud's initial contributions, the value of his psychoanalytic *method* of investigating "unconscious" mental processes remains unquestioned. No other approach to the understanding of what goes on *at a psychological level* in the "black box" of the human information-processing apparatus has been able to equal the psychoanalytic method of open-ended verbal communication ("free association") and painstaking exploration of dreams, fantasies, parapraxes, and the like. It is my conviction that when the final chapter of the history of psychiatry is written, the development of this methodological tool will be recognized as having been Freud's greatest contribution.

However, classical psychoanalysis as a *theory* of human behavior has not equally withstood the test of time; but this statement requires qualification. I do not wish to imply that all of Freud's views have become valueless. Certain of his basic constructs, such as those of conflict, repression, transference, and the "unconscious," still constitute an extremely effective foundation for an understanding of human behavior and psychopathology *despite the fact that the data upon which they were based can be dealt with just as effectively within other frames of reference, such as those of communication theory or learning theory.* What has become obsolete has been the cumbersome metapsychological superstructure that Freud erected upon these fundamental concepts—notably his theory of instincts, of libido, of the tripartite structure of the psyche, and of psychic energy. This "mythology" of psychoanalysis, as Freud once called his theory of instincts, has been rendered untenable by newer developments and findings in the behavioral sciences.

Even more regrettable is the fact that the high promises once held forth by psychoanalysis as a *technique* of *therapy* have failed to materialize. In retrospect, and with the benefit of hindsight, we ought not be surprised at this. Freud's method arose primarily out of his efforts *to understand* the meaning and origins of his patients' disturbances. There is no good reason a priori why a technique of investigation necessarily should be at the same time a good method of therapy. I suspect that it was largely the historical accident that Freud was attempting to earn a living as a psychiatric practitioner that drove him to utilize his investigative tool simultaneously as a therapeutic instrument. Indeed, compared to the then existent crude techniques of direct suggestion, hypnosis, electrotherapy, and repression, Freud's method of *involving* himself with the patient and the patient's life problems did have much to offer. Moreover, the fact that he brought elements of rational understanding and organization into an area that hitherto had been full of vast confusion lent a certain persuasiveness to the nineteenth-century rationalistic expectation that if the patient could but understand what his symptoms meant and from whence they came, this in itself would be enough to cure him.

Today, we have learned the difficult lesson that rational understanding alone is not enough; that people can understand why they behave in certain ways and yet be unable to alter their unsatisfactory patterns. The problem of modifying behavior has many parameters other than that of cognitive awareness (Marmor, 1962a, 1966a).

Freud's requirement that the patient appear daily at the therapist's office and open his heart and mind to him without holding anything back inevitably results in a powerful intensification of relationship between the patient and the help-giving person. Little wonder that Freud said in later years that although his initial problem had been one of getting patients to come to him, his eventual difficulty was in getting them to leave him. Kubie (1967) has pointed out that in his experience, under current analytic practices, the vast majority of analytic patients are left with unresolved transference patterns in relation to their analysts. In an earnest effort to deal with this problem, he began casting about for devices that might facilitate the "dissolution" of the transference, and ended by suggesting that the problem might be solved by a cautious socializing with patients during the termination phase, or by the utilization of a second therapist at that time, either alone or conjointly. What Kubie refused to see, however, was the fact that the problem that he was describing was inherent in the therapeutic method employed, and *was an iatrogenic artifact*.

The patient who seeks psychiatric therapy always brings with him certain basic distortions in his perceptions and feelings. These have been shaped and "learned" in the course of his early personality development in relationship to the significant people in his life. These distortions, which are the essence of the transference phenomenon, were not invented by Freud; they exist not only in the psychoanalyst's office, but in every significant human relationship. Freud's great contribution in this area was that he not only recognized transference as a factor of paramount importance, but also identified its historical sources and discovered its value in the therapeutic transaction. One of the unique aspects of psychoanalytically oriented psychotherapies is that transference reactions are consciously and deliberately used for the purpose of confronting the patient with the unreality of his interpersonal perceptions and reactions. The ultimate goal of such interpretations and confrontations is to enable the patient to become more realistic and adaptive in his interpersonal relationships. An important consequence of this should be that the patient ultimately perceives himself as more mature and is able to interact with authority figures with self-respect and on a greater basis of equality. The dissolution of the transference, therefore, should mean that the patient terminates his analysis with more comfortable feelings *not only toward the analyst but toward all authority figures.*

As I have indicated, however, the classical psychoanalytic relationship, by its very nature, tends to foster rather than resolve this core problem. Especially when the analyst adopts the model of the "neutral mirror" and carefully protects his "analytic incognito," these regressive patterns in the patient are enormously magnified. Under such circumstances, the patient tends to "perceive" the analyst as an olympian, omniscient, God-like person in comparison to whom the patient feels less adequate than ever (Marmor, 1953). Many classical analysts believe that this regressive reaction is a basic prerequisite for good analytic therapy, and have laid down the dictum—one that Freud himself never formulated—that no psychoanalytic procedure is adequate if it has not produced in the patient a regressive "transference neurosis," which then has to be "worked through."

There is an intriguing parallel between this transaction of classical psychoanalytic technique and that which takes place between Zen masters and their pupils. In the Zen relationship the master's impersonality, strictness, and frustrating responses ultimately provoke in his pupil a regressive state akin to depersonalization. The "ego boundaries" of the Zen pupil then seem to dissolve and he experiences a sense of "oneness with the universe" that leads him to the longed-for state of "satori" (insight). In classical psychoanalysis, the patient asks questions and also is met with silence, reaches out for a relationship and also is rebuffed. The progressive frustration and helplessness that this kind of relationship produces ultimately provoke a similar kind of regressive reaction (Marmor, 1962b).

When, over the years, progressive psychoanalysts have argued that a more human kind of transaction seemed to produce better therapeutic results, the argument of the classicists has always been that such results were imperfect as compared with the profound characterological transformation that presumably emerged from the working through of the transference regression. I can only say, after many years of experience with both techniques, that this conviction on the part of classical psychoanalysts is more an article of faith than a matter of fact. The therapeutic results of the classical psychoanalyic method simply do not warrant this assumption.

Where, then, are the newer system-centered psychodynamic concepts leading us, therapeutically speaking?

At the level of individual therapy, the emphasis is changing from one in which the therapist does something to the patient by "analyzing" him, to an examination of the nature of the reciprocal interaction between therapist and patient. The nature and quality of this transactional system is now seen as the crucial factor in achieving therapeutic progress, rather than the former assumption that what was crucial was the nature of the repetitive insights that the analyst gave to the patient. As a consequence, the therapist is no longer viewed as a neutral, impersonal conveyor of interpretations, but rather as an active human participant in a verbal and nonverbal, affective as well as cognitive, reciprocal interaction in which *both* participants "change" over the course of time. In this view the personality of the therapist is seen as an important factor which needs to be evaluated and understood just as fully as that of the patient (Strupp, 1968). Moreover, in recognition of the fact that both patient and therapist, as open systems, are products of their surrounding media, an understanding of class differences, value systems, group-linked verbal and behavioral patterns and the like becomes highly relevant and indeed essential for optimal therapeutic effectiveness (Minuchin, 1968; Kluckhohn, 1956).

Within this context, modern psychoanalytic therapists in increasing numbers have been breaking away from blind adherence to many of the traditional technical and ritualistic demands of classical analysis. The use of the couch, for example, is recognized as a tool which may be useful and necessary under some circumstances, not under others. There has been increasing experimentation with modifying the frequency of visits, also with interruptions of therapy and

irregularity of appointments to see whether the finding in learning
theory experiments that intermittent reinforcements of learning are
more effective than regularly scheduled ones are applicable to efforts
at modification of human behavior (Marmor, 1964). The long-standing shibboleth about the necessity for the patient's making a financial
"sacrifice" in order for therapy to be successful has faded away
in the light of experience with low-cost psychoanalytic clinics. The
application of psychodynamic insights to various other modifications
of therapeutic approach such as crisis-oriented therapies and short-
term therapeutic approaches has also become more widespread.

The system-orientation of modern psychodynamics has led also
to an increasing interest in the possibility of dealing with other
factors within the patient's transactional life-system. Child analysts
recognized early that psychoanalysis of the individual child was often
an unnecessarily long, arduous, and circuitous approach to helping
the child, and that more expeditious and effective help could be
forthcoming by working with the child's parents, whose participation
and influence in the child's life-space, after all, were considerably
greater than those of the analyst could possibly be. This led to
a concern with the dynamics of the entire family system, and in
recent years family therapy has become an area of interest for
increasing numbers of psychoanalysts who deal with children and
adolescents. Similarly, conjoint therapy of marital partners in conflict
has begun to be employed, in contrast to the traditional approach
of separate therapists treating each partner without communicating
with each other. Although many of these changes are now taken
for granted, it cannot be strongly enough emphasized how great
a break this kind of approach represents from the early classical
psychoanalytic techniques. The student who entered psychoanalytic
training in the 1930's was strongly impressed with the dangers implicit
in any contact with a family member, even over the telephone,
as though somehow the purity of the analyst's relationship with
his patient would thereby be contaminated. As a consequence, the
valuable assistance that could have been provided by enlisting the
help of cooperative relatives was foregone, as well as the ability
to correct some of the distortions inevitably inherent in the patient's
perceptions of his milieu. Often, too, under those circumstances,
the refusal of the analyst to have anything to do with the relatives

unnecessarily created in them feelings of distrust and hostility that were destructive to the patient's progress.

I must emphasize here that such opening up of technical procedures to include other people in the patient's life-system has not meant a lessening of concern with individual intrapsychic mechanisms. On the contrary, a proper awareness of the transactional operations in the patient's life-system is extremely helpful in enabling the psychoanalytically trained psychiatrist to achieve a more sophisticated understanding of his patient's psychodynamics.

Similar considerations have played a role in the development of analytic group psychotherapy. Although family therapy was extremely useful in the problems involving children and adolescents, and in marital conflicts, it did not lend itself as well to problems of the individual adult with emotional difficulties. In the therapies of such individuals, analytic group psychotherapy offered an additional dimension which could supplement or at times replace individual therapy as might be indicated. As a result of the transference aspects of the dyadic process, the therapist becomes directly aware of the way the patient relates to authority surrogates, but many other aspects of the patient's interpersonal life—his behavior toward colleagues, juniors, members of the same and opposite sex, and the like—are presented through the spyglass of the patient's own perceptions and are consequently subject to considerable distortion which the analyst may or may not be able correctly to evaluate. In a group situation, on the other hand, the therapist has the opportunity to perceive these other transference patterns directly, and thus to evaluate the patient's perceptions of them more objectively.

As analysts have become increasingly aware of how aspects of the external environment are dynamically interwoven into the patient's intrapsychic reactions, there has been growing concern also with understanding the cultural milieu of the patient, and the technical demands that this imposes on therapeutic method. Spiegel (1959) was one of the first to call attention to the effect of class differences on transference-countertransference problems. Hollingshead and Redlich (1958) have noted that class position plays an important role in determining even what is defined as psychiatric illness, and whether or not psychodynamic psychotherapy will be prescribed for the patient.

The relationship of schizophrenic disturbances to cultural milieu and socioeconomic levels has been frequently noted. More relevant to our psychoanalytic interests, however, are the fascinating studies of Lidz (1963), Wynne and Singer (1963), Jackson (1957), and their various co-workers in demonstrating the way in which communication difficulties, ambiguities, and contradictions among family members of schizophrenics contribute to the development of schizophrenic disturbances.

As psychoanalysts have broadened their awareness of the relevance of the nature of the social system to individual psychopathology, their interest in the institutional structures of society has also grown. The educational system, employment opportunities, racial segregation and prejudice, housing and the like are no longer considered matters just of sociological concern. Their effects on personality development, ego strengths, social competence, and mental health have become increasingly apparent. Some of the ways in which psychoanalytic understanding is beginning to be applied to this growing field of community psychiatry have been ably documented by Duhl and Leopold (1968).

The interests of modern psychoanalysts have not been limited to psychosocial areas. In the fields of ethology (Masserman, 1968), neurophysiology (Weinstein, 1968), psychophysiological medicine (Engel, 1968), and psychopharmacology (Mandell, 1968), there are numerous evidences of new levels of both theoretical and clinical sophistication. Similar refinements are taking place in the application of psychoanalytic insights to the areas of sociology and anthropology (Scotch and Levine, 1968), the creative arts (Edel, 1968), law (Freedman, 1968), and political science (Rogow, 1968).

What does the long-range future hold for psychoanalysis and psychoanalysts? I believe it is inevitable that its traditional forms will continue to be altered in the years to come (Marmor, 1966b). Psychoanalytic theory will not only move further away from Freudian metapsychology but will gradually begin employing more and more of the common language of the other behavioral sciences: the language of adaptation, learning theory, communications, and information theory. The beginning efforts to find certain theoretical common denominators that cut across all organic systems will undoubtedly continue at an enhanced rate, and the search for uniform theories of behavior, as encompassed within general systems theory, will go on. We can also anticipate new breakthroughs in neurophysiology and neuropharmacology, the implications of which will have to be integrated with psychodynamic theory.

As mental health care becomes more available to all who need it under the rapidly burgeoning mental health center programs, our society will be forced to dispense with the wasteful and inequitable luxury of having a highly trained specialist devote most of his professional life to the treatment of a handful of middle- or upper-class people while the vast majority of those in need of psychiatric care are consigned to second-class treatment or none at all. Psychoanalytically trained psychiatrists will continue increasingly to utilize their specialized skills in the various modifications of therapy in order to help greater numbers of people. The distinction between psychoanalysis and psychodynamic psychotherapy will continue to fade away. Ultimately there will evolve only one psychotherapy which will rest, as Knight once predicted, "on a basic science of dynamic psychology" (Knight, 1949, p. 101). Psychoanalysis itself as a formal, technical procedure will become more and more restricted, I suspect, to its investigative and training potentials; that is to say, it will be used either for purposes of research in unique and unusual problems of psychopathology, or it will be employed on a limited scale for the purpose of training psychiatrists to use it as an investigative tool.

As psychodynamic theory and practice, with the assistance of psychoanalysts, become more and more integrated into psychiatric residency programs (Marmor, 1961), we may anticipate that the current trend of diminishing numbers of applicants to psychoanalytic training institutes will continue. Conceivably, in time, the independent psychoanalytic institute—which after all was a kind of anachronism forced upon psychoanalysis by the original antagonism to it in organized medical and academic circles—may disappear from the scene and its role be taken over by postgraduate training in medical schools, universities, and residency training programs. Psychiatrists with special interests in intensive psychotherapy will probably continue to seek personal analyses for themselves, although in all likelihood the rather rigid requirements of the "didactic analysis" in terms of minimum hours, frequency of visits, and so forth, which characterize contemporary psychoanalytic training, will become modified in terms of techniques that are more flexibly oriented to the actual clinical needs of each individual psychiatrist-in-training. Psychotherapy with other human beings, regardless of what form it takes, is one of the most emotionally and ethically demanding functions that one human being can take on in relationship to another. Its seductive potentials as well as its stresses are far greater than those in almost any other field of therapeutic practice, and I firmly believe that personal intensive psychotherapy aimed at removing, insofar as possible, the personal weaknesses, blind spots, and emotional immaturities of the would-be psychotherapist should be an essential aspect of his training.

The problem of whether or not this kind of intensive psychotherapeutic practice should be confined only to members of the medical profession will continue to be a knotty one. My guess is that in the years to come, as lines of clinical practice become increasingly blurred, it will become a greater source of controversy rather than a lesser one. There is ample justification for those who argue that, since mind and body are one, a thorough knowledge of both is essential for those who would deal with disorders of the human mind. Certainly as our knowledge of how to integrate the uses of various drugs with intensive psychotherapeutic approaches increases, the value of a medical degree in this area of functioning cannot be dispensed with. And yet, assuming that a medically trained person has ruled out any causative somatic factors, can one honestly argue that *competently trained* nonmedical psychotherapists cannot, under usual circumstances, perform a psychotherapeutic function for most people equally well? In any event, the combination of shortage of adequately trained personnel plus the enormous psychiatric needs of our complex society will put ever growing pressure on the dispensers of mental health care to widen the circle of those who provide it. Indeed many are already pointing out that even present paramedical personnel—psychologists, psychiatric social workers, psychiatric nurses, and so on—will not be enough to provide sufficient care and that some kind of training for specially qualified laity may be essential in the future. Perhaps one path out of this difficult dilemma may ultimately lie in some variation of Kubie's creative suggestion (1954) which has never been given an adequate trial: the formation of a new specialty of medical psychotherapy which will dispense with much of the prolonged medical training which psychiatrists now must undertake and enable them to focus more thoroughly on only those aspects of physiology, pharmacology, psychology, sociology, and anthropology which are relevant to their future work.

There will be those who argue that this apparently inevitable dilution of the intensive one-to-one involvement in psychotherapy will constitute a tragic loss; that the uniquely humanistic aspect of devoting one's life, regardless of cost, to the improvement of another human being ought never to be sacrificed. There is indeed an important value here which must be cherished, but may we not succeed in finding other ways of retaining it? I cannot believe that it is any less humanistic to be concerned about many individuals than about only a few. We have the opportunity in the years ahead to broaden our humanistic horizons to a scale never before possible in human history. This is a challenge worth rising to; surely our generation of psychoanalysts and those who will follow us cannot fail to meet it!

REFERENCES

DUHL, L. J., AND LEOPOLD, R. L. "Relationship of Psychoanalysis with Social Agencies." In J. Marmor (ed.), *Modern Psychoanalysis*, New York: Basic Books, 1968. Pp. 577–597.

EDEL, L. "Psychoanalysis and the 'Creative' Arts." In J. Marmor (ed.), *Modern Psychoanalysis*, 1968. Pp. 626–641.

ENGEL, G. L. "The Psychoanalytic Approach to Psychosomatic Medicine." In J. Marmor (ed.), *Modern Psychoanalysis*, 1968. Pp. 251–273.

FREEDMAN, L. Z. "Psychoanalysis, Delinquency, and the Law." In J. Marmor (ed.), *Modern Psychoanalysis*, 1968. Pp. 642–662.

HOLLINGSHEAD, A. B., and REDLICH, F. C. *Social Class and Mental Illness.* New York: Wiley, 1958.

JACKSON, D. D. "The Question of Family Homeostasis." *Psychiatric Quarterly Supplement*, 31 (1957), 79–90.

KLUCKHOHN, FLORENCE. "Dominant and Variant Value Orientations." In C. Kluckhohn and H. A. Murray (eds.), *Personality in Nature, Society, and Culture.* New York: Alfred A. Knopf, 1956. Pp. 342–357.

KNIGHT, R. P. "A Critique of the Present Status of the Psychotherapies." *Bulletin of the New York Academy of Medicine*, 25 (1949), 100–114.

KUBIE, L. S. "The Pros and Cons of a New Profession: A Doctorate in Medical Psychology." *Texas Reports in Biological Medicine*, 12 (1954), 692–737.

KUBIE, L. S. "Unsolved Problem Concerning the Resolution of the Transference:

Who Can and Who Cannot Resolve It?" Presented at the annual meeting of the American Psychoanalytic Association, Detroit, May 1967.

LIDZ, T. *The Family and Human Adaptation*. New York: International Universities Press, 1963.

MANDELL, A. J. "Psychoanalysis and Psychopharmacology." In J. Marmor (ed.), *Modern Psychoanalysis*, 1968. Pp. 274–292.

MARMOR, J. "The Feeling of Superiority: An Occupational Hazard in the Practice of Psychotherapy." *American Journal of Psychiatry*, 110 (1953), Pp. 370–376. (Chapter 21, this volume.)

MARMOR, J. "Psychoanalysis and Psychiatric Practice." In J. H. Masserman (ed.), *Current Psychiatric Therapies*. New York: Grune & Stratton, 1961. Pp. 131–138. (Chapter 14, this volume.)

MARMOR, J. "Psychoanalytic Therapy as an Educational Process." In J. H. Masserman (ed.), *Science and Psychoanalysis*, Vol. 7. New York: Grune & Stratton, 1962. Pp. 286–299. (a). (Chapter 15, this volume.)

MARMOR, J. "A Reevaluation of Certain Aspects of Psychoanalytic Theory and Practice." In L. Salzman and J. H. Masserman (eds.), *Modern Concepts of Psychoanalysis*. New York: Philosophical Library, 1962. Pp. 189–205. (b).

MARMOR, J. "Psychoanalytic Therapy and Theories of Learning." In J. H. Masserman (ed.), *Science and Psychoanalysis*, Vol. 7. New York: Grune & Stratton, 1964. Pp. 265–279. (b). (Chapter 16, this volume.)

MARMOR, J. "The Nature of the Psychotherapeutic Process." In G. L. Usdin (ed.), *Psychoneurosis and Schizophrenia*. Philadelphia: Lippincott, 1966. Pp. 66–75. (a). (Chapter 23, this volume.)

MARMOR, J. "Psychoanalysis at the Crossroads." In J. H. Masserman (ed.), *Science and Psychoanalysis*, Vol. 10. New York: Grune & Stratton, 1966. Pp. 1–9. (b). (Chapter 17, this volume.)

MASSERMAN, J. "The Biodynamic Roots of Psychoanalysis." In J. Marmor (ed.), *Modern Psychoanalysis*, 1968. Pp. 189–224.

MINUCHIN, S. "Psychoanalytic Therapies and the Low Socioeconomic Population." In J. Marmor (ed.), *Modern Psychoanalysis*, 1968. Pp. 532–550.

ROGOW, A. A. "Psychiatry, History, and Political Science." In J. Marmor (ed.), *Modern Psychoanalysis*, 1968. Pp. 663–691.

SCOTCH, N. A., and LEVINE, S. "The Import of Psychoanalysis on Sociology and Anthropology." In J. Marmor (ed.), *Modern Psychoanalysis*, 1968. Pp. 598–625.

SPIEGEL, J. P. "Some Cultural Aspects of Transference and Countertransference." In J. H. Masserman (ed.), *Science and Psychoanalysis*, Vol. 2. New York: Grune & Stratton, 1959. Pp. 160–182.

STRUPP, H. H. "Psychoanalytic Therapy of the Individual." In J. Marmor (ed.), *Modern Psychoanalysis*, 1968. Pp. 293–342.

WEINSTEIN, E. A. "Symbolic Neurology and Psychoanalysis." In J. Marmor (ed.), *Modern Psychoanalysis*, 1968. Pp. 225–250.

WYNNE, L. C., and SINGER, M. T. "Thought Disorder and Family Relations of Schizophrenics." *American Medical Association Archives of General Psychiatry*, 9 (1963), 191–198.

20

LIMITATIONS OF FREE ASSOCIATION
(1970)

One of the most sacred tenets in the psychoanalytic tradition—one to which I subscribed unquestioningly during most of my professional life—is that regardless of what other limitations might exist in the method of psychoanalysis, the technique of free association was without a doubt the best and most dependable avenue that had yet been devised for bringing into consciousness the unconscious sources of the patient's neurotic difficulties. This conviction rested on certain fundamental cornerstones of psychoanalytic thought—the concepts of psychic determinism, repression, and resistance. The basic assumptions involved were that psychic processes are not capricious in nature and are subject to the fundamental laws of cause and effect. Therefore, bypassing the defensive resistances of the patient by having him say everything that went through his mind meant that whatever he was unwittingly repressing would sooner or later come into consciousness like a cork bobbing to the surface of water and then could be articulated.

Actually, this is often the case and it can hardly be denied that the method of free association has given us unique insights into the roots and meanings of men's fantasies and parapraxic distortions. Nevertheless, the conviction has slowly grown upon me, in the course of over 30 years of clinical experience, that there are serious limitations to the free-associational method that have gone largely unrecognized and which have an important bearing on certain shortcomings of classical psychoanalysis *as a therapeutic method.*

One of the clinical facts that has forced itself strongly upon my awareness has been the repeated observation of people who have undergone prolonged and painstaking analyses and yet have been left with clear-cut residual patterns of narcissism, exploitativeness, social aggression, rigidity, compulsiveness, and other similar characterological attitudes. One might reasonably explain this away in many patients on the basis of the fact that either the analyst or the patient had decided to give up the work short of an optimum goal; but when one sees such patterns also present in analysts who have undergone thoroughgoing and demanding didactic analyses, the former explanation no longer sounds convincing. The suspicion then begins to grow that perhaps there is something in the method itself that in some cases, at least, is failing to get at some of these fundamental personality patterns.

In considering this problem, one is reminded of Ferenczi's reproaching his analyst, Freud, for not having adequately analyzed his (Ferenczi's) repressed hostility. It will be recalled that Freud referred to this incident in his paper on "Analysis Terminable and Interminable" in the following words:

> The man who had been analyzed adopted an antagonistic attitude to his analyst and reproached him for having neglected to complete the analysis. "The analyst," he said, "ought to have known and to have taken account of the fact that a transference-relation could never be merely positive; he ought to have considered the possibilities of a negative transference." The analyst justified himself by saying that, at the time of the analysis, there was no sign of a negative transference. But even supposing he had failed to observe some slight indication of it . . . it was still doubtful, he thought, whether he would have been able to activate a psychical theme or . . . "complex," by merely indicating it to the patient, *so long as it was not at that moment an actuality to him* [italics mine]. Such activation would certainly have necessitated real unfriendly behavior on the analyst's part. (1).

Here we see one of the basic shortcomings in the method of free association; a shortcoming, it seems to me, that has not been adequately recognized in the theoretical preconceptions that have surrounded it. *The fact is that the patient cannot report, even by the method of free association, that which has never actually registered itself on his perceptions, consciously or unconsciously.* In his *Autobiographical Study*, Freud stated that the free-associational method "achieved what was expected of it, namely, the bringing into consciousness of the *repressed material which was held back by the resistances*" (2) [italics mine]. Clearly then, if material has never been registered and therefore is not repressed, the free-associational method will not bring it into consciousness. The importance of this fact, as we shall see, is that this may apply to some of the most fundamental aspects of the patient's character structure.

A second basic assumption about the method of free association that Freud explicitly advanced was that it "guarantees to a great extent that . . . nothing will be introduced into it by the expectations of the analyst" (2). Clinical experience has demonstrated that this simply is not so and that the "free" associations of the patient are strongly influenced by the values and expectations of the therapist. As I have stated elsewhere:

> These inevitably become communicated to our patients in what we choose or do not choose to interpret, in the kinds of questions we ask, in what we implicitly approve of as "healthy" or focus upon as "unhealthy" and even in our nonverbal mannerisms. In face-to-face transactions the expression on the therapist's face, a questioning glance, a lift of the eyebrows, a barely perceptible shake of the head or shrug of the shoulder all act as significant cues to the patient. But even *behind* the couch, our "uh-huhs" as well as our silences, the interest or the disinterest reflected in our tone of voice or our shifting posture all act like subtle radio signals influencing the patient's responses, reinforcing some responses and discouraging others. (3)

That this actually occurs has been confirmed experimentally by numerous observers (4–6).

As a result, depending on the point of view of the psychoanalyst, patients of every psychoanalytic school tend, *under free association,* "to bring up precisely the kind of phenomenological data which confirm the theories and interpretations of their analysts! Thus each theory tends to be self-validating. Freudians elicit material about the Oedipus complex and castration anxiety, Adlerians about masculine strivings and feelings of inferiority, Horneyites about idealized images, Sullivanians about disturbed interpersonal relationships, etc. The fact is that in so complex a transaction as the psychoanalytic therapeutic process, the impact of patient and therapist upon each other, and particularly of the latter upon the former, is an unusually profound one" (3).

Freud himself was not unaware of this fact. In the same article in which he asserts that free association "guarantees . . . that . . . nothing will be introduced . . . by the expectations of the analyst" he states: "We must, however, bear in mind that free association is not really free. The patient remains under the influence of the analytic situation. We shall be justified in assuming that nothing will occur to him that has not some reference to that situation" (2). What Freud did not realize was that the nonverbal *expectations and values* of the analyst, as revealed in all the subtle ways to which I referred earlier, are a basic part of the analytic situation.

To return to my basic theme, the significant fact that has been overlooked in most psychoanalytic theory is that *material of which the patient is unconscious does not necessarily always reside in the patient's "unconscious."* There are many aspects of a patient and his character structure that he has never repressed because he has never been aware of them, even subliminally. This is particularly true of characterological attitudes, which, as has been pointed out by countless analysts beginning with Wilhelm Reich, are usually experienced as ego-syntonic by the patient.

It might be argued that such patterns always will emerge behaviorally in the transference relationship with the analyst; indeed many of them often do and thus become subject to interpretation and confrontation. However, one must not forget that the relationship to the analyst is a special kind of relationship. The analyst is a help-giving, prestigious, parental surrogate whom the patient is usually eager to please and to whom he frequently relates on the basis of the expectations that are communicated within the structure of their transaction. Thus, a patient who is always reasonably objective and cooperative in working with an analyst may be quite another kind of person entirely in working with colleagues or subordinates *and yet be totally unaware of this.* Such characterological contradictions may never be brought out in the analytic transaction itself unless the patient's attitudes actually involve him in objective difficulties with other people. Moreover, even if they do involve him in such difficulties, he may not have the slightest perception of *why* this is happening and neither free association nor his transference behavior within the analytic situation may shed any light on the matter.

An analytic colleague (G. Sayer, personal communication, 1967) reported a case that beautifully highlights this point. A female patient with whom he worked for a number of years was doing extremely well in the analysis but continued to report interpersonal difficulties which seemed to be totally unprovoked by her. Baffled, the analyst finally decided to put her into group therapy. Within a few sessions the mystery was solved. The woman, who in the dyadic relationship with the analyst had been a "perfect patient," utilizing free association easily and continuously, was observed in the group situation to be a controlling, dominating female who talked incessantly and found it difficult to listen quietly to the others in the group! The qualities that had made her a good patient in the analytic situation—in which she was expected to do all the talking and the analyst all the listening—were the very ones that were creating difficulties for her in other interpersonal relationships in which the rules of the "game" were different. Yet she was quite unaware of this pattern in herself and it never came up in her free associations. Thus certain significant information about the patient may never be brought into the analysis no matter how optimal the use of free association may be within the dyadic analytic relationship.

Indeed, classical psychoanalytic technique has tended to exclude such information by its interdiction of contact with other significant people in the patient's life. However, any analyst who is willing to be "flexible" enough to have interviews with such "significant others" cannot but be struck by the profoundly different way in which an identical situation often may be reported by such an other, in contrast to the patient's version. By exposing himself to such additional sources of information, the analyst's view of his patient is considerably enriched and he is enabled to bring into the context of his work with his patient material that might otherwise never be touched upon.

In making this point, I do not wish to imply that insight alone—whether "cognitive" or "emotional"—is the central factor in the psychotherapeutic process of the psychoanalytic method. I recognize—and have stressed elsewhere (3,7)—that the quality of the *relationship* between analyst and patient is at least as important, and perhaps even more so. This includes such factors as the patient's expectations, his faith and trust in the analyst, his unconscious identification with the analyst (what Strachey has called the "dosed introjection of good objects"), and the corrective emotional experiences (Alexander) that he has in the course of the analysis as a result of the analyst responding differently to him than the significant others of his childhood did. Granting all of this, the fact remains that unless all of the basic maladaptive defenses and reactions of the patient are brought into the analytic situation and into the patient's field of awareness, there is a strong likelihood that those which are not may remain unaltered. My thesis is that the method of free association alone, in an exclusively dyadic relationship with an analyst, may not be sufficient to accomplish our therapeutic objective.

What does all of this add up to? Does it mean that free association is without value? By no means! To draw such a conclusion would be to completely misinterpret the impact of this communication. Free association is still the best methodological tool we have—our Royal Road—for exploring a person's subjective feelings and perceptions and for bringing into awareness that which he has repressed. It has brought us invaluable insights into the nature and meaning of man's dreams, fantasies, and parapraxes. As a technique of investigation it still remains one of the brightest stars in Freud's shining galaxy of achievements.

What I am endeavoring to call attention to, however, are its limitations when it is depended on as an *exclusive* instrument in a dyadic psychotherapeutic procedure. What follows from this is that it is of utmost importance that the psychotherapist retain the utmost flexibility in his therapeutic techniques in order to maximize every possibility of bringing to light all facets of his patient's characterological problems. This includes not only the willingness to glean information by interviewing significant others in his patient's life, but also the willingness and ability to alter the therapeutic field itself from an exclusively dyadic one to others such as conjoint marital, family, or group, *if or as it seems indicated.* Within these varied field models other aspects of the patient's transference distortions and behavioral patterns—toward siblings, subordinates, peers, and members of the same and opposite sex—may be brought into play in ways that often do not emerge at all in the exclusively dyadic analytic situation. These comments should not be misinterpreted as advocating an indiscriminate form of "shotgun therapy" utilizing all kinds of techniques for all cases. The therapist, with his psychodynamic knowledge, has the responsibility of deciding which techniques, in which cases, *will best serve his analytic objectives.* My plea is only that he not feel restricted, by virtue of his self-image as an analyst, from being as flexible as his patients' problems require.

In terms of modern field and communication theory, we must recognize that *any* change in the field situation is apt to change both the input and the output of the analytic transaction. Classical analysts themselves have implicitly recognized this when they occasionally recommend a second analysis with a different analyst or with an analyst of the other sex on the grounds that a different kind of transference will thus develop. When Freud said in the Ferenczi case that "activation" of the negative transference would "have necessitated real unfriendly behavior on the analyst's part," he was also recognizing that the real behavior of the analyst plays a role in determining what kind of unconscious material will emerge. Ferenczi's setting of a termination date in order to mobilize separation anxiety and Alexander's alterations in frequency or duration of interviews were such efforts to influence the patient's "free" associations and bring certain kinds of unconscious material into the forefront of the analytic transaction. For many years I have made a practice of almost never terminating an analysis with the patient on the couch. To do so, I am convinced, is to leave untouched important transference reactions which emerge when the patient is forced to look directly at the analyst after being on the couch for several years.

From such modifications within the dyadic pattern, the introduction of significant others into the transaction between the patient and analyst in order to heighten or bring out other kinds of transference patterns is not such a revolutionary or "unanalytic" procedure as might be thought. Recently, a young analyst, a member of one of the constituent societies of the American Psychoanalytic Association, was turned down for membership in that national association on the grounds that his submitted cases included situations in which he had put his analytic patients into group therapy to supplement his continuing dyadic work with them. His rationale was that although his patients were doing quite well in their analyses, he wished to see whether other transference patterns might emerge in the group relationships that he might then work through with them dyadically. This is precisely what happened, but the august elders of the Board of Professional Standards decided that this constituted an improper modification of psychoanalytic technique and ordered this very competent analyst to take another analytic case and bring it to termination under supervision without utilizing any such "improprieties." Only then would his application be reconsidered. It seems to me that this kind of official reaction confuses the essence of psychoanalysis with a set of narrow, ritualistic formalities. As Alexander has put it, this is "a deification of technique as an aim in itself, as the essence of psychoanalysis, instead of making technique a servant of its goals" (8). If an essential goal of psychoanalysis is broadening the patient's understanding of his unconscious defenses and resistances, then we must seek to identify what is unconscious by whatever means we can. Since, as I have shown, what is unconscious to the patient is not always within his "unconscious," we cannot depend upon free association alone to achieve this analytic objective. What this analyst was attempting to do was to *broaden the field of his analytic work* with his patient, in order to uncover more of what was unconscious than the dyadic free-associational technique alone had been able to do. He should have been commended for this rather than censured!

Let us be honest with ourselves. Although it has been a longstanding shibboleth in psychodynamic circles that the formal method of psychoanalysis is the ultimate and best psychotherapeutic weapon at our disposal if we are aiming at really deep characterological changes, many of us who have utilized this method for years cannot but be aware of the fact that our therapeutic intentions have often outstripped our actual achievements. The *goals* of psychoanalytic therapy have indeed been superior to that of other techniques. The psychoanalyst is not content to achieve symptomatic improvement—he aims at nothing less than a major characterological overhaul, ending in "genitality" and full emotional maturity. Yet over and over again we have seen a situation occurring that is typified in the well-known ironic riddle which psychoanalysts themselves often bandy about among themselves:

QUESTION: "What happens when you analyze a schmoe?"

ANSWER: "You get an analyzed schmoe."

The limitations of classical psychoanalytic therapy have not been in intent but in technique. A method that restricts itself strictly to a dyadic relationship, utilizing free association as its major tool, will indeed uncover a great deal—far more, I am convinced, than any nonpsychodynamic technique—but runs the risk of also missing a great deal.

In terms of game theory, all psychotherapeutic methods constitute a kind of "game" played by the participants. Both therapist and patient can learn to play the psychoanalytic "game" superbly and sincerely without achieving their professed goals. The implications of this are particularly significant not only in clinical psychoanalytic practice but also in the training of psychiatrists and psychoanalysts. I fully subscribe to the importance of trying to achieve maximum self-understanding and emotional maturity in all persons who intend to practice psychotherapy. Not only is our ability to understand others limited by our own blind spots, but also any persistent characterological immaturities are subject to enormous stress in the caldron of intense psychotherapeutic relationships. The propensities and temptations toward "acting out" with patients, often rationalized as being in the patient's interest, are all too well known and, unfortunately, all too often manifested in the field of psychotherapy.

Yet in our efforts to help psychiatric trainees achieve full self-knowledge and maturity, we have relied primarily on dyadic techniques of therapy that often fail to achieve the desired result. This is best exemplified in current patterns of psychoanalytic training. It has long been known in most psychoanalytic institutes that the way to "beat the rap and graduate" is "not to make waves." This has meant learning, in the didactive analysis, to play the "game" of free association well; to "accept" supervision (which means not contradicting the supervising analyst and dutifully following his instructions); to avoid calling too much attention to oneself in seminars; and finally to produce a safe, conservative "graduation thesis" in which one carefully plays back all the things one has been taught in the preceding four or five or six years. The result is that those candidates who tend to be most conforming and least original in their thinking get through the training system with the fewest difficulties, and eventually become teachers themselves, thus perpetuating the cycle. The original thinker, the nonconformist, is apt to be charged with "resistance" and may have far greater difficulties in completing his training.

If this all sounds rather cynical, this is not my intention. I do not mean to impugn the sincerity of either the training analysts or candidates involved in this process. What I am trying to indicate is that in the very nature of such a process, a subtle self-deception tends to take place on both sides. In the intensive interaction that takes place between therapist and patient, and teacher and pupil, over the course of years, a significant transference-countertransference reaction takes place between them in which they both become deeply committed to the "truth" of what they are doing. The fault is not in their vision but in the blinders that the limitations of their method impose upon them.

Such a consequence could be avoided if our training techniques become more flexible. To rely only on the royal road of free association and transference interpretations within its context is not enough. I believe that all psychiatric and psychoanalytic trainees should have the benefit of exposure to group therapeutic experiences as well as individual therapy and that, wherever possible, auxiliary avenues to understanding their personality patterns, such as family or conjoint marital interviews, should be utilized. Interviews with "significant others" in the trainee's life should not only be permitted, they should be mandatory!

Will this produce more mature psychotherapists? Perhaps not. But it will certainly make us more aware of the complexity of the problems with which we are dealing, and make us less smug and complacent about our therapeutic potentialities. If it does no more than that, it will serve as an impetus for striving to find the better answers that we and our patients so sorely need.

SUMMARY

The method of free association has offered unique insights into the nature and meaning of human fantasy life and parapraxic distortions. Without gainsaying this fact, this article is an effort to examine some of its limitations.

One basic factor is that what the patient is unconscious of does not necessarily always reside in the patient's "unconscious." Free association can only bring into consciousness what is repressed. Information about himself that the patient has never registered is not repressed and will not be brought into the psychotherapeutic transaction by free association. Secondly, free association is never truly "free." It is strongly influenced by the therapeutic situation and by the expectations and communications of the therapist.

The exploration of this problem leads to the question of under what circumstances the dyadic relationship itself is or is not an optimum model for psychotherapeutic change. Certain implications in the training of psychotherapists are also touched upon.

REFERENCES

1. FREUD, S.: "Analysis Terminable and Interminable," in *Collected Papers,* London: Hogarth Press, 1950, vol 5, pp 322–323.
2. FREUD, S.: *An Autobiographical Study,* London: Hogarth Press, 1946.
3. MARMOR, J.: "Psychoanalytic Therapy as an Educational Process," in Masserman, J. (ed.): *Science and Psychoanalysis,* New York: Grune & Stratton, Inc., 1962, vol 5, pp 286–299. (Chapter 15, this volume.)
4. KRASNER, L.: Studies of the Conditioning of Verbal Behavior, *Psychol. Bull.* 55:148–170, 1958.
5. MANDLER, G., and KAPLAN, W. K.: Subjective Evaluation and Reinforcing Effect of a Verbal Stimulus, *Science* 124:582–583, 1956.
6. SALZINGER, K.: Experimental Manipulation of Verbal Behavior, *J. Gen. Psychol.* 61:65–94, 1959.
7. MARMOR, J.: "Psychoanalytic Therapy and Theories of Learning," in Masserman, J. (ed.): *Science and Psychoanalysis,* New York: Grune & Stratton, Inc., 1964, vol 7, pp 265–279. (Chapter 16, this volume.)
8. ALEXANDER, F.: *The Western Mind in Transition,* New York: Random House, Inc., 1960, p 209.

Part III

PSYCHOTHERAPY

Part III

PSYCHOTHERAPY

21

THE FEELING OF SUPERIORITY:
AN OCCUPATIONAL HAZARD IN THE
PRACTICE OF PSYCHOTHERAPY
(1953)

In 1913 Ernest Jones published an article entitled "The God Complex" (1) in the course of which he suggested that an unconscious identification with God, when sublimated, was one of the factors which might lead people to a strong interest in psychology and psychiatry. His formulation was based upon the assumption that individuals with this type of character formation had strong exhibitionistic trends, with the usual counterpart of strong scoptophilia and curiosity concerning the private life of others.

The purpose of the present article is to examine the hypothesis that *whether or not* unconscious feelings of superiority have been part of the psychiatrist's original make-up, certain factors peculiarly inherent to the practice of psychotherapy have a tendency to foster such feelings.

There is no single type of motivation, nor any single type of character, that leads to the practice of psychotherapy. There are as many varying personalities among psychotherapists as there are in any other professional group. Some are unconsciously motivated primarily by an effort to solve inner psychological conflicts of their own; others by prestige values (particularly since the increase in the status of psychiatry in recent years); others by needs to "mother" or "father" other people; others, as Jones has suggested, by sublimation of strong curiosity about the private affairs of other people; still others by combinations of these and many other determinants.

279

There are others whose entrance into the profession has been determined more by accidental environmental factors than by inner needs. Choice of occupation is rarely determined by inner psychological factors alone, but rather by a combination of these with external factors. The same psychological needs that motivate a person to become a doctor might, in a different social setting, lead him to become a priest, a businessman, or a teacher.

The important factor relevant to the present discussion is that *the constant exercise of authority carries with it the occupational hazard of tending to create unrealistic feelings of superiority in the authority figure.* This problem may be seen not only in psychotherapists, but in a wide variety of occupations that involve some relationship of authority over other people, e.g., doctors, lawyers, clergymen, teachers, business executives, political and military leaders, etc. In the practice of psychotherapy, however, there are special conditions that make this hazard particularly operative.

It is of special concern in the practice of psychotherapy, moreover, because its implications involve not merely the psychotherapist, but all of his patients. Unconscious arrogance and grandiosity must inevitably interfere with the capacity for good psychotherapy. It is inherent and implicit in the nature of modern dynamic psychotherapy that the therapist is trying to help people develop emotional maturity, to become free from oedipal fixations, and to acquire a sense of self-respecting adulthood. It must be apparent that any therapist who consciously or unconsciously assumes an attitude of authoritarian superiority over his patients will be less able to establish the kind of psychotherapeutic relationship with them that will enable them to give up their immature transference attitudes.

The psychotherapist pursues an unusually isolated kind of practice. He sits alone in his office for a large part of each day and works with a succession of individuals, most of whom have come to him only after vainly trying other solutions. The majority of these patients, sooner or later, tend to relate to the therapist as though he were a parent-figure, and to idealize him much as the young child does the parent—this regardless of the actual physical or intellectual attributes of the therapist. Such "transference" reactions, moreover, may come from people of considerable achievement themselves—particularly when the therapist begins to acquire prestige. The seductive influence of an abundant flow of transference admiration from such sources may be considerable.

This is particularly so since there is a reality factor operative in addition to the transference distortion. The therapist, in a real sense, *is* an important person to his patients. They come to him in need and he is trying to help them. The tendency for the therapist to feel that his patients are dependent upon him for their functioning rests, therefore, upon a small grain of truth, which adds to the danger of occupational arrogance. This hazard will, of course, be greater for those therapists who utilize an authoritarian, directive approach rather than a nondirective one.

Another contributory element is the fact that what goes on between the therapist and his patients is peculiarly personal and unique. Without in any way minimizing the scientific basis that underlies good psychotherapeutic technique, in practice it is inevitably colored by the therapist's individual personality and his unique manner of expressing himself. Psychotherapy is not like a surgical procedure which can be standardized, studied, observed, and carried out almost identically by a score of different surgeons. There is rarely but one way of handling a psychotherapeutic problem. Many different approaches may "work" equally well for the patient. The therapist rich in literary background may express himself in literary allusions; the "serious minded" therapist may utilize a direct, literal approach; still a third may use wit effectively. When a therapist's technique is reasonably effective, his professional isolation and inability to observe directly the techniques of others may in time lead to a tendency to overestimate the virtue of his own particular approach and ability in contrast to those of his colleagues. It may be worth considering to what extent such factors contribute to the ardor and conviction with which various "schools" of thought in psychiatry proclaim their superiority over rival schools.

It is not only the reactions of his patients that tend to foster "God-like" feelings in the psychotherapist. The attitude of the lay public is equally significant in this regard. When a psychotherapist is identified as such in a social gathering the reaction that is often elicited is one compounded of awe and distrust. The psychotherapist has become the shaman of our society, the all-seeing father with the Cyclopean eye. He is endowed with God-like perceptiveness.

"I'd better be careful or you'll read my thoughts," is a constantly encountered reaction. The assumption that the psychotherapist merely by a glance can understand any variety of dream, behavior problem, or emotional disturbance is one that is often shared by patients and public alike. Not infrequently a patient will say to a therapist who is straining to understand something, "Of course *you* know exactly what the trouble is, but you're just trying to make me find out for myself."

Another aspect of this overvaluation of the psychotherapist appears in the way he is portrayed in literature, on the screen and stage, or in popular magazines. He is either the omniscient embodiment of God himself, as in Eliot's *Cocktail Party*, or a malevolent but powerful fraud, such as the quack psychologist in the book, *Nightmare Alley*. He is either Deity or Devil, but rarely is he portrayed as he really is—a person with special training and ability, with human strengths and human frailties. Psychodynamically, we can recognize in this the pattern of emotional ambivalence that characterizes the attitude of the child to the father-figure, who is the presumptive source both of support and frustration. Since the concept of God Himself, as Freud has pointed out (2), is a projection of this father symbol, we see in this pattern a fertile soil for the development of a God complex in the psychotherapist.

The factors that we have been discussing thus far have been chiefly *external* factors in the environment of the psychotherapist. Let us now consider some of the *internal* factors within the psychotherapist which may predispose him to the development of an unconscious attitude of superiority.

A feeling of grandiosity, like any other character trait that involves some distortion of reality, must be, in part at least, a result of an ego-defense against anxiety. What is the source of anxiety in the practice of psychotherapy? Disregard, for the moment, the obvious example of the therapist who is incompetent or poorly trained. It is obvious that the need to take refuge behind a wall of conscious or unconscious arrogance is bound to be greater the more inadequate the therapist feels himself to be. The well-trained psychotherapist rarely lays claim to the omniscience that the quack or the amateur "parlor psychologist" so readily assumes.

There are factors inherent in the practice of psychotherapy, however, that are capable of producing anxiety even in the most competent and well-trained therapist. Consider the human material with which he deals. It is infinitely variable, complex, confusing, and often distressing. The happiness not merely of individuals, but often of entire families, hinges on the outcome of his work. There are few professions that present their practitioners with so challenging a series of daily trials and responsibilities. No conscientious therapist can be unconcerned in dealing, for example, with the danger of suicide or of aggressive acting-out on the part of a patient.

Moreover, the evaluation of what goes on in a psychotherapeutic relationship is further complicated by the variability of the human observers themselves. No two therapists studying the same individual come up with identical findings. What the therapist sees, recognizes, emphasizes, and how he interprets it is always, at least in part, dependent on his "personal equation." Every human being's perceptions in this area are bound to be colored by his own developmental history, personal experiences, social position, and cultural background. Although theoretically many dynamic psychotherapists try to be free from value judgments, in actual fact this is an ideal impossible of attainment. Value systems of one sort or another inevitably enter into every psychotherapeutic relationship—into the choice of patients, into the concept of what is psychologically healthy or unhealthy, into the very selection of what is interpreted or not interpreted.

All of these factors, then—the lack of fixed standards, the necessity of adapting to constantly changing and shifting problems, the complexity of the material, the realistic difficulties involved in achieving success, the constant need to make corrections for subjective blind spots, the disparity between the therapist's human limitations and the expectations of his patients and the public—are a constant potential source of anxiety to the psychotherapist and may create in him defensive tendencies to bolster his threatened ego by maximizing his successes, by minimizing his shortcomings and in extreme cases by taking refuge in the character traits of the God complex.

For despite occasional brash claims to the contrary, the fact is that we are far from knowing all the answers in this field. In spite of continuing progress, our techniques of treatment still lag behind our understanding of the forces that make people ill. As psychotherapists we are faced with the problem of trying to help people live with a minimum of tension in a world that is insecure, complex, and contradictory. In a conflict-ridden society such as ours which spawns mental illness with fearful fecundity, the efforts of the psychotherapist seem at times as futile as those of Canute, ordering the waves of the ocean to recede!

Let us now examine some of the actual manifestations of this syndrome, keeping in mind that we are particularly concerned with how it may reflect itself among psychotherapists. We turn to Jones' original formulations (1). He says:

> These first manifestations (of the God Complex) like those through the whole complex, are most typically reaction-products. Thus obvious self-conceit or vanity is not so frequent or characteristic as an excessive self-modesty, which at times is so pronounced as to be truly a *self-effacement*. . . . [There is] a tendency to aloofness. . . . [The man] makes himself as inaccessible as possible, and surrounds his personality with a cloud of mystery. . . . Even the most trivial pieces of information about himself, those which an ordinary man sees no object in keeping to himself, are invested with a sense of high importance, and are parted with only under pressure. . . . He rarely expresses his thought clearly and directly. Very characteristic is a lengthy, involved and circuitous form of diction. . . . Such men are both unsociable and unsocial, in the wider sense. They adapt themselves with difficulty to any activity in common with others, whether it be of a political, scientific or business kind. . . . One of the most distressing character traits . . . is the *attitude of disinclination towards the acceptance of new knowledge*. This follows quite logically from the idea of omniscience, for anyone who already knows everything naturally cannot be taught anything new; still less can he admit that he has ever made a mistake in his knowledge. . . . The resentment with which these men observe the growing prominence of younger rivals forms a curious contrast to another character trait, namely, their *desire to protect*. They are fond of helping, of acting as patron or guardian, and so on. All this, however, happens only under the strict condition that the person to be protected acknowledges his helpless position and appeals to them as the weak to the strong.

This brief excerpt from Jones' keen clinical description (which deserves to be read in its entirety) contains a number of elements that can be identified with traits sometimes associated with psycho-therapists. Consider, for example, the tendency to cloak oneself in mystery. It will be recognized that one of Freud's early formulations concerning psychoanalytic technique was precisely that the therapist *should* remain "impenetrable to the patient, and like a mirror, reflect nothing but what is shown to him" (3). As time has gone on in the development of psychoanalytic technique there has been a tendency to modify this original formulation of Freud's. This is not the place in which to argue the various pros and cons of this technical problem. What concerns us here is the importance of the therapist's realizing that an element in the need to maintain an air of mystery about himself may be a defense against his own anxiety in relation to his patient. If the therapist is truly convinced that for sound technical reasons he should not reveal any or all aspects of his personal life, that is well and good. He needs to look constantly within himself, however, to check whether or not the retreat behind a cloak of mystery is a defense against anxiety, a fear of being unable to deal with an emotional relationship with a patient, or perhaps a manifestation of an unconscious attitude of superiority, as though to say, "The patient doesn't have to know anything about me. We live in different worlds."

Another aspect of the psychotherapist's surrounding himself in mystery is that it tends to intensify the idealizations of him by his patients. The less they see him as an ordinary human being, the greater the tendency to assume that he is, indeed, perfect. Patients under such circumstances will often say: "I am sure *your* relationship with *your* wife must be wonderful," or "Of course, *you* probably never have such problems with *your* children," or, "It must be wonderful to know how to handle every kind of situation." Thus there is a tendency to increase the unrealistic aspects of the transference and to foster an unconsciously authoritarian parent-child relationship. It might be well for psychotherapists to reconsider whether or not "trivial pieces of information . . . those which an ordinary man sees no object in keeping to himself," really must be kept inaccessible to the patient. This is not in any way to negate the technical importance of always at the same time trying to understand any unconscious significance which may exist behind a patient's curiosity.

Occasionally, however, the feeling of superiority expresses itself in a diametrically opposite way, namely, in terms of communicating *too much* about oneself to the patient. This can be equally damaging to the therapeutic goal. The therapist who does this is often unconsciously setting himself up as a model for the patient, and implying to the patient: "Try to do as I do." Even though patterning himself after the therapist might afford a patient temporary relief from anxiety, it obviously fails to meet the basic need of achieving the kind of emotional maturity that will enable him to develop independent standards of thought and behavior. Such transference improvement, which is usually based on pleasing the therapist, is almost always transitory, since it carries with it no real character growth on the part of the patient.

Jones' description of the attitude towards younger colleagues strikes another reminiscent note when one considers the field of psycho-therapy. Aggressiveness to one's competitors is, of course, not confined to the field of psychotherapy, but the need of occasional outstanding leaders in the field to surround themselves with disciples rather than with independent-thinking colleagues is worth noting. As Jones has indicated, this is really a way of disarming a rival, the unconscious formula being, "I will love you and protect you if you accept my domination." The disciple thus gets the vicarious glory of being associated with the leader, while the leader whose "godliness" is accepted is protected from the threat of competition.

Similar patterns can be observed also in the fields of psychology and social work. When one examines more closely the psychodyna-mics of the relationship between a supervising teacher and a younger colleague, some of the reasons for this become apparent. The supervising therapist, whether he is aware of it or not, usually operates under an inner need to demonstrate his superior knowledge or experience, since his sense of usefulness as a supervisor is largely dependent on his ability to point out errors of omission or commission to the student. Thus the supervising therapist has a double occupa-tional hazard. Not only is he exposed to the idealization of his own patients, but he also receives frequent deference from colleagues who are themselves usually extremely competent and intelligent people. Moreover, the potential anxiety to which the psychotherapist is exposed is even greater for the supervising therapist who is expected, often on the basis of inadequate material, to understand all the complexities that his colleagues are failing to grasp.

Another common occurrence in our field is the tendency to be destructively critical of other colleagues. Trigant Burrow, in discussing this problem among psychoanalysts (though it is equally pertinent to other psychotherapists), said: "Let any two psychoanalysts get together long enough for a heart-to-heart talk and before parting they will have damned the methods of every other psychoanalyst extant" (4). It must be emphasized that such tendencies, where they do exist, do not indicate that psychotherapists as a group are less tolerant or more aggressive than are other people. It is precisely that the hazards and insecurity of their work, plus its ego-seductive aspects, plus its isolationism, tend to foster such defensive arrogance to a greater extent perhaps, than do many other professions.

Another phenomenon is the degree of separatism and mutual hostility that exists between the adherents of different schools of thought in this field. The same dynamic tendencies that predispose the psychotherapist to the development of defensive feelings of superiority also tend to foster strong in-group formations. By being part of a group that lays claim to possessing the Only True Theory, the therapist's ego finds additional security against the constant challenges that the complex realities of his practice present to his theories and his methods. It is a manifestation of all in-group thinking to believe that one's own group has some quality or virtue that makes it superior to all the out-groups. Behind this is usually some latent insecurity that manifests itself by one's feeling comfortable only with members of his own group, with people who presumably think and do as he does. This leads not only to an increasing isolationism but often even to increasingly esoteric private languages. Thus the communication between the groups grows ever more difficult.

This isolationism, moreover, has a tendency to cause the different groups to become increasingly cult-like, self-contained, and immune to outside influences. All facts are made willy-nilly to fit the framework of one's own viewpoint, and there is a defensive reluctance to examine or accept concepts that do not fit. Thus the unconscious feeling of superiority of each group tends to be constantly reinforced.

What safeguards can the psychotherapist exercise to protect himself against this occupational hazard? The following suggestions come to mind:

(1) The greater the emotional security of the therapist, the less susceptible will he be to the blandishments and anxieties that promote unconscious grandiosity. Assuming that one has not had the rare good fortune of growing up without neurotic distortions of personality, a good personal analysis still remains, theoretically at least, one of the best ways of achieving such security. Freud's original comments about this are as pertinent today as when they were first published in 1912:

> If the physician is to be able to use his own unconscious in this way as an instrument in the analysis, he must fulfill one psychological condition in a high degree. He may tolerate no resistance in himself which would withhold from his consciousness what is perceived by his unconscious. . . . It is a justifiable requisition that he should . . . become aware of those complexes in himself which would be apt to affect his comprehension of the patient's disclosures. Every unresolved repression in the physician constitutes what W. Stekel has well named a 'blind spot' in his capacity for analytic perception. (3)

In this connection it is perhaps well to point out, however, that even the most successful of personal analyses never represents the completion of one's emotional growth, but merely a phase of growth. The successfully analyzed person is one who has acquired sufficient understanding of his motivations and character traits to enable him to continue to change and develop as a person for the balance of his life. The analyzed individual who utilizes his analysis to justify an attitude of smug superiority over others thereby reveals an island of unresolved insecurity in himself. Strictly speaking, a good analysis is never really completed—it merely continues to operate as a "self-analysis" without requiring the assistance of a psychoanalyst.

(2) Next to personal analysis, the importance for the psychotherapist of an adequate period of supervised work cannot be too strongly emphasized. With all of its limitations (the gaps in the student's reporting, the variable adequacy of supervisors, etc.) it still remains the most important method by which the student in this field can get some objective appraisal of what he is doing.

Presenting a case over a long period of time to a group of colleagues ("continuous case seminar") is an equally valuable experience for the student; and more use could and should be made of recording devices for teaching purposes, even if only an occasional hour were recorded.

(3) The psychotherapist in practice needs to be constantly on guard against the defensive tendency of the ego to take refuge in arrogance. It is as natural for the ego to minimize its failures and cherish its successes as it is for the abdominal musculature to become rigid when a tender area is touched. The perceptive psychotherapist must correct against this tendency by not letting himself forget his errors and striving ceaselessly to learn from them. It is important to be able to admit errors and human weaknesses to patients also, and not to foster in them the illusion that the therapist is the embodiment of perfection. The therapist has to be as objective about the hostile comments of patients as about their flatteries of him. It is too easy to attribute such comment always to "negative transference," although this is undoubtedly ego-protective. Criticisms of the therapist by the patient may be based on real deficiencies in the former, and the therapist whose mind is open to such possibilities cannot but benefit from such increased awareness of himself. Moreover, the psychotherapist is in actual fact always learning from every patient. Since every patient's problem is, at least in part, a unique one, the working through of every problem is part of the psychotherapist's research as well as his continuing education.*

The willingness to admit, not only to patients but to the world at large, the limitations of our knowledge is important. I am not advocating any false modesty, however. We need not minimize the progress that is constantly being made in our knowledge and methods, but our very security in the scientific base of our techniques should protect us against the necessity of claiming omniscience.

---

*I am indebted to Frieda Fromm-Reichmann for reminding me of the value of having psychotherapeutic experience with schizophrenic patients. Not only do schizophrenic patients have a greater ability than most therapists to interpret the language and symbolism of the unconscious, but they also often put their fingers with penetrating keenness on weaknesses and pretensions in the therapist's personality.

(4) There should be increasing emphasis on interdisciplinary contacts, not only between psychiatrists, psychologists, and psychiatric social workers, but also with physicians in general as well as with anthropologists, sociologists, and social philosophers. Every effort should be made to avoid being isolated into narrow in-groups. It would also have a salutary effect upon our science if we tried to express ourselves in terms that can be universally understood rather than in language that only the "indoctrinated" can understand. This tendency to esoteric expression is something that people outside the field of psychotherapy have justly criticized. There is no valid reason why concepts in our field cannot be presented in terms that are intelligible to all physicians and allied social scientists.

(5) Every psychotherapist ought to reserve some portion of his time for outside work that brings him into contact with other colleagues, where mutual experiences can be shared, discussed, and criticized.

(6) Relationships with people outside one's own field are equally important. One too often sees an unhealthy limitation of social and professional life to members of a psychotherapist's in-group.

(7) Finally, a constant cherishing of, and working toward, a democratic kind of interpersonal relationship with all people—patients, friends, relatives, and strangers—is an essential safeguard against the God complex. The need for deference is always an expression of unconscious arrogance and an underlying anxiety and insecurity. Authoritarianism is psychologically unhealthy for those who dominate as well as for those who are dominated. Only in an atmosphere of democratic interrelationships can both the psychotherapist and his patients achieve their fullest development.

REFERENCES

1. JONES, ERNEST. The God Complex. Essays in Applied Psychoanalysis. Vol. II:244. Hogarth Press, London, 1951.
2. FREUD, SIGMUND. The Future of an Illusion. Hogarth Press, London, 1934.
3. FREUD, SIGMUND. Recommendations for Physicians on the Psychoanalytic Method of Treatment. Coll. Papers Vol. II:323. Hogarth Press, London, 1924.
4. BURROW, TRIGANT. Psychoanalytic improvisations and the personal equation. Psychoan. Review 13:178. 1926.

22

THE DOCTOR-PATIENT RELATIONSHIP
IN PSYCHOTHERAPY
(1955)

Any discussion of the patient-physician relationship in dynamic psychotherapy inevitably brings up two terms which have come from psychoanalytic theory—*transference* and *countertransference*. Unfortunately there is much confusion about these terms because they are sometimes used in a highly specific sense, while at other times they are used very loosely. Thus the term "transference" may be employed to include all of the emotionally-tinged attitudes that a patient may have toward a therapist. If he likes the therapist, it is called "positive transference," if he dislikes him it is "negative transference." Such use of the term transference leaves no room for the realistic aspects of the patient-physician relationship. If a patient reacts positively to a therapist who is friendly and warm, or negatively to one who appears cold or disinterested, this is not necessarily a transference reaction. It may be, and often is, a perfectly valid and realistic judgment on the part of the patient.

Much semantic confusion would be avoided, in my opinion, if the terms "transference" and "countertransference" were used only to refer to the *irrational* aspects of the patient-physician relationship, and if different terms, such as "rapport" and "empathy," were utilized for its rational aspects. Thus transference, positive or negative, would designate attitudes toward the therapist—expectations, fears, idealizations or hostilities—which are rooted in the patient's previous life experiences and unwarranted in the light of the actual facts of the current relationship. It is for this reason, of course, that positive transference, which early in analytic therapy is utilized to advance the therapeutic objectives, sooner or later presents an obstacle to therapy and must be dissolved for the analysis to achieve its optimum goals.

Similarly, the term countertransference should be reserved for a therapist's irrational attitudes toward his patient, attitudes which have grown out of *his* previous life experiences and are not justified by the realities of the therapeutic situation. In this sense, *all manifestations of countertransference represent "blind spots" on the part of the therapist which interfere with accurate perception or optimum therapeutic relationship with the patient.*

Although it is true that a countertransference reaction, like a faulty interpretation, may occasionally have an unexpectedly salutary effect upon a patient, this fact should no more be used to justify countertransference behavior than it should encourage faulty interpretations. As scientists, we must seek to discover the underlying laws that govern such unexpected therapeutic reactions and to bring them under rational and conscious control. To do less than this, to allow countertransference reactions (in the sense in which I have defined them) free play, is to throw darts haphazardly with a blindfold on, while hoping that somehow, somewhere, they will hit the target.

It is true, unfortunately, that we are still far from achieving the goal of a completely scientific and objective psychotherapy. Psychotherapy is still largely an art as well as a science. It is extremely difficult to measure objectively all the subtle nuances and nonverbal interplay that go on between a patient and therapist in the psychotherapeutic relationship. The fact that therapists of many different schools, often employing widely varying techniques, report similar therapeutic successes adds to the complexity of the problem.

Nevertheless, we must not make the mistake of throwing up our hands in despair and confusing the difficult with the impossible. I am firmly convinced that ultimately we shall be able to extrapolate out of all of the diverse and multitudinous approaches which are included under the broad concept of psychotherapy, those common denominators which are the specific therapeutic factors. I would venture the prediction, furthermore, that when we do we shall find that the most significant factors lie not in the area of verbal interpretations made to our patients but, more importantly, in the area of the interpersonal relationship between the therapist and the patient. It is for this reason, I believe, that the subject under discussion here is one of the more significant and important areas in the entire field of psychotherapy.

Is it possible to set down rules for the psychotherapist in his relationship to the patient? Should he be directive or nondirective, silent or talkative, reserved or friendly? I do not believe that generalizations can be made which will be universally applicable. The relationship of the therapist to the patient must inevitably vary with the dynamic needs of the patient, and with the nature of the therapeutic goal. Frieda Fromm-Reichmann and others have demonstrated that the psychotherapy of the psychotic patient requires different technique from that of the neurotic. It also makes a difference whether the goal is merely the immediate removal of a symptom, or personality reintegration. Counseling may require one type of relationship to a patient, analytically oriented therapy another.

Still another factor enters into the entire problem of the patient-therapist relationship: the question of values. We are indebted to Karen Horney for being one of the first to challenge the traditional assumption that the psychotherapist was free from value judgments. Although, theoretically, many psychoanalysts seek to disclaim any adherence to value judgments, in actual fact this is an impossible objective. Value systems are an inevitable and integral part of every psychotherapeutic relationship. The choice of patients, the concept of what is psychologically healthy or unhealthy, the very selection of the material to be interpreted all involve a greater or lesser degree of evaluative judgment. This fact notwithstanding, there was an important germ of truth in the traditional effort to avoid value judgments, which should not be lost sight of in our belated recognition that value judgments enter into the psychotherapeutic relationship. That germ of truth was an awareness that even within the framework of inevitable values there is still a wide latitude for self-determination for our patients, and that it is in the interest of the patient's healthy maturation that he be encouraged to make his own choice within that latitude.

This point touches on one of the most fundamental aspects of the patient-doctor relationship in psychotherapy, namely, the importance of the physician's genuine regard and respect for the patient's own personality and its innate potential for growth and health. This fundamental regard is probably the sine qua non which underlies all successful psychotherapy, whether directive or nondirective, if we define successful psychotherapy as one which encourages a patient's growth and self-realization.

One of the interesting developments in psychotherapeutic literature in recent years has been this increasing appreciation of the positive potentials that exist in even the sickest of patients, and at the same time an increasing recognition of the importance of self-understanding on the part of the therapist himself. Elsewhere (1) I have discussed the occupational hazard inherent in the very process of psychotherapy, which by reason of its tensions, the complexity of the problems dealt with, the isolationism of its practice, and a number of other factors, often tends to create in the psychotherapist the defensive pattern of a feeling of superiority. Quite apart from the damage this does to the personality of the psychotherapist himself, it creates a real barrier toward the performance of effective psychotherapy, since it must inevitably interfere with what Whitehorn calls the "genuine attitude of respect and consideration" for the patient, which is an essential ingredient of good psychotherapy. If the core of the psychotherapeutic process is, as increasing evidence seems to indicate, the patient-doctor relationship, then this increasing focus upon the self-understanding of the psychiatrist must continue to be one of our major preoccupations. The personal analysis of the psychotherapist, the prolonged period of postgraduate study, and the years of case supervision, which our present standards require, must remain important elements in the structure upon which a truly scientific psychotherapy will eventually be established. Perhaps then we shall achieve that ideal of the psychotherapist which Nathaniel Hawthorne expressed so brilliantly a decade before Freud was born: "If the (physician) possess native sagacity, and a nameless something more—let us call it intuition; if he show no intrusive egotism, nor disagreeably prominent characteristics of his own; if he have the power . . . to bring his mind into such affinity with his patient's, that this last shall unawares have spoken what he imagines himself only to have thought; if such revelations be received without tumult, and acknowledged not so often by uttered sympathy as by silence, an inarticulate breath, and here and there a word, to indicate that all is understood; if to these qualifications of a confidant be joined the advantages afforded by his recognized character as a physician—then, at some inevitable moment, will the soul of the sufferer be dissolved, and flow forth in a dark, but transparent stream, bringing all its mysteries into the daylight." (2)

REFERENCES

1. MARMOR, JUDD: "The Feeling of Superiority: An Occupational Hazard in the Practice of Psychotherapy," Amer. J. of Psychiatry, 110, 5, 1953. (Chapter 21, this volume.)
2. HAWTHORNE, NATHANIEL: *The Scarlet Letter* (2nd Ed., 1850), New York: Pocket Books, 1952, 127–128.

23

THE NATURE OF THE
PSYCHOTHERAPEUTIC PROCESS
(1964)

The helping process in psychiatry has two fundamental goals. It may concern itself with efforts either to modify the environmental stresses which have disrupted the individual's psychic equilibrium, or else to improve the individual's adaptive capacity to these stresses, or both. In the discussion that follows, I shall concern myself primarily with the process involved in endeavoring to improve an individual's ego-adaptive capacity.

Psychotherapy, in its broadest sense, may be defined simply as a method of modifying an individual's symptoms, feelings, thought processes, or behavior by means of communication in an interpersonal relationship. Drugs may or may not be utilized as secondary adjuvants to facilitate this process, but not for the primary purpose of altering the patient's inner reactions or outer behavior. If drugs are used for this latter purpose, we are then dealing with pharmacotherapy rather than psychotherapy. A physician may, however, choose to combine both therapeutic approaches for certain conditions.

I shall begin with two major premises. The first of these is that all of the major psychotherapeutic approaches have essentially similar objectives, although they may attach different names to these objectives and although their approaches may rest on differing theoretical frameworks. Thus, Freudians may talk of genitality, Adlerians of social interest, Rankians of active, creative will, Jungians of the full development of the self, Sullivanians of an integrated self, Horneyites of self-realization, Frommians of the productive

296

personality, and eclectics of improved adaptation or emotional maturity—all, however, are talking of helping an individual to have meaningful and satisfying interpersonal and sexual relationships, to work effectively, and to be a socially responsible and productive human being within the limits of his capacity. These objectives, it should be noted, represent normative standards in our culture and are not unique to psychotherapy. What is unique in modern dynamic psychotherapy is not its *objective*, but rather its *method* of attempting to make an individual aware of his previously unconscious thoughts, feelings, and motivations, and its deliberate and controlled utilization of the patient-therapist relationship for therapeutic purposes.

My second major premise is that, by and large, mature and experienced therapists of different theoretical orientations achieve comparable results. Admittedly, reliable statistics concerning this point are difficult to come by, but I know of no convincing evidence to the contrary—if we omit the personal conviction of each individual therapist that his results are better (9) than anyone else's! Over the past twenty-eight years I have had the opportunity of working closely with, and of observing the work of, therapists of most of the leading psychodynamic schools of thought, and my experience has been fully in agreement with the findings of Fiedler (4) and Heine (5) that favorable psychotherapeutic results are less dependent on the theoretical inclination of the therapist than they are on his personal characteristics, empathic capacity, and clinical maturity.

But how is this possible? How can approaches based on different theoretical orientations be equally efficacious for the patient? The inference is justified that if this is so there must be some common denominator which underlies these diverse approaches. This brings us to a consideration of the fundamental nature of the psychotherapeutic process.

Up until relatively recently, the most prominent assumptions concerning what happens in psychotherapy were outgrowths of psychoanalytic theory. The first of these dealt with the effect of emotional release (abreaction), and the second was based on the role of insight.

The assumption that abreaction—the liberation of repressed emotions or memories—is the core of the psychotherapeutic process was an outgrowth of Breuer and Freud's famous studies in hysteria (2). This assumption, however, has not been borne out by clinical experience, except in some cases of acute traumatic hysteria where recovery of the repressed memory of the traumatic incident will often cause dramatic disappearance of the hysterical *symptom*. In most instances, however, although the release of repressed emotion may result in transitory feelings of improvement, it does not in itself bring about lasting personality changes. Moreover, as Franz Alexander pointed out as long ago as 1930 (1), the recovery of repressed memories is often a *result* rather than a *cause* of therapeutic change in the patient. Because the theory of abreaction is such a dramatic one, however, it has taken a powerful hold on the imagination of the public, and has become the basis of innumerable movies, plays, and television dramas, where the doctor, at the appointed minute (just prior to the final commercial or the closing curtain) elicits the crucial concealed memory or emotion, and presto, the patient is magically cured! The lay public may be forgiven for this wishful thinking, but what is harder to understand is the fact that this theory is still clung to by many psychiatrists, who ought to know better. Freud himself discarded this theory more than fifty years ago, yet numerous modern psychiatrists working with such tools as hypnosis, or with drugs such as pentothal, CO_2, or LSD, continue to assume that whatever therapeutic results they are achieving are on the basis of the release of repressed memories or feelings!

The second major assumption concerning the psychotherapeutic process has been that it is based primarily upon the insight that is acquired by the patient. What is insight, however? When we begin to examine it carefully, we find that it is a highly complex phenomenon. To begin with, it is necessary to distinguish between insight as it is given by the therapist, and insight as it is perceived by the patient. Insight as given by the therapist is defined differently by practitioners of differing schools of thought, and each school gives its own brand of understanding. The remarkable fact, however, is that patients treated by members of each school seem to respond with more or less equal effectiveness to the insights they are given. But even more remarkably, patients of each school seem to bring up precisely the kind of phenomenological data that confirm the theories and interpretations of their therapists! The patients of classical Freudians bring in dreams and material about Oedipus complexes and castration anxiety; the patients of Jungians, about archetypes; the patients of Adlerians, about masculine strivings and feelings of inferiority; the patients of Rankians, about separation anxiety; the patients of Horneyites, about idealized images; and so forth. What this indicates is that the material in which the therapist shows interest, the kinds of questions he asks, the kinds of data to which he reacts or that he chooses to ignore, and the nature of the interpretations that he makes, all exert a subtle but significant impact upon the patient to bring forth certain kinds of data in preference to others. I shall return to this point a little later in this discussion. What I wish to suggest at this point is that *what we call insight as given by the therapist is essentially the conceptual framework by means of which a therapist establishes, or attempts to establish, a logical relationship between events, feelings, or experiences that seem unrelated in the mind of his patient.* It thus constitutes the rationale on the basis of which the therapist hopes that the patient will accept the model of more "mature" or "healthy" behavior that therapists of all schools, *implicitly* or *explicitly,* hold out to him. Since interpretations in different frames of reference seem to be equally effective for the patient, it seems obvious that the *specific* insight given cannot be the fundamental or exclusive basis for the therapeutic reaction.

In saying this, I do not wish to imply that insights given by therapists of different schools are capriciously variable, or that they bear no relationship to the actual realities of the patient's life and behavior. On the contrary. Interpretations given by ethical practitioners of different schools all bear a definite relationship to clinical reality and all fit the observable facts to a reasonable degree, although each school, of course, believes that its approach constitutes the most valid frame of reference. I can illustrate this point by a simple clinical example. Consider a young man whose basic behavioral patterns are those of passive dependency. The classical Freudian will make interpretations revolving around concepts of fixation at an oral receptive level, and of an unresolved Oedipus complex; the Adlerian will talk of expectations of being taken care of, and of a "life style" of passivity and helplessness; a Horneyite might confront the patient with his neurotic need for affection and with his patterns of "moving toward" people; a Rankian might talk primarily about separation anxiety and the patient's defenses against it; a Jungian might speak of striving for reunion with an archetypal mother; a Sullivanian might make reference to oral dynamisms and disturbances in interpersonal relationships. All of these interpretations, however, deal with essentially the same behavioral problem, and the implicit or explicit message in all the interpretations is also the same—namely that the patient ought to become more self-assertive, autonomous, and mature. Similar parallel interpretations can be demonstrated with other personality patterns, such as aggressivity, withdrawal, compulsiveness, etc.

If now we turn to a consideration of the problem of insight as it is perceived by the patient, we run into difficulties also. The literature of psychoanalysis is quite confusing with regard to this point. Sometimes the insight referred to is purely cognitive. It is then described as "intellectual insight." If, however, the insight is associated with a simultaneous release of emotion, it is then referred to as "emotional insight." Generally, it is assumed that "emotional" insight will be therapeutically more effective than "intellectual" insight. Experienced clinicians know, however, that even so-called emotional insight does not necessarily lead to more mature patterns of behavior. There are, it is true, occasions in which a patient will have a sudden acquisition of insight with what Karl Bühler (3) has referred to as an "a-ha" feeling and thereafter is able to modify a particular pattern of neurotic behavior in all of its ramifications, very much the way Yerkes' and Kohler's apes were able to do once they grasped the gestalt of the test situation. Such persistent changes of behavior following upon insight, however, are the exception rather than the rule. The important point to note here is that whatever therapeutic effect any given insight may have upon a patient depends fundamentally on how it is perceived by the *patient*, not as it is given by the *therapist*.

As an example of this point, in 1947 Rosen (12) reported some striking remissions in schizophrenic patients by a technique that he called "direct analysis" in which he made direct interpretations of the patient's supposed incestuous fantasies, castration anxieties, and similar "deep" material. Although Rosen attributed the remissions that he obtained to the "insights" he was giving his patients, most modern students of schizophrenia would agree that what was really producing these remissions was not these "deep" interpretations given by the therapist but rather what was being perceived by the patients; namely, that here was a doctor who cared deeply and passionately about them, who spent an inordinate amount of time with them, and who absolutely refused to permit them to retreat into their autistic worlds.

What then is the nature of the therapeutic process? I submit that fundamentally it is a kind of learning experience (10, 11) that takes place in a number of different ways. One basic difference between psychotherapeutic learning and any de novo learning situation, however, is that in psychotherapy the previously learned behavior (the neurotic pattern) is particularly resistant to change. It was this stubborn fact that forced Freud to abandon his initial hopes that insight alone could dramatically cure his patients, and to emphasize instead the much more arduous, time-consuming, and difficult process of "working through." This process of working through is the core of the long-term psychotherapeutic process.

Let us consider the factors involved in a typical psychotherapeutic relationship. (1) There is a patient, whose discomfort, maladjustment, or unfulfilled needs *motivate* him to seek therapy. (2) The patient brings with him something else, however, which is very important— not only a *motivation* for therapy, but also *faith, hope,* and *expectancy* that therapy will help him. (3) There is a therapist, who by virtue of his *social and professional role* is endowed by the help-seeking patient with qualities of knowledge, prestige, authority, and help-giving potential. (4) There are the *real attributes* of the therapist—his actual knowledge, self-confidence, intelligence, objectivity, integrity, and empathy. Here we must also include the therapist's own needs and ambitions as they enter into the therapeutic transaction. The real attributes of the therapist have often been minimized in the psychiatric literature, as though the therapist's personality was of no real significance and as though he were as "neutral" and standardized a factor as a surgical instrument might be. This has often led to the tendency to interpret all positive and negative reactions of the patient toward the therapist as though they were aspects of positive and negative "transference" and to ignore the reality factors that may be involved in a patient's reaction to a therapist. When a patient dislikes a therapist, it is not always negative transference—it can be a reaction to certain real deficiencies in the therapist's personality. Similarly, a patient's liking for a therapist is not necessarily always positive transference, but may be a realistic response to positive attributes in the therapist's personality. It would be useful in this regard to make a distinction between "rapport" as a response to the therapist's real attributes, and "transference" as a response which is based not on the therapist's real attributes but on experiences and reactions with significant figures in the past. (5) Finally (although this does not necessarily exhaust the list of variables in the therapeutic transaction) there are the *value-systems* of the therapist. All therapists are purveyors of certain mores of their culture, and these values are inevitably transmitted to the patient in terms of what the therapist considers healthy or unhealthy, properly masculine or properly feminine, "normally" aggressive, emotionally mature, etc.

Given the above five factors, a number of things begin to happen more or less simultaneously but in varying degrees. First, the patient experiences some initial relief, as a rule, not only by virtue of his faith, hope, and expectancy, but also by being able to confide in a trusted and respected authority figure. This latter element involves the principle of catharsis and serves as a tension-reducing phenomenon. Second, the therapist begins to convey to the patient his therapeutic objectives and values in a series of interpretations, confrontations, and questions, by virtue of what the therapist chooses to focus on, by what he chooses to ignore, and *by his nonverbal as well as verbal reactions.* The importance of the therapist's nonverbal reactions is something that has been generally overlooked in the literature. This is understandable when one realizes that all reports of the therapeutic process have hitherto always been made by the therapist himself. As one of the participants in the transaction, the therapist could hardly be expected to be aware of everything that he was doing, particularly his nonverbal reactions. In the five-year study of the nature of the psychotherapeutic process* in which

*This study was financed by the Ford Foundation, and was carried out at Mount Sinai Hospital in Los Angeles. The voluminous data are still being processed.

I participated with Dr. Franz Alexander and other colleagues, I had a unique opportunity to observe many psychotherapeutic and psychoanalytic hours through a one-way screen, and to witness the impact of the therapist's nonverbal reactions upon the patient. When therapist and patient are in a face-to-face position, these nonverbal reactions, of course, are quite apparent to the patient. The therapist's facial expressions, a questioning glance, a lift of the eyebrows, a barely perceptible nod of the head, or a shrug of the shoulders, are all capable of being eloquent bits of communication to the patient. But even with the therapist sitting behind a couch, when and how often he says his "mm-hmms," the length and patterns of his silences, the degree of interest or distinterest in his voice, his shifting movements—all act as cues to the patient whose highly sensitive antennae are alerted to even the tiniest signal of approval or disapproval, interest or disinterest, on the part of the therapist. That these cues are capable of influencing the actual content of a patient's communication has been clearly demonstrated in a number of experimental studies by Mandler and Kaplan (8), Krasner (7), and others. These investigators have shown that the "mm-hmms" of a therapist can be used to actually manipulate the content of a patient's "spontaneous" communications. Thus if a therapist says "mm-hmm" every time the patient talks about his past and is silent when he talks about his present, the patient will begin in a short while to talk considerably more about his past than about his present. If now the therapist shifts the emphasis of his "mm-hmms" to the present, the content of the patient's communications can be reversed! Thus the cues act as a kind of reward-punishment operant conditioning system in which the communication and behavior that the therapist approves of is reinforced and that which he disapproves of is discouraged.

In addition, however, the therapist's interpretations actually *do* teach the patient and clarify things for him. One might make a crude analogy between what goes on in the psychotherapeutic process and learning to play golf. The golf pro* begins by confronting

---

*Parenthetically, anyone who has taken golfing lessons knows that different golfing teachers belong to different "schools" of theory, no less than do different psychoanalysts!

the patient with what he is unconsciously doing wrong. The interpretation, in effect, says, "Look what you are doing," and implicitly or explicitly offers a more suitable model of functioning. Over a period of time, however, the patient tends to fall back again and again on the old patterns of behavior ("resistance") and the golf pro makes repeated "confrontations" which, in effect, say, "There you go again." Eventually, the student begins to become aware of his own errors as he makes them and is able to say, in effect, "There *I* go again." Finally the student is able to anticipate his errors and not make them, and thus he eventually begins to develop new and more effective patterns of functioning. This, in greatly oversimplified form, of course, is the essence of the working-through process. Therapeutic change does not always, however, follow this slow and tortuous pattern. Occasionally a bit of insight may, as indicated above, result in rapid modifications of patterns of behavior through a kind of gestalt learning. Obviously, also, the "faith" of the student in the teacher, as well as the empathic support of the therapist-teacher and his belief in the patient-student's ability to change, are important elements in helping the student to persist in the often painful and difficult process of learning new patterns of adaptation.

Still another factor in the psychotherapeutic process is the fact that the therapist's reactions, by being different from what the patient has previously experienced from authority figures, become an important additional basis for the reconditioning of the patient. What has been called the corrective emotional experience is essentially a kind of reconditioning process in which the patient encounters understanding, approval, support, or consistent firmness and dependability in place of the criticism, disapproval, disinterest, or inconsistencies that he has experienced with the significant authority figures of his past life.

Finally, the therapist, largely by virtue of the patient's positive transference reaction, unwittingly becomes a model to the patient, after whom the latter consciously or unconsciously patterns himself. This is a process of unconscious imitation which psychoanalysts call "identification" and is a very important element in every psychotherapeutic process. It tends to take place in a climate of rapport and positive transference whether or not the therapist consciously intends it.

We can now summarize the main factors in the psychotherapeutic process. They are:— (1) *Release of tension* through catharsis and by virtue of the patient's hope, faith, and expectancy. (2) *Cognitive learning,* both of the trial-and-error variety and of the gestalt variety. (3) Reconditioning by virtue of *operant conditioning,* by virtue of subtle reward-punishment cues from the therapist, and by corrective emotional experiences. (4) *Identification* with the therapist. (5) Repeated *reality testing,* which is the equivalent of *practice* in the learning process. These five elements encompass the most significant factors on the basis of which change takes place in a psychotherapeutic relationship.

A number of questions present themselves, however. (1) Does defining psychotherapy as a learning experience minimize the importance of the patient-therapist relationship? My reply to this would be an emphatic "no." The patient-therapist relationship is not a matter of mystique, although existential psychoanalysts tend to write of it as though it were. It is simply *the matrix* in which the learning process takes place and as such it is a tremendously important element. If the therapist's relationship to his patient is one of gentleness, understanding, and empathy, and if the patient has hope and faith in the therapist, the learning process is thereby facilitated. If there is a less favorable emotional climate between them, the learning process will be retarded or even totally inhibited. (2) A more fundamental question, however, is whether structuring the psychotherapeutic process in these terms does not imply that the patient is being pressed into a mold of the therapist's making, with no free choice of his own. My answer to this would again be strongly in the negative. We must remember, first, that the therapist's goal is, as a rule, the patient's also. Secondly, even though the therapist is indeed trying to move the patient along the road toward emotional maturity, his method, if it is a nonauthoritarian one, permits the patient to follow his own paths toward that goal. The psychoanalytic concept of the dissolution of the transference, which is one of the prerequisites to a successful termination of therapy, implies helping the patient to achieve autonomy in his relationship to *all* authority figures *including the therapist.* This is an important difference between directive and nondirective techniques of therapy. Although these are obviously relative terms, the more authoritarian the therapist is in relationship to the patient, the more difficult it is for the patient to achieve genuine autonomy even though he may relinquish his symptoms in deference to the therapist. As Klein (6) aptly has put it, the nondirective therapist, like the progressive teacher, "permits the student to set his own goals, encourages independent and spontaneous expression, shows respect for the pupil's worth and promise, prefers a democratic to an authoritarian learning atmosphere, and abhors techniques of domination and coercion." (3) Still a third question that presents itself is, where does suggestion enter in the psychotherapeutic process? As I have indicated, the therapist's value-system is implicit, if not explicit, in every interpretation he makes, in the things he shows interest in, in the things he treats as normal, and the things he treats as neurotic. These reactions of the therapist are inevitably communicated to the patient, implicitly or explicitly. Therefore suggestion is part of every psychotherapeutic process, even the most nondirective ones. Obviously those patients who have the greatest need to please the therapist are going to be most "suggestible."

Finally, a word would seem to be in order concerning the so-called "behavioral therapies" which are coming increasingly into vogue and which utilize constructs of learning theory such as counter-conditioning, extinction, operant conditioning, and reciprocal inhibition as their basic therapeutic maneuvers. This school of therapists, exemplified by Eysenck in England and Bandura and Wolpe in the United States, tends to focus only on the patient's external behavior and symptomatology and considers irrelevant the subjective, cognitive, or emotional processes that go on within the patient. They argue that all that is necessary in psychotherapy is to recondition the patient's external behavior, and his internal processes will then remedy themselves automatically. It is significant that most of the cases reported by the members of this school deal with phobias and circumscribed symptom complexes rather than personality disorders.

The chief defect of this approach, it seems to me, is that it ignores the whole complex area of symbolic abstraction that plays so important a part in human behavior and that distinguishes man from all other animals. To base a psychotherapeutic approach on animal conditioning experiments is to ignore the tremendously important and unique role that symbols play in human behavior, and to return to a kind of renascent Watsonian behaviorism. Can anyone doubt that there is a vast difference between a socially adjusted but delusional schizophrenic who behaves normally to all outward appearances, and a nonschizophrenic whose external behavior is essentially the same? Moreover, we have had decades of experience with counterconditioning therapy of alcoholism, and even where such techniques are successful in temporarily eliminating the desire for alcohol, their failure to eliminate the underlying tension and anxiety of the alcoholic is well known. It is highly significant that Wolpe himself in extolling the value of his reciprocal inhibition therapy, states that it is "applicable. . . . to almost any source of neurotic anxiety not involving inadequacies in the handling of interpersonal relationships" (13). One can only be astonished that Wolpe does not realize how stringently his statement limits the applicability of these techniques! There are very few neurotic conflicts indeed that do not involve "inadequacies in the handling of interpersonal relationships."

I do not wish to imply, however, that these behavioral therapies are of no value at all. I believe that they are particularly useful for symptom disorders in which the therapeutic goal is a limited one; that is, restricted to the amelioration of symptoms rather than to the modification of the patient's adaptive capacity. It should not surprise us that some techniques work better than others with certain types of patients and problems. Just as there is no single best way of teaching all people and all subjects, there is no single best way of treating all patients and all illnesses. To assume, however, that basic personality abnormalities and maladaptive techniques that have been subtly inculcated by many years of daily disturbances in interpersonal relationships with resultant complex perceptual and symbolic distortions can be totally eradicated by a dozen or two counterconditioning sessions aimed at some specific behavioral symptom, is simply to misjudge the complexity of the problems that are being dealt with.

In conclusion, a brief word about the relationship of drugs to psychiatric practice in the mid-sixties may be in order. There is no doubt whatever that drugs have made an enormous contribution in recent years to modern psychiatric practice. They have transformed our mental hospitals and given us invaluable assistance in controlling and modifying many of our patients' symptoms. Psychiatric practice would be vastly more difficult without them. However, the fantasy of the magic pill or drug that will some day cure all mental illness is, I believe, a fantasy based on wishful thinking, and will never materialize. The origin of most psychoneurotic disorders will continue to lie in the life experiences and early interpersonal relationships that have distorted the perceptions and the ego-integrative mechanisms of the people we see as patients. In a very fundamental sense, therefore, the heart of psychiatric practice will always be the psychotherapeutic process. The better we understand the nature of that process, the better our chances of helping those who turn to us for this critical assistance.

REFERENCES

1. ALEXANDER, F. The development of psychoanalytic therapy, in *Psychoanalytic Therapy* (F. Alexander & T. M. French, Eds.), New York, Ronald Press, 1946, p. 20
2. BREUER, J. & FREUD, S. *Studies on Hysteria* (1893–1895), New York, Basic Books, 1957
3. BUHLER, K. *Die Krise der Psychologie*, (2nd ed.), Jena, Gustav Fischer, 1929, p. 136
4. FIEDLER, F. E. A comparison of therapeutic relationships in psychoanalytic, nondirective, and Adlerian therapy. J. Consult. Psychol. 14: 436–445, 1950
5. HEINE, R. W. A comparison of patients' reports on psychotherapeutic experience with psychoanalytic, nondirective and Adlerian therapists. Am. J. Psychother. 7: 16–23, 1953
6. KLEIN, D. B. *Abnormal Psychology*, New York, Holt & Co., 1951, p. 521
7. KRASNER, L. Studies of the conditioning of verbal behavior. Psychol. Bull. 55: 148–170, 1958
   _____: The therapist as a social reinforcement machine. Presented at Second Conference on Research in Psychotherapy. Univ. North Carol., Chapel Hill, May 17–20, 1961
8. MANDLER, G. & KAPLAN, W. K. Subjective evaluation and reinforcing effect of a verbal stimulus. Science 124: 582–583, 1956
9. MARMOR, J. The feeling of superiority: an occupational hazard in the practice of psychotherapy. Am. J. Psych. 110: 370–376, 1953 (Chapter 21, this volume.)
10. MARMOR, J. Psychoanalytic therapy as an educational process, in *Science & Psychoanalysis* (J. Masserman, Ed.), Vol. V, New York, Grune & Stratton, 1962, pp. 286–299 (Chapter 15, this volume.)
11. MARMOR, J. Psychoanalytic therapy and theories of learning, in *Science & Psychoanalysis* (J. Masserman, Ed.), Vol. VII, New York, Grune & Stratton, 1964, pp. 265–279 (Chapter 16, this volume.)

12. Rosen, J. N. The treatment of schizophrenic psychosis by direct analytic therapy. Psychiat. Quart. 21: 3–37, 117–119, 1947
13. Wolpe, J. Quantitative relationships in the systematic desensitization of phobias. Am. J. of Psychiatry, Vol. 119, May 1963, p. 1063

24

DYNAMIC PSYCHOTHERAPY AND
BEHAVIOR THERAPY
Are They Irreconcilable?
(1971)

In the course of psychiatric training and practice our professional identities become so intimately linked to what we have learned and how we practice that we are prone to extol uncritically the virtues of our own techniques and to depreciate defensively those techniques that are different. The dialogue that has gone on between most behavior therapists and dynamic psychotherapists has been marred by this kind of bias, and claims as well as attacks have been made on both sides that are exaggerated and untenable. Science is not served by such emotional polemics but rather by objective efforts to evaluate and extend our knowledge.

Part of the confusion that exists in discussing these two basic approaches to therapy is that they are often dealt with as though each group represents a distinct entity when, in fact, they are anything but monolithic. The various schools of thought among dynamic psychotherapists are too well known to require elaboration. They cover a wide range from classical Freudians, to adherents of other major theorists, to eclectics who borrow from all of them, to still others who try to adapt their concepts to correspond with modern learning theories, information theory, game theory, or general systems theory.

What is less well known is that among behavior therapists also there is a broad range of differences, from adherents of Pavlov and Hull, to Skinnerians, to eclectics, and to those who lean toward information theory and general systems theory. At one end of each spectrum the theories of behavioral and dynamic psychotherapists tend to converge, while at the other end their divergence is very great. It is because adherents of these two approaches tend to define each other stereotypically in terms of their extremes that so much misunderstanding and heat are often generated between them.

It would further serve to clarify the discussion of this problem if we distinguish between investigative methods, therapeutic techniques, and theoretical formulations. A good investigative technique is not necessarily a good therapeutic technique, nor is the reverse true. By the same token, as we have long known, the success of a psychotherapeutic method for any particular condition does not in itself constitute a validation of its theoretical framework; indeed, exactly why and how any particular psychotherapeutic method works, and what it actually accomplishes within the complex organization of drives, perception, integration, affect, and behavior that we call personality, is itself a major research challenge.

In the remarks that follow, therefore, I shall not concern myself with the knotty issues of the comparison of results between behavior and psychodynamic therapies or of their validation. The problem of how to measure or evaluate psychotherapeutic change is still far from clear, and a matter for much-needed research. Moreover, comparisons of results between these two approaches are unsatisfactory because different criteria of efficacy are applied, and different techniques of investigation are employed, even if complete objectivity on the part of the various protagonists could be assumed—which is doubtful!

In addition, I shall not get into the oft-argued issue of whether or not simple symptom removal inevitably leads to symptom substitution. Long before behavior therapists began to question this hoary assumption, hypnotherapists had presented evidence that symptom substitution did not always take place when a symptom was removed by hypnosis (1). Indeed, I would agree, on purely theoretical grounds, that symptom substitution is *not* inevitable. Earlier psychoanalytic assumptions concerning symptom substitution were based on what we now know was an erroneous closed-system theory of personality dynamics. If the conflictual elements involved in neurosis formation are assumed to be part of a closed system, it follows logically that removal of the symptomatic consequences of such an inner conflict without altering the underlying dynamics should result in some other symptom manifestation. If, however, personality dynamics are more correctly perceived within the framework of an open system, then such a consequence is not inevitable. Removal of an ego-dystonic symptom may, on the contrary, produce such satisfying feedback from the environment that it may result in major constructive shifts within the personality system, thus leading to modification of the original conflictual pattern. Removal of a symptom also may lead to positive changes in the perception of the self, with resultant satisfying *internal* feedbacks, heightening of self-esteem, and a consequent restructuring of the internal psychodynamic system.

Psychodynamic theorists have been aware of this possibility for many years, dating back at least to 1946 when Alexander and French (2) published their book entitled *Psychoanalytic Therapy.* In this volume a number of cases of brief psychotherapy are described, some of them involving only one to three interviews, following which the patients were not only dramatically relieved of their presenting symptoms but were then able to go on to achieve more effective adaptive patterns of functioning than they had previously displayed. In the years that followed this important publication, dynamic psychotherapists have become increasingly involved with techniques of brief psychotherapy and of crisis intervention, with a growing body of evidence that in many instances such interventions can have long-lasting positive consequences for personality integration.

Where I part company with most behavior therapists is not in questioning their therapeutic claims—although I would offer the caution that many of them are repeating the error of the early psychoanalysts of promising more than they can deliver—but in what I consider to be their oversimplified explanations of what goes on in the therapeutic transaction between patient and therapist. The explanations to which I refer are those which assume that the essential and central core of their therapeutic process rests on Pavlovian or Skinnerian conditioning and, incidentally, is therefore more "scientific" than the traditional psychotherapies. With these formulations often goes a conception of neurosis that seems to me to be quite simplistic. Thus, according to Eysenck, "Learning theory [note that he uses the singular—actually there are many theories of learning] regards neurotic symptoms as simply learned habits; there is no *neurosis* underlying the symptom but merely the symptom itself. *Get rid of the symptom and you have eliminated the neurosis"* (3). Such an explanation is like evaluating the contents of a package in terms of its wrapping, and represents a regrettable retrogression from the more sophisticated thinking that has begun to characterize dynamic psychiatry in recent years; an approach that recognizes that "psychopathology" does not reside solely in the individual but also has significant roots in his system of relationships with his milieu and with other persons within his milieu. Hence the growing emphasis on family therapy, on conjoint marital therapy, on group therapy, and on dealing with the disordered socioeconomic conditions which constitute the matrix of so many personality disorders. To see the locus of psychopathology only in the individual leads to an emphasis on techniques of adjusting the individual to his environment regardless of how distorted, intolerable, or irrational that environment might be. Such an emphasis brings us uncomfortably close to the dangerous area of thought and behavior control.

However, I do not wish to overemphasize this ethical issue. The fact that a technical method may lend itself to being misused does not constitute an argument against its scientific validity. My major point is that the *theoretical* foundation of Eysenck's formulation is scientifically unsound. Even if we deliberately choose to restrict our focus only to what goes on within the individual himself, the Eysenckian point of view has profound limitations. It overlooks all of the complexities of thought, symbolism, and action which must be accounted for in any comprehensive theory of psychology and psychopathology. To assume that what goes on subjectively within the patient is irrelevant and that all that matters is how he behaves is to arbitrarily disregard all of the significant psychodynamic insights of the past 75 years. In saying this, I am not defending all of psychoanalytic theory. I have been as critical as anyone of certain aspects of classical Freudian theory and I am in full accord with those who argue that psychodynamic theory needs to be reformulated in terms that conform more closely to modern theories of learning and of neurophysiology. Current researches strongly suggest that the brain functions as an extremely intricate receiver, retriever, processor, and dispatcher of information. A stimulus-response theory of human behavior does not begin to do justice to this complex process. It is precisely what goes on in the "black box" *between* stimulus and response that is the central challenge of psychiatry, and no theory that ignores the complexities of the central processes within that "black box" can be considered an adequate one. It is to Freud's eternal credit, regardless of the limitations of some of his hypotheses, that he was the first to develop a rational investigative technique for, and a meaningful key to, the understanding of this uncharted realm that exerts so profound an influence on both our perceptions and our responses.

Evidence from learning theories themselves reveals that neurotic disorders are not necessarily the simple product of exposure to traumatic conditioning stimuli or to the operant conditioning of responses. The work of Pavlov, Liddell, Masserman, and others has clearly demonstrated that neurotic symptoms can ensue when an animal is faced with incompatible choices between simultaneous approach and avoidance reactions, or with confusing conditioned stimuli which it is unable to differentiate clearly. This corresponds to the psychodynamic concept of conflict as being at the root of the vast majority of human neurotic disorders. Once such a neurotic conflict is set up in a human being, secondary elaborations, defensive adaptations, and symbolic distortions may become extensively and indirectly intertwined with almost every aspect of the individual's perceptual, cognitive, and behavioral process.

A behavioral approach alone cannot encompass these complexities. Granting that Skinnerians include verbal speech as an aspect of behavior that may require modification, what shall we say about subjective *fantasies,* concealed *thoughts,* and hidden *feelings?* Are they totally irrelevant? What about problems involving conflicts in value system, disturbances in self-image, diffusion of identity, feelings of anomie, or even concealed delusions and hallucinations? Are they less important than specific symptom entities of a behavioral nature? No comprehensive theory of psychopathology or of the nature of the psychotherapeutic process can properly ignore these aspects of man's subjective life.

To illustrate my point that much more goes on between therapist and patient than most behavior therapists generally recognize, I should like now to briefly focus on three constrasting behavioral therapeutic approaches: (1) Wolpe's technique of reciprocal inhibition, (2) aversive conditioning treatment of homosexuality, and (3) the Masters and Johnson technique of treating sexual impotence and frigidity. In discussing these three approaches, I wish to emphasize that it is not my intention to denigrate their usefulness as therapeutic modalities or to question their results, but solely to present some of the diverse variables that I believe are involved in their therapeutic effectiveness.

Wolpe has elaborated his technique in many publications as well as in at least one film that I have seen. Although he considers the crux of his technique to be the development of a hierarchical list of graded anxieties which are then progressively dealt with by his technique of "reciprocal inhibition," the fact is that a great deal more than this takes place in the patient-therapist transaction in the Wolpe technique. Most significantly, in the orientation period of the first session or two the patient is not only informed of the treatment method per se, but also of the fact that it has yielded successful results with comparable patients, and it is indicated implicitly, if not explicitly, that the patient can expect similar success for himself if he is cooperative. Wolpe, moreover, is warm, friendly, and supportive. At the same time he is positive and authoritative in such a way as to reinforce the patient's expectations of therapeutic success. During this introductory period a detailed history is taken and even though the major emphasis is on the symptom with all of its manifestations and conditions for appearance, a detailed genetic history of personality development is usually taken also.

Following this a hierarchical list of the patient's anxieties is established. The patient is then taught a relaxation technique which is remarkably similar to what is traditionally employed in inducing hypnosis. After complete relaxation is achieved, the patient is instructed to create in fantasy these situations of graded anxiety beginning at the lowest level of anxiety, and is not permitted to go to the next level until he signals that he is completely relaxed. This procedure is repeated over and over again in anywhere from 12 to 60 or more sessions until the patient is able to fantasy the maximally phobic situation and still achieve muscular relaxation.

Throughout this procedure the patient receives the strong implication, either explicitly or implicitly, that this procedure will cause
his symptoms to disappear.

Wolpe attributes the success of his technique to "systematic desensitization" and explains it on the basis of Pavlovian counterconditioning. He asserts that any "activities that might give any grounds
for imputations of transference, insight, suggestion, or de-depres-
sion" are either "omitted or manipulated in such a way as to render
the operation of these mechanisms exceedingly implausible" (4).
This kind of claim that Wolpe repeatedly makes in his writings
clearly reflects his failure to appreciate the complexity of the variables
involved in the patient-therapist transaction. I cannot believe that
anyone who watches Wolpe's own film demonstration of his technique would agree that there are no elements of transference, insight,
or suggestion in it. Indeed, one could make as plausible a case
for the overriding influence of suggestion in his technique as for
the influence of desensitization. In saying this I am not being
pejorative about Wolpe's technique. Suggestion, in my opinion, is
an integral part of every psychotherapeutic technique, behavioral
or psychodynamic. It need not be overt; indeed, it probably works
most potently when it is covert. Suggestion is a complex process
in which elements of transference, expectancy, faith, and hope all
enter. To the degree that a patient is receptive and perceives the
therapist as a powerful help-giving figure, he is more likely to accept
the suggestions he is being given and to try to conform to them.
This process is most obvious in hypnosis but it is equally present
in all psychotherapeutic techniques, where the suggestion is usually
more covert. Wolpe's technique abounds in covert as well as overt
suggestion. It is questionable, moreover, whether the fantasies that
Wolpe has his patients create are actual substitutes for the phobic
reality situations, as he would have us believe. It may well be that
what is really taking place is not so much desensitization to specific
stimuli, as repeated reassurance and strong systematic suggestion,
within a setting of heightened expectancy and faith.

However, even the combination of *desensitization* (assuming that
it is taking place) and *suggestion* do not begin to cover all the elements
that are present in the Wolpe method. There is also the *direct
transmission of values,* as when Wolpe says to a young patient, "You

must learn to stand up for yourself." According to Ullman and Krasner (5), Wolpe hypothesizes that if a person can assert himself, anxiety will automatically be inhibited. (Parenthetically, one might question whether this is inevitably so. One frequently sees patients who assert themselves regularly, but always with enormous concomitant anxiety.) In any event, Ullman and Krasner say: "The therapist provides the motivation by pointing out the irrationality of the fears and encouraging the individual to insist on his legitimate human rights" (5). Obviously this is not very different from what goes on in dynamic psychotherapy and it is not rendered more scientific by virtue of the fact, according to Ullman and Krasner, that it is "given a physiological basis by Wolpe who refers to it as excitatory" (5). Still another variable which cannot be ignored is Wolpe's manner, which, whether he realizes it or not, undoubtedly facilitates a "positive transference" in his patients. In his film he is not only kindly and empathic to his female patient, but occasionally reassuringly touches her. Does Wolpe really believe that a programmed computer repeating his instructions to a patient who had had no prior contact with the doctor himself would achieve the identical therapeutic results?

The second behavioral technique that I would like to briefly consider is that of the aversion treatment of homosexuals. I had occasion to explore this technique some time ago with Dr. Lee Birk, of the Massachusetts Mental Health Center, who was kind enough to demonstrate his technique and go over his results with me.

Dr. Birk's method is based on the anticipatory avoidance conditioning technique introduced by Feldman and MacCulloch (6). The patient is seated in a chair in front of a screen with an electrode cuff attached to his leg. The method involves the use of patient-selected nude and semi-nude male and female pictures which are flashed onto the screen. The male pictures (and presumably the fantasies associated with them) become aversive stimuli by linkage with electric shocks which are administered to the leg whenever these pictures appear on the screen. On the other hand, the female pictures become discriminative stimuli signaling safety, relief, and protection from the shocks.

In Dr. Birk's hands, as in others, the use of this method has apparently produced a striking reversal of sexual feelings and behavior in more than one half of the male homosexuals so treated.

On the face of it, this would seem to be the result of a relatively simple negative conditioning process to aversive "male" stimuli, with concomitant positive conditioning to "female" stimuli.

Closer inspection will reveal, however, that the process is considerably more complex. I wonder whether most psychiatrists realize what is actually involved in such aversive conditioning. I know that I, for one, did not, until I asked Dr. Birk to permit me to experience the kind of shock that he administered to his patients—the least intense, incidentally, of the graded series that he employed. I can only say that if that was a "mild" shock, I never want to be subjected to a "severe" one! I do not have a particularly low threshold for pain, but it was a severe and painful jolt—much more than I had anticipated—and it made me acutely aware of *how strongly motivated toward change a male homosexual would have to be to subject himself to a series of such shocks visit after visit.*

The significance of this variable cannot be ignored. Once it is recognized, the results of aversive therapy, although still notable, become less remarkable. The fact is that if other forms of psychotherapy were limited only to such a select group of exceptionally motivated homosexuals, the results also would be better than average. Although one might assume that in dynamic psychotherapies the cost of therapy in itself should insure equally good motivation, this is not always the fact. Costs of therapy may not be sacrificial, or they may be borne or shared by others, but no one else can share the pain involved in the aversive conditioning process.

Again, then, it becomes clear that we are dealing with something that is much more complicated than a simple conditioning process. The patient's intense wish to change, and his faith and expectation that this very special technique will work for him—as the doctor himself implicitly or explicitly suggests—are important factors in the total therapeutic gestalt of this aversive technique, as they are in successful dynamic psychotherapies also.

But more than this, the transference-countertransference transaction between therapist and subject is also of paramount importance. Dr. Birk communicated two interesting experiences he had which underline this point. Two of his subjects who had had very favorable responses to the "conditioning" procedure suffered serious relapses immediately after becoming angry at him. The first patient became upset because of what he considered a breach in the privacy of his treatment. Before this, he had not only been free from homosexual contacts for the first time in many years, but also of conscious homosexual urges. When he became angry, he immediately went and sought out a homosexual partner because he wanted to see "how really good" the treatment was. Dr. Birk was aware that his patient obviously wanted to show him up and prove that the treatment was no good. Although the patient remained improved as compared to his previous homosexual behavior, *he was never again,* despite many more conditioning treatments, completely free from conscious homosexual urges and continued to act them out although less frequently than in the past. The second patient became angry with Dr. Birk because he concluded that the therapist seemed to be more interested in the results he was obtaining than he was in the patient as a person. Immediately after expressing this irritation the patient regressed to a series of homosexual encounters.

These striking examples illustrate that a simple conditioning explanation does not fit the complex process that goes on in such techniques of therapy. Aversive conditioning that has been solidly established would not be expected to disappear on the basis of such experiences unless there is something that goes on centrally in the patient that is a very important factor in the therapeutic modifications achieved. A basic aspect of this central process is in the patient-physician interpersonal relationship and it cannot and must not be ignored even in behavior therapies. I have recently encountered a number of instances where patients who were referred to behavior therapists failed to return to them after the initial sessions because the behavior therapists involved ignored this essential factor and related to the patients as though they were dealing with experimental animals.

Let us now turn to a consideration of the Masters and Johnson (7) technique of treating disorders of sexual potency. In many ways this technique falls midway between a behavioral and a psychodynamic approach and illustrates one of the ways in which a fusion of both can be successfully employed. The Masters and Johnson technique is behavioral in the sense that it is essentially symptom-focused, and that one of its most important technical tools is desensitization of the performance anxieties of the patients.

Conceptually, however, the Masters and Johnson approach to their patients goes considerably beyond simple conditioning or desensitization processes. For one thing, Masters and Johnson recognize that the problem of impotency or frigidity does not exist merely in the symptomatic individual but in his relationship with his partner. Therefore, they insist on treating the couple as a unit, and the symptom as a problem of the unit. This constitutes a systems approach in contrast to a strictly intrapsychic or behavioral one.

Secondly, Masters and Johnson are acutely aware of the influence of psychodynamic factors on the sexual behavior of their couples. In their preliminary interviews they carefully assess and evaluate the importance of these factors, and if they consider the neurotic components or interpersonal difficulties to be too great, they may refuse to proceed with their method and will refer the couple back to their physicians for appropriate psychotherapy.

This kind of selective procedure has an effect, of course, on their percentage of successful results, as does the high degree of motivation that their patients must have to come to St. Louis (who, after all, goes to St. Louis for a two-week vacation?) and to commit themselves to the considerable expense and inconvenience that is involved.

The fact, also, that Masters and Johnson insist that the therapeutic team consist of a man and a woman reveals their sensitivity to the transference implications of their relationship to their couples. They function as a sexually permissive and empathic mother-surrogate and father-surrogate who offer not only valuable technical advice and suggestions concerning sexual behavior, but also a compassion and understanding that constitute a corrective emotional experience for their patients.

Finally, the tremendous charisma and authority of this highly publicized therapeutic team must inevitably have an enormous impact on the expectancy, faith, and hope with which their patients come to them. This cannot help but greatly accentuate the suggestive impact of the given instructions in facilitating their patients' therapeutic improvement. This improvement is then reinforced by subsequent follow-up telephone calls which, among other things, confirm to the patient the empathic interest, concern, and dedication of these parent-surrogates.

I am all too aware that these brief and summary remarks cannot begin to do justice to the three above-mentioned behavioral techniques. I hope, however, that I have succeeded in making the point that in each of these instances, complex variables are involved that go beyond any simple stimulus-response conditioning model.

The research on the nature of the psychotherapeutic process in which I participated with Franz Alexander beginning in 1958 has convinced me that all psychotherapy, regardless of the techniques used, is a learning process (8–10). Dynamic psychotherapies and behavior therapies simply represent different teaching techniques, and their differences are based in part on differences in their goals and in part on their assumptions about the nature of psychopathology. Certain fundamental elements, however, are present in both approaches.

In any psychotherapeutic relationship, we start with an individual who presents a problem. This problem may be in the form of behavior that is regarded as deviant, or it may be in the form of subjective discomfort, or in certain distortions of perception, cognition, or affect, or in any combination of these. Usually, but not always, these problems motivate the individual or someone in his milieu to consider psychiatric treatment. This decision in itself establishes an *expectancy* in the individual which is quite different than if, say, "punishment" rather than "treatment" were prescribed for his problems. This expectancy is an essential part of *every* psychotherapeutic transaction at its outset, regardless of whether the patient presents himself for behavioral or dynamic psychotherapy. The patient, in other words, is *not* a neutral object in whom certain neurotic symptoms or habits have been mechanically established and from whom they can now be mechanically removed.

Expectancy is a complex process. It encompasses factors that Frank (11) has demonstrated as being of major significance in psychotherapy—the degree of faith, trust, and hope that the patient consciously or unconsciously brings into the transaction. It is based in large part on previously established perceptions of authority or help-giving figures, perceptions that play a significant role in the degree of receptivity or nonreceptivity that the patient may show to the message he receives from the psychotherapist. Psychoanalysts have traditionally referred to these presenting expectations as aspects of "transference," but regardless of what they are called, they are always present.

Transference is not, as some behavior therapists seem to think, something that is "created" by the therapist—although it is true that transference distortions may be either increased or diminished by the technique the therapist employs. The way in which the therapist relates to the patient may reinforce certain maladaptive perceptions or expectations, or it may teach the patient that his previously learned expectations in relation to help-giving or authority figures are incorrect. The latter teaching is part of what Alexander and French (2) called the "corrective emotional experience."

Even in "simple" conditioning studies, experimenters like Liddell, Masserman, and Pavlov have called attention to the significance of the relationship between the experimental animal and the experimenter. In humans the problem is more complex, however. Thus, a therapist who behaves in a kindly but authoritarian manner may confirm the patient's expectancies that authority figures are omnipotent and omniscient. This increases the patient's faith and may actually facilitate his willingness to give up his symptoms to please the powerful and good parent-therapist, but it does *not* alter his childlike self-image in relation to authority figures. Depending on the therapist's objectives, this may or may not be of importance.

What I am indicating, in other words, is that a positive transference facilitates symptom removal, but if the patient's *emotional maturation, rather than just symptom removal, is the goal of therapy,* what is necessary eventually is a "dissolution" of this positive transference—which means teaching the patient to feel and function in a less child-like manner, not only in relation to the therapist but also to other authority figures.

Closely related to and interacting with the patient's motivations and expectancies is the therapist's social and professional role, by virtue of which the help-seeking patient endows him with presumptive knowledge, prestige, authority, and help-giving ptoential. These factors play an enormous role in strengthening the capacity of the therapist to influence the patient, and constitute another element in the complex fabric that makes up the phenomenon of positive transference.

Also, the *real persons* of both patient and therapist, their actual physical, intellectual and emotional assets and liabilities, and their respective *value systems* enter into the therapeutic transaction. Neither the patient nor the therapist can be regarded as stereotypes upon whom any particular technique will automatically work. Their idiosyncratic variables are always an important part of their transaction.

Given the above factors, a number of things begin to happen more or less simultaneously, in varying degrees, in behavior therapies as well as in dynamic psychotherapies. I have discussed these factors in detail elsewhere and will merely summarize them here. They are:

> (1) *Release of tension* through catharsis and by virtue of the patient's hope, faith, and expectancy. (2) *Cognitive learning,* both of the trial-and-error variety and the gestalt variety. (3) Reconditioning by virtue of *operant conditioning,* by virtue of subtle reward-punishment cues from the therapist, and by corrective emotional experiences. (4) *Identification* with the therapist. (5) Repeated *reality testing,* which is the equivalent of *practice* in the learning process. These five elements encompass the most significant factors on the basis of which change takes place in a psychotherapeutic relationship. (10)

As I have mentioned above, suggestion takes place in all of these, covertly or overtly. Furthermore, as can be seen, a conditioning process takes place in dynamic psychotherapies as well as in behavior therapies, except that in the latter this process is intentional and more structured, while in the former it has not been generally recognized. In focusing on this conditioning process, behavior therapists have made a valuable contribution to the understanding of the therapeutic process. It is the thrust of this paper, however, that in so doing they have tended to minimize or ignore other important and essential elements in the therapeutic process, particularly the subtle but critical aspects of the patient-therapist interpersonal relationship.

In the final analysis, the technique of therapy that we choose to employ must depend on what aspect of man's complex psychic functioning we address ourselves to. If we choose to focus on the patient's overt symptoms or behavior patterns, some kind of behavior therapy may well be the treatment of choice. On the other hand, if the core of his problems rests in symbolic distortions of perception, cognition, affect, or subtle disturbances in interpersonal relationships, the source and nature of which he may be totally unaware, then the more elaborate reeducational process of dynamic psychotherapy may be necessary.

Moreover, indications for one approach do not necessarily rule out the other. Marks and Gelder (12,13) and Brady (14), among others, have demonstrated that the use of both behavior therapy and dynamic therapy with the same patient either concurrently or in sequence often brings about better therapeutic results than the use of either approach alone. Indeed, many dynamic psychotherapists have for years been unwittingly using such a combination of approaches when they prescribe drugs for the direct control of certain symptoms while concurrently pursuing a psychotherapeutic approach.

To conclude, then, in my opinion behavior therapies and dynamic psychotherapies, far from being irreconcilable, are complementary psychotherapeutic approaches. The line of demarcation between them is by no means a sharp one. As Breger and McGaugh (15) and others have shown, behavior therapists do many things in the course of their conditioning procedures that duplicate the activities of dynamic psychotherapists including ". . . discussions, explanation of techniques and of the unadaptiveness of anxiety and symptoms, hypnosis, relaxation, 'nondirective cathartic discussions,' and 'obtaining an understanding of the patient's personality and background'" (15). The process in both approaches is best explicable in terms of current theories of learning which go beyond simple conditioning explanations and encompass central cognitive processes also. The fact that in some disorders one or the other approach may be more effective should not surprise us and presents no contradiction. Just as there is no single best way of teaching all pupils all subjects, there is no single psychotherapeutic technique that is optimum for all patients and all psychiatric disorders.

Within this total context, it seems to me that behavior therapists deserve much credit for having opened wide the armamentarium of therapeutic strategies. By so doing they have forced dynamic psychotherapists into a reassessment of their therapeutic techniques and their effectiveness—a reassessment that in the long run can only be in the best interests of all psychiatrists and their patients. The psychotherapeutic challenge of the future is to so improve our theoretical and diagnostic approaches to psychopathology as to be able to most knowledgeably and flexibly apply to each patient the particular treatment technique and the particular kind of therapist that together will most effectively achieve the desired therapeutic goal.

Since completing this paper, I have come across the excellent article by Klein et al (16) in which many of the conclusions I have set forth are confirmed by them as a result of five days of direct observation of the work of Wolpe and his group at the Eastern Pennsylvania Psychiatric Institute. The authors also point out that as a consequence of their increasing popularity, behavior therapists are now beginning to treat a broader spectrum of more "difficult" patients (complex psychoneurotic problems, character neuroses, or borderline psychotic problems) with the result that their treatment procedures are "becoming longer and more complicated, with concomitant lowering of success rates."

REFERENCES

1. WOLBERG, L. R.: Hypnotherapy, in McCary, J. L. (ed): *Six Approaches to Psychotherapy.* New York, Dryden Press, 1955, pp. 63–126.
2. ALEXANDER, F., FRENCH, T. M., et al: *Psychoanalytic Therapy.* New York, Ronald Press Co, 1946.
3. EYSENCK, H. J. (ed): *Behavior Therapy and the Neuroses.* New York, Pergamon Press, 1960.
4. WOLPE J.: *Psychotherapy by Reciprocal Inhibition.* Stanford, Calif, Stanford University Press, 1958.
5. ULLMAN, L. P., KRASNER, L. (eds): *Case Studies in Behavior Modification.* New York, Holt Rinehart & Winston Inc, 1965.
6. FELDMAN, M. P., MacCULLOCH, M. I.: The application of anticipatory avoidance learning to the treatment of homosexuality. *Behav Res Ther* 2:165–183, 1965.
7. MASTERS, W. H., JOHNSON, V. E.: *Human Sexual Response.* Boston, Little Brown & Co, 1965.
8. MARMOR, J.: Psychoanalytic therapy as an educational process, in Masserman J., Salzman, L. (eds): *Modern Concepts of Psychoanalysis.* New York, Philosophical Library Inc., 1962, pp 189–205. (Chapter 15, this volume.)
9. MARMOR, J.: Psychoanalytic therapy and theories of learning, in Masserman, J. (ed): *Science and Psychoanalysis.* New York, Grune & Stratton Inc, 1964, vol 7, pp 265–279. (Chapter 16, this volume.)
10. MARMOR, J.: The nature of the psychotherapeutic process, in Usdin, G., (ed): *Psychoneurosis and Schizophrenia.* New York, J. B. Lippincott Co, 1966, pp 66–75. (Chapter 23, this volume.)
11. FRANK, J. D.: *Persuasion and Healing.* Baltimore, Johns Hopkins Press, 1961.

12. MARKS, I. M., GELDER, M. G.: A controlled retrospective study of behavior therapy in phobic patients. *Brit J Psychiat* 111:561–573, 1965.
13. MARKS, I. M., GELDER, M. G.: Common ground between behavior therapy and psychodynamic methods. *Brit J Med Psychol* 39:11–23, 1966.
14. BRADY, J. P.: Psychotherapy by a combined behavioral and dynamic approach. *Compr Psychiat* 9:536–543, 1968.
15. BREGER, L., McGAUGH, J. L.: Critique and reformulation of learning theory approaches to psychotherapy and neurosis. *Psychol Bull* 63:338–358, 1965.
16. KLEIN, M. H., DITTMAN, A. T., PARLOFF, M. B., et al: Behavior therapy: Observations and reflections. *J Consult Clin Psychol* 33:259–266, 1969.

25

SEXUAL ACTING-OUT IN
PSYCHOTHERAPY
(1972)

Erotic transference reactions on the part of patients and problems dealing with seductive female patients have been dealt with frequently in psychiatric and psychoanalytic literature. There has been relatively little written, however, about seductive psychotherapists and *counter-transference* sexual acting-out. Masters and Johnson make passing references to sexual relations between patients and therapists (5), and more recently Dahlberg (1) and Marmor (4) independently have dealt with this issue.

Although no profession involving intimate contacts with clients or patients of the opposite sex is immune to heterosexual temptation, psychoanalysts and psychotherapists are put to the test more often and more stringently than most because, by its very nature, an intensive psychotherapeutic transaction over a long period of time tends to foster a special quality of emotional intimacy.

The erotized idealization of the therapist that often develops in the course of such a transaction can be a heady wine (3), and when combined with a physically attractive patient of the opposite sex, often creates a powerfully seductive mixture.

For his own part, the psychoanalyst or psychotherapist is himself beset by deeply rooted, often unconscious, needs that tend to foster or stimulate impulses toward physical closeness towards his patients. First, there is the obvious factor of the strength of his own biological needs. These are by no means constant, and will vary in urgency at any point in time, depending on a number of factors such as age, physical health, the satisfactory or unsatisfactory state of his own sex life and marriage, recency of drive satisfaction, and the relative attractiveness and/or seductiveness of his patient. Second, the therapist's psychological need to be a helping figure (a factor in his choice of profession) is reinforced by the actual needs and dependency of his help-seeking patient. Thus, just as the patient often reacts to the therapist in the transference as a wise, good and loving father-figure, the therapist's countertransference may stimulate him to respond as a loving and affectionate "parent" to his deprived "child."

An interesting note in the early history of psychoanalysis exemplifies this point. In the late 1920's Ferenczi, one of Freud's most devoted friends and disciples, began to experiment with more "active" techniques of analysis because of his dissatisfaction with the therapeutic results of the classic method. One of these techniques—based on his ideas about the central importance of infantile traumas, and especially parental unkindness, in the genesis of neurosis—involved his acting the part of a loving parent, even to the point of showing physical affection, so as to presumably neutralize the early unhappiness and emotional deprivation of his patients. Ferenczi communicated his technical ideas to Freud, who responded to them as follows, in a letter dated December 13, 1931:

". . . You have not made a secret of the fact that you kiss your patients and let them kiss you; I had also heard that from a patient of my own. Now when you decide to give a full account of your technique and its results you will have to choose between two ways: either you relate this or you conceal it. The latter, as you may well think, is dishonorable. What one does in one's technique one has to defend openly. Besides, both ways soon come together. Even if you don't say so yourself it will soon get known, just as I knew it before you told me.

"Now I am assuredly not one of those who from prudishness or from consideration of bourgeois convention would condemn little erotic gratifications of this kind. And I am also aware that in the time of the Nibelungs a kiss was a harmless greeting granted to every guest . . . But that does not alter the fact . . . that with us a kiss signifies a certain erotic intimacy. We have hitherto in our technique held to the conclusion that patients are to be refused erotic gratifications . . .

"Now picture what will be the result of publishing your technique. There is no revolutionary who is not driven out of the field by a still more radical one. A number of independent thinkers in matters of technique will say to themselves: Why stop at a kiss? Certainly one gets further when one adopts 'pawing' as well, which after all doesn't make a baby. And then bolder ones will come along who will go further, to peeping and showing—and soon we shall have accepted in the technique of analysis the whole repertoire of demiviergerie and petting parties, resulting in an enormous increase of interest in psychoanalysis among both analysts and patients. The new adherent, however, will easily claim too much of this interest for himself; the younger of our colleagues will find it hard to stop at the point they originally intended, and God the Father Ferenczi, gazing at the lively scene he has created will perhaps say to himself: Maybe after all I should have halted in my technique of motherly affection before the kiss." (2)

Freud's misgivings concerning Ferenczi's technical innovations proved to be prophetic. Over the course of the succeeding decades, various "more radical" colleagues have indeed extended Ferenczi's ideas step by step to a point at which some psychotherapists have attempted to rationalize various forms of erotic interplay and even intercourse with their female patients on grounds of offering restitutive emotional experiences, or of providing a learning experience for naive or virginal patients. As might be expected, no figures are available concerning the relative frequency or infrequency of such practices. My impression is that such behavior is limited to a very small segment of practicing psychotherapists. Nevertheless, because its potential for harm, not only to the patient but also to the practice of psychotherapy, is far-reaching, it should not be ignored.*

A significant psychoanalytic figure in these extensions of Ferenczi's ideas was Wilhelm Reich. Although Reich never openly advocated sexual acting-out with patients, his theoretical views lend themselves, at the very least, to patient-therapist interactions that greatly increase

---

*I shall not deal in this paper with the various types of erotized "group therapy" which seem to be increasing in frequency and popularity in recent years, although some of the issues I shall be raising may have relevance to them also. An important difference, however, is that individuals participating in such group interactions for the most part are *consciously* seeking erotic experiences and have some idea of what they are getting into. This is not usually true of the patient seeking psychotherapy.

the temptation towards such behavior. Reich's views carried Freud's libido theory to a reductio ad absurdum, in which achieving the capacity for satisfactory sexual release (as the ultimate expression of "genital object libido"), became the prime measure of mental health. "The goal of analytic therapy," according to Reich, "is that of crystallizing out the genital object libido, of liberating it from repression and from its admixture with narcissistic, pre-genital and destructive impulses . . . The task in handling the transference is that of *concentrating all object libido in a purely genital transference*" [italics are Reich's] (9). Reich considers the following as signs that the "sensual genital striving" has been liberated from repression—a prime criterion, in his judgment, for a successful analysis:

"1. *Genital masturbation without guilt feeling,* with genital transference phantasies and corresponding gratification . . .
"2. *Phantasies of incest without guilt feeling* . . .
"3. *Genital excitation during the analysis,* indicating that the castration anxiety has been overcome." [italics are Reich's] (10)

Exactly what techniques Reich employed to achieve these goals is not explicitly stated, but according to McCartney (see below), who claims to have talked with some of Reich's students and analysands, "they related that he required each to disrobe and to respond to their instinctual needs. He physically manipulated the patient to appropriate response, concentrating on the erotic zones until the orgasm was reached" (7).

It is difficult to know, since McCartney is no longer living (he died in 1969), whether this report of his had any validity or not. Since the publication of my first article on this subject (4), however, I have received a communication from a group of "orgonomic" psychiatrists, followers of Reich, who strongly deny that this was his practice. What is important in the context of my present thesis, however, is not whether or not this *was* Reich's practice, but that McCartney used Reich's theories to rationalize the most extreme form of sexual acting-out with patients that has ever, to my knowledge, been reported in the psychiatric literature.

In a paper published in 1966 (7) McCartney reported that during the last forty years of his practice he had conducted "over 1500 psychoanalyses." This would mean that he "completed" an average of more than thirty-seven analyses a year; yet, according to him, these represented only twenty-six percent of all the psychiatric patients that he saw! His concept of psychoanalysis may be better understood when it is realized that many of his "analyses" consisted of about 30 hours over an 8-month period, and that their overall average was 89 hours. (I need hardly add that as far as I have been able to ascertain, McCartney belonged to no accredited psychoanalytic society and that his "training" evidently consisted of some relatively brief contacts with Carl Jung, and with Ben Karpman, a Stekelian, who worked at St. Elizabeth's Hospital in Washington, D.C., for most of his professional life.) McCartney goes on to state that of his 825 adult woman "analysands," "thirty percent expressed some form of overt transference as sitting on the analyst's lap, holding his hand, hugging or kissing him," and that about ten percent "found it necessary (sic!) to act out extremely, such as mutual undressing, genital manipulation, or coitus" (8). McCartney's rationalization for this form of "therapy" is that "in working through Overt Transference the analyst should allow himself to be reacted to as though he were a parent. As the analysand progresses through the various stages of psychosexual development, she at first expresses infantile strivings and adolescent needs but, if she is to achieve full heterosexual maturity, she must be able to work through both libidinal and aggressive urges which the analyst must help her to understand and normally express" (8).

McCartney's recognition that there is a parent-child element to the transference relationship between therapist and patient is indeed correct, but the logic by which he then proceeds to justify an overt sexual relationship between the "parent" and the "child" is little short of remarkable. *It is precisely because this kind of unconscious relationship exists between patient and therapist that an erotic exchange between them cannot be ethically or psychotherapeutically justified.* Since when is it necessary for a parent to have sexual intercourse with his children in order to enable them to achieve sexual and emotional maturity? Such behavior between the therapist and patient has all the elements of incest at an unconscious psychodynamic level, and represents an equivalent dereliction of moral responsibility.

Therapists who ignore the transference-countertransference implications of such behavior and attempt to rationalize it on other grounds, such as the importance of establishing "contact" with their patients, or of removing the sexual inhibitions or fears of "intimacy" of their patients simply betray an ignorance of unconscious psychodynamics. Moreover, depite all of the "technical" explanations that these therapists may attach to their erotic exchanges with their patients, the fact is that the vast majority of patients invest such intimacies with reality connotations, and develop hopes and expectations that are doomed to disappointment. As every experienced psychotherapist knows, erotized fantasies of transference-love often develop in female patients, but when the therapist lends reality to these fantasies by his overt behavior, he fosters a serious confusion between reality and fantasy in such patients. The ultimate consequences are inevitably anti-therapeutic.

The essential foundation on which the patient-therapist relationship rests in psychotherapy is that of a *basic trust*. On the implicit and explicit assumption that this trust will not be betrayed, the patient is encouraged to set aside her customary psychological defenses and open herelf completely to the presumably benign and therapeutic influence of the therapist's professional skill. The ethical psychotherapist cannot and must not exploit the positive transference that develops under such circumstances. Any therapist who insists that this method helps his patients has the burden of proof to demonstrate that they *could not have been equally helped in any other way*. Otherwise the suspicion will always remain that such therapists are using their techniques to mask and rationalize their own countertransference needs.*

Moreover, in the interests of scientific integrity, any therapist using such techniques should publicly affirm that this is how he works so that patients going to him may be fully aware that this is the technique to which they may be subjected, *before* they are

---

*It is not my purpose in this brief essay to expound on the variety of inner needs that may be involved in such countertransference behavior. Suffice it to say that they are not all necessarily erotic in nature. Unconscious hostility towards women, reaction-formations against feelings of masculine inadequacy or against unconscious fears of homosexuality are other factors that may be encountered. Obviously, none of these are mutually exclusive.

caught in the emotional web of a positive transference. To patients who will nevertheless choose to go to such a therapist, one can only say, "caveat emptor"! I have yet to see a woman who became involved in an erotic relationship with a therapist who did not subsequently end up resenting him and feeling betrayed by him. Some of these patients were actually precipitated into psychotic decompensation by these experiences. The counterclaim can be made, of course, that, after all, the consulting psychiatrist comes into contact with only those cases that have gone awry. Perhaps so, but the psychodynamics of these situations leave little doubt in my mind that the negative effects must inevitably outweigh any positive ones. Those who argue to the contrary have a professional obligation to publish their "favorable" results and expose them to the consensual validation of their peers.

Still another element involved, of course, is the threat that such behavior poses to the professional status of the psychotherapist himself. I still recall the tragic end to the brightly promising career of that gifted psychiatrist, W. Beran Wolfe, who had to flee the country in the 1930's when he was charged with "impairing the morals" of an adolescent girl whom he had had under treatment. Wolfe subsequently was killed in an auto accident in Europe while traveling with another patient of his.

It is, of course, possible for a therapist to genuinely fall in love with his patient. After all, therapists are human beings and are not immune to such feelings. If and when such an event should take place, however, there is a primary obligation on the part of the therapist to immediately discontinue his therapy and thereafter relate to his patient simply as one human being to another. Any further treatment that she receives should be at the hands of another therapist. Having said this, however, I must still affirm my clinical conviction that the therapist to whom this happens has failed in his primary responsibility to the woman who came to him as a patient. I make this statement in full knowledge of the fact that a number of prominent psychiatrists and psychoanalysts have married former patients. How many others, who did not reach this honorable end-point, have nevertheless rationalized their loss of self-control on the basis of "falling in love" with their patients I do not know.

My point, however, is that such a rationalization should not obscure the fact that whenever this happens, the psychotherapist has not been able to master his countertransference feelings.

Although up to this point this article has ben written primarily within the context of the male therapist-female patient relationship, it should not be assumed that sexual acting-out is restricted only to this pattern. In their volume on *Human Sexual Inadequacy,* Masters and Johnson report obtaining histories of sexual exchange between patients and therapists from every conceivable level of professional discipline involved in the counseling or treatment of sexually inadequate individuals, including theologians and lawyers as well as physicians and psychologists. Although the most frequently encountered pattern was that of seduction of females by male therapists, they have also recorded histories of male patients seduced by male therapists, of female patients seduced by female therapists, and of "two female therapists who have joined male patients in sexual intercourse" (6).

It is interesting to note that seduction of male patients by female therapists, although not unknown, seems to occur much less frequently than the reverse pattern. There are a number of probable reasons for this. For one thing, women in our culture are conditioned from an early age not to take the initiative sexually, and thus generally are more able than men to control their sexual impulses. Within the same cultural context, women are reared to consider it ego-syntonic and virtuous to reject a male's sexual advances but our sexual double standards provide much less of a protective superego barrier to the male faced with a seductive female. Finally, of course, in almost all societies, the incest taboos between mothers and sons are more powerful than those between fathers and daughters. Thus within the parent-child transference of the therapeutic interaction, the barriers toward sexual acting-out between female therapist and male patient tend to be stronger on both sides.

One final consideration: Can the "laying on of hands" ever be considered a useful therapeutic adjuvant? My answer to this would be a qualified yes—in highly specific clinical situations. In an anaclitic therapeutic approach to seriously ill psychosomatic patients, such as those with ulcerative colitis, or status asthmaticus, a "maternal" holding or stroking of hands may be both helpful and justified.

Similar behavior may be indicated and useful with regressed psychotic patients. Nonerotic holding or hugging of preadolescent children, especially autistic and withdrawn ones, may even be essential to their therapy.

With most patients with neurotic and personality disorders, however, in my opinion, the psychotherapist should be extremely wary with regard to physical contacts if there is the slightest possibility that they might be interpreted or responded to as erotic. Once therapist and patient have gotten to know each other well, and a complete sense of mutual trust and security has been established between them, a friendly or reassuring pat on the shoulder may be a useful bit of nonverbal communication. But the therapist who does this must be quite sure of his own motives and feelings in so doing. If there is any hidden erotic element in such a gesture, the patient's unconscious will usually pick it up—to the detriment of the therapeutic process. The cardinal rule of all medical therapy applies here as elsewhere—*above all else, do not harm your patient. Primum non nocere!*

REFERENCES

1. DAHLBERG, C. C., "Sexual Contact Between Patient and Therapist," *Contemporary Psychoanalysis*, 6:107–124, 1970.
2. JONES, E., *Life and Work of Sigmund Freud*, Vol. 3, Basic Books, Inc., New York, 1957, pp. 163–164.
3. MARMOR, J., "The Feeling of Superiority: An Occupational Hazard in the Practice of Psychotherapy," *Amer. J. of Psychiat.* Vol. 110, No. 5, 370–373, Nov. 1953. (Chapter 21, this volume.)
4. MARMOR, J., "The Seductive Psychotherapist," *Psychiatry Digest* 31: 10–16, 1970.
5. MASTERS, W. & JOHNSON, V., *Human Sexual Inadequacy*, Little, Brown & Co., Boston, 1970.
6. _____ op. cit., p. 390.
7. McCARTNEY, J., "Overt Transference," *J. Sex Research*, 2:227–237, November 1966, p. 230.
8. _____ op. cit. p. 236.
9. REICH, W., *Character-Analysis*, Orgone Institute Press, New York, 1945, pp. 126–127.
10. _____ op cit. p. 133.

26

CHANGING TRENDS IN
PSYCHOTHERAPY
(1973)

Most psychiatric historians trace the beginnings of dynamic psychotherapy to the currents initiated by Mesmer in the late eighteenth century, currents which made the first substantial inroads into the then prevailing approaches based on somatic supremacy. By the time Freud opened his office in Vienna in 1886, a considerable development was already beginning to take place in the treatment of neurotic disorders. The Nancy school under Bernheim had coined the term "psychotherapeutics," and strongly emphasized the importance of suggestion in the treatment process. Under the influence of this school, a variety of psychotherapies were developed over the next decade by French psychiatrists, all emphasizing techniques of suggestion, persuasion, and indoctrination. Pierre Janet described unconscious psychodynamic mechanisms and developed a system which he called "psychological analysis." In Switzerland, Paul Dubois achieved considerable prominence and success with a method that he called rational psychotherapy, in which he specifically abjured "authority, suggestion, and suggestibility" which he considered to be only of temporary effect. He believed in "curing the will through self-education," and his method was based on modifying "the erroneous ideas that the patient has allowed to creep into his mind." He recognized, he said, "but one means of education, persuasion by means of proof, by demonstration, by logical induction, and by reason which touches the heart" (1).

Thus the method of treating neurosis that Sigmund Freud gradually evolved in the 1890's and early 1900's was not entirely a unique one. His special genius was that in addition to a well-organized therapeutic method, he also evolved an original and creative psychological theory resting on developmental concepts. He was the first to emphasize the importance of sexuality, especially infantile sexuality, in human behavior, and the first to recognize and identify the phenomenon of transference and its significant implications in the psychotherapeutic process. Freud believed that most psychoneurotic disorders could be traced back to the experiential vicissitudes of the first six years of childhood, and his psychoanalytic method was based on the assumption that if patients could be enabled to recall and "work through" the repressed memories of these early experiences, they would ipso facto be cured of their disorder.

It is an ironic paradox, that Freud, who more than any other man in history is credited with shattering man's belief in his rationality by emphasizing the degree to which man is driven by blind, irrational forces outside of his awareness, nevertheless put his own ultimate faith in man's reason. "We may insist as much as we like (he wrote) that the human intellect is weak in comparison with human instincts, and be right in doing so. But, nevertheless, there is something peculiar about this weakness. The voice of the intellect is a soft one, but it does not rest until it has gained a hearing" (2). Freud regarded the analytic treatment of neurotics as a process whereby "the consequence of repression [is replaced] by the results of rational mental effort" (3). "Where id was, there shall ego be" (4).

It is worth noting that despite the sometimes bitter disputes that have arisen between the Freudian and other psychoanalytic schools of thought—from the earliest Adlerian and Jungian variations through the diverse neo-Freudian groups, to the current Kleinian vogue—this basic premise of Freudian psychotherapy has never really been seriously questioned by these other schools. Differences have been principally over what constituted the best or most "correct" interpretation of the underlying psychodynamics, but all psychoanalytic schools have shared the assumption that making the correct cognitive interpretation to the patient is the core factor in the therapeutic process.

As the years have passed, however, the classical psychoanalytic model has undergone a number of modifications, and the sharp line of demarcation between psychoanalysis and other forms of dynamic psychotherapy has become blurred (5). Although there are still some who adhere rigidly to the original therapeutic technique recommended by Freud, more and more psychoanalysts have begun to modify their techniques in a number of ways. Thus they often see their patients two or three times weekly, instead of four or five. Many more patients are seen sitting up, with less rigid insistence on the use of the couch. Relatives are interviewed and occasionally even seen conjointly with the patient instead of being strictly excluded as they were formerly. In contrast to the old dictum that no major life changes were to be permitted for the duration of the analytic process, many analysts not only allow their patients but even encourage them to make basic changes in their life patterns when these changes seem rational and constructive. Finally, many psychoanalysts have begun to feel freer in general to enter into active communicative exchanges with patients instead of remaining bound to the classical incognito "neutral mirror" model of relative silence and impassivity.

One important consequence of this trend toward increasing flexibility in technique has been a growing interest in the *process* of the psychotherapeutic transaction, in contrast to the former preoccupation with its ideational or verbal content. Research into the nature of the psychotherapeutic process (6,7,8) has begun to make it increasingly clear that although cognitive understanding as administered via interpretive psychodynamic "insight" is a valuable adjuvant and facilitator of therapeutic change, it is by no means a sine qua non for such change. Considerable evidence has accumulated to indicate that the psychotherapeutic process is a learning process; what is most relevant to this process, however, is not so much specific historical correlations between past experiences and current reactions, as it is the acquisition of new models of behavior, thinking and feeling. Moreover, these new models are not always achieved cognitively and consciously, but as often as not are acquired subtly, as a result of overt or covert suggestion, unconscious identification with the therapist, corrective emotional experiences in the interaction with him and a kind of operant conditioning via implicit or explicit expressions of his approval or disapproval. In this process the nature and quality of the patient-therapist interaction, the real personalities of both patient and doctor, and the degree of faith, hope, trust, and motivation to change that the patient brings to the therapeutic situation are of paramount importance in enabling the new learning to take place successfully. These factors obviously also encompass the transference and countertransference aspects of the psychotherapeutic relationship. It should be noted, too, that in contrast to the early views of psychotherapy, in which the patient was regarded as an essentially passive object to whom the therapist applied certain objective skills and powers, the newer views take cognizance of the active and mutual transaction between patient and therapist.

Contemporaneously with the growing awareness on the part of many dynamic psychiatrists of these learning aspects of the psychotherapeutic process, a major new trend in psychotherapy, explicitly rooted in theories of learning, began to make its appearance in the 1950's. The best known of these was Wolpe's "reciprocal inhibition" therapy, based on the assumption that if anxiety-provoking situations or fantasies were associated with complete muscular relaxation, the anxiety would be inhibited and the capacity of the situation to provoke anxiety would be rapidly extinguished (9). Wolpe's reported successes by this technique quickly brought in its wake a host of other technical psychotherapeutic innovations, all presumptively based on Pavlovian, Hullian, or Skinnerian theories of conditioning behavior. Aversive conditioning techniques of many types, operant conditioning methods utilizing varying forms of reward and punishment, desensitization, social reinforcement, training and rehearsal techniques and the like have been developed and reported in great profusion, all claiming a high rate of success.

It is worth noting that most of these techniques, in contrast to the dynamic psychotherapies, tend to eschew cognitive awareness. The emphasis in them is strictly on altering behavioral manifestations, and the subjective problems, feelings or thoughts of the patient are considered, if not unimportant, at least irrelevant to the psychotherapeutic process.

Still another major trend in psychotherapy also began to emerge in the 1950's—a trend which focused *neither* upon cognitive awareness, *nor* upon behavior, but rather on the *feeling states* of the patient. Perhaps the earliest examplar of this approach was Carl Rogers, who advocated a technique of therapy based primarily on reflecting the patient's feelings back to him (10). From these modest beginnings a wide spectrum of techniques has gradually emerged, designed to heighten emotional awareness and encourage the expression of feelings. These techniques are usually employed with groups, and involve such approaches as sensitivity training, so-called gestalt therapy, as well as various forms of bodily contact, and marathons—nude or otherwise—all designed to break down both rational and conventional controls and to intensify emotional and sensate experience. The past decade has seen an enormous profusion of public offerings of such therapies, some leaning heavily on erotic overtones, others moving toward transcendental meditation, Zen, Yoga, and the like.

A more recent trend, which represents a kind of marriage between the scientism of the behavioral techniques and the inward focus of the feeling-oriented therapies, has been the proliferation of therapeutic approaches based on biofeedback mechanisms and aiming at the relief of anxiety by the promotion of the relaxation thus achieved.

However, all this does not even begin to exhaust the list of therapeutic offerings that have emerged in the last few decades. I have referred above to the diverse group settings in which many of the feeling-oriented therapies have taken place. But group therapies in themselves have occupied an important role in the psychotherapeutic armamentarium for the past 25 years at least, and have been used within psychodynamic frameworks, as well as behavioral ones. Analytic group therapy has been conducted within Freudian, neo-Freudian, and Kleinian orientations; other approaches have invoked psychodrama, sociodrama, transactional game-therapy, and behaviorally-oriented role-playing or rehearsal in groups. There have been small-group and large-group therapies; conjoint marital therapies, and multiple marital groups; single-family and multiple-family groups; groups for adolescents, for the elderly, for divorcees, for parents without partners, for accident-prone individuals, for drug addicts, for alcoholics, for criminals, for people with sexual inadequacies, and for homosexuals.

The 1950's also witnessed the dramatic emergence of Dianetics, initially as a hoax, then as a fantastic merchandising operation when to its founder's surprise the public took it seriously. After a few years of widespread popularity it underwent a rapid demise, only to reemerge a decade or so later in the pseudo-religious garb of Scientology, under which it is experiencing a mild renascence. A somewhat related approach presently enjoying some popularity on the West Coast is Primal Scream Therapy, which also employs the technique of regression (not to the intra-uterine state, as in Dianetics—merely to the moment of birth!) but combines it with an emphasis on the noisy release and dramatic acting out, in both dyadic and group settings, of presumably buried early infantile angers and anguishes.

These latter approaches, of course, are variations on the abreaction theme in psychotherapy, based on Freud's early belief that the release of repressed childhood memories with their attached affects would bring about a discharge of fixated libido that would automatically cure the patient. Freud abandoned this approach when he found that the abreaction effect was only a transitory one, and replaced it with the more tedious, far less dramatic, technique of "working through" resistances. The dramatic appeal of a sudden cure by abreaction, however, continues to hold sway in the popular mind, and reappears periodically not only on stage and screen, but also in a variety of therapeutic techniques like the foregoing. The sudden and rapid "cures" (where are they all now?) of life-long personality disorders by LSD and other psycho-active drugs (the amphetamines, the barbiturates, CO_2, etc.) in 5 or 10 dramatic sessions, that were being widely reported a few years ago, were based on the abreaction hypothesis also.

Quite a different approach which has achieved some popularity in recent years is the so-called reality therapy of William Glasser. This technique ignores unconscious and developmental psychodynamic factors and places great emphasis on conscious personal responsibility for one's actions. It is a kind of "Dutch Uncle" approach to psychotherapy and is a throwback to the exhortatory and persuading techniques of the 19th century. Originally employed in relationship to adolescent delinquents in a controlled environment where it proved useful, it appears quite simplistic when Glasser attempts to apply it to the understanding and treatment of severe psychoneurotic and psychotic disorders.

* * *

It should be quite apparent even from this cursory survey that the past twenty-five years have witnessed the emergence of an enormous array of psychotherapeutic techniques, each with its own group of devoted adherents, and each trumpeting its superiority over all others. What are we to make of them?

It seems to me that despite the enormous profusion of psychotherapeutic techniques that we have been witnessing in the past few decades, a careful look at what has been happening will reveal that the pattern is not as haphazard as might appear on first sight. Indeed, there is reason to surmise that the character of these therapies is related to certain significant trends in our contemporary culture, trends that are operating simultaneously, even though often at cross-purposes.

The first of these is a strong current of anti-intellectualism—a current which has been described in detail in Roszak's *The Making of the Counter Culture* (11). This is, I believe, a reaction to a widespread disenchantment with, and unconscious fear of, the results of scientific technology. The increasing complexity and tensions of urban life, the pressures toward conformity imposed by standardized mass communication media, the background menace of nuclear annihilation and ecological spoliation—these and other factors beyond the scope of this paper—all have contributed to a mounting sense of helpnessness, alienation, and distruct of science and technology in large numbers of the American people. It is not surprising therefore that psychotherapeutic techniques have arisen which are responsive to these feelings, and that these techniques have flourished expansively. Particularly representative in this regard are the various sensitivity-type group therapies, all avoiding cognitive insights, and focusing instead on emotional expressiveness and physical contact (with or without erotic elements). Also part of this trend have been the therapies based on transcendental meditation and on Eastern philosophies (a rejection of the "technological West"). Thus it is not accidental that we find both the sensitivity groups and the Eastern philosophy approaches usually offered at the same "Institutes." Another expression of this anti-intellectual pattern is the extraordinary resurgence of astrology, with its combination of quick psychological diagnosis and facile psychotherapeutic guidance. Numerology, witchcraft, and spiritualism are other aspects of the same trend which have been reappearing. Perhaps it is unfair to put parapsychological research in the same category inasmuch as a number of sincere and dedicated scientists have been devoting themselves to a legitimate exploration of this field. Nevertheless, the emotional pull of this field for many of its devotees stems from a similar search for answers beyond the realm of science and bordering on the supernatural.

The second major contemporary cultural current stands in direct contrast to the one just described. It is the remarkable advance in technological and communicative techniques as they apply to the sources of human behavior. As might be expected, many therapists have seized on these technologies and have attempted to adapt them to the modification of human behavior. Thus we have witnessed a growing use of tape recorders, movies, videotapes, computers, and various electrotherapeutic devices. Growing sophistication concerning psychopharmacological agents has led to their increased use also as adjuvants to psychotherapy. Presently biofeedback techniques are being widely developed to facilitate control of both voluntary and autonomic nervous system mechanisms.

The third, and in some ways the most far-reaching in its ultimate effects, of the major cultural factors impinging on psychotherapeutic change has been the rapidly burgeoning societal demand for more economical and more equitable distribution of health care, and the shortage of trained professional personnel to meet this demand. As a result there has been increasing pressure on the psychiatric profession to abandon its emphasis on costly long-term one-to-one psychotherapeutic techniques, and to replace them with more economical short-term or group approaches.

Psychoanalysis found its earliest applications in the treatment of middle- and upper-class individuals, primarily because only they could afford such therapy. It found a receptive haven, and enjoyed its greatest popular acceptance, on American soil, despite Freud's derogation and distrust of this country, because only an affluent nation such as ours could afford to cultivate and utilize so expensive a technique on a broad scale. It is ironic to note that in a way it was precisely the success and popularity of psychoanalytic psychiatry in the United States both during and after World War II that paved the way for the forces that began to undermine it in the succeeding decades. As the mental health movement grew stronger, and more and more people became aware of what dynamic psychotherapy could offer, there was an increasing demand for such treatment from people of more modest means. This became an important factor in the tendency of analytically trained psychiatrists to begin seeing patients fewer times weekly, and to begin experimentation with short-term therapies as well as with group therapies. (After all, it may not be unfair to speculate that Freud's insistence upon daily visits with his patients may have been at least partially influenced by the fact that in the initial years of his practice he had a great deal of open time in his schedule!)

The point is, of course, that both theory and practice, in any field, are never independent of their sociocultural milieu, and what we are witnessing today in psychotherapy is that profound socioeconomic pressures are rapidly modifying its forms and modes of operation.

The advent of third-party payments, for example, has had a major impact by bringing insurance companies and governmental agencies into the picture as standard-setters and evaluators for psychotherapeutic practice. Despite the fact that the two major national psychoanalytic organizations—the American Psychoanalytic Association and the American Academy of Psychoanalysis—are making valiant efforts to have psychoanalytic therapy included in any national health insurance program, the sheer logic of cost analysis makes it highly unlikely that a technique involving 4–5 expensive visits per week for an indeterminate (and sometimes "interminable"!) number of years can be included in such a program. At best any viable insurance program will have to set some fiscally tolerable limit on the number of psychotherapeutic visits per year that it can subsidize, and that limit will almost surely be considerably below a 4–5 time per week, 50 week per year frequency.

It may be argued that this will represent a serious loss for psychiatry and will deprive some patients of the opportunity to achieve maximum or optimum therapeutic benefit for their problems. The bias of my own psychoanalytic training might lead me to lean somewhat in this direction. And yet in all candor I am forced to admit that such a conviction is more an article of faith than a matter of fact. I know of no satisfactory hard data to support the conclusion that long-term 4–5 time a week psychoanalytic treatment produces superior ultimate results in terms of emotional growth and motivation than does long-term 2–3 time a week analytically oriented psychotherapy. Indeed, at least as far as the treatment of certain phobic and sexual dysfunctional disorders are concerned, the present evidence seems to be that some behaviorally oriented procedures of relatively short duration are considerably more effective than standard psychoanalytic treatment.

On many grounds, therefore, it seems safe to predict that the coming decades will see a continuation of the trend to more active, shorter-term psychotherapeutic techniques, as well as an expanding use of group therapies. As experience has grown with group psychotherapy, both on a short-term and long-term basis, it has proven to be a highly effective technique for mobilizing behavioral change, and, of course, it has the advantage of lower unit-costs as well as of making more efficient use of psychotherapeutic person-power. This is not the occasion for a discussion of the indications and contraindications for group therapy versus individual psychotherapy. Each approach has therapeutic values which are indicated in specific instances, and at times both may be indicated. What we shall be seeing more of, therefore, as time goes on, I suspect, is the expansion of a trend that has already begun, that is, of combining individual with group therapy. More and more young psychiatrists are acquiring skills in both modalities and are able to use either technique or both as the indications call for them.

Indeed, many psychiatric residency programs today are training their graduates to be capable of utilizing a broad-spectrum psychotherapeutic approach encompassing behavioral *as well as* psychodynamic techniques, in both individual and group contexts—although there is still much to be desired in this respect, particularly with regard to conjoint marital and family therapies.

Obviously in some instances, alternative therapeutic options may be available, since some patients can be equally helped by diverse approaches. In such cases the therapist's choice of technique will continue as now to be determined in part by his own idiosyncratic characterisics—his training, his professional identification models, as well as his personality make-up and system of values—which make him feel more comfortable with some approaches than with others. Also it is only fair to point out that it is highly unlikely that any one psychiatrist can be expected to acquire superior skills in all psychotherapeutic techniques.

I believe that behavioral therapy methods are here to stay, but that as times goes on, its practitioners will become increasingly aware of the interpersonal and subjective variables operating between them and their patients, and will be able to incorporate these variables in their approaches. Some behavioral therapists, such as Lazarus and his students, have already moved in this direction (12).

By the same token, dynamic psychotherapists will no longer, in justice to their patients, be able to continue to ignore the short cuts to symptom-amelioration offered by behavioral techniques, and will have to learn to make use of them when indicated. Thus we can anticipate, in the decades ahead, techniques that will attempt to combine the two basic approaches into new technical forms. Behavior therapists like Brady (13) and Marks and Gelder (14) have begun to attempt this, as have dynamic therapists like Feather and Rhoads (15). The latter two therapists have recently reported on a method of ingeniously combining psychoanalytic concepts with behavior therapy by desensitizing, not the external anxiety-producing stimuli—as is usually done in behavioral therapies—but rather the underlying unconscious conflictual drives and impulses from which the patient's symptoms are presumably derived. Their reported successes certainly merit further explorations along such lines.

I would predict also that the taboo on the adjunctive use of psychopharmacological agents that has characterized the practice of many psychoanalytically oriented psychiatrists will become a thing of the past. This is not to say that some of the concerns upon which this taboo was based were without merit. The too-liberal use of such agents can all too easily become an avenue toward narcotizing patients into a deceptive kind of anxiety-free apathy without the therapists' having to face up to the more difficult task of helping their patients learn to cope more effectively with their life problems. It can also serve to mask emotions which need to be worked through therapeutically, or to facilitate denial or avoidance reactions on the part of the patient. On the other hand, there is no doubt that excessive anxiety or depression on the part of a patient may constitute an impenetrable obstacle to psychotherapy, and it is both inhumane and inefficient to allow such patients to continue to suffer because of a blanket therapeutic taboo against the use of medication. The judicious use of medication in properly selected cases, far from interfering with the psychotherapeutic process, can facilitate it.

It would be too much to expect that the present profusion of polymorphic therapies will not continue in the future, although we can anticipate that those fringe therapies whose results are essentially dependent on the placebo effect of their novelty will be dropped by the wayside as this effect wears off. However, they will almost inevitably be replaced by new ones, promising equally miraculous results. The hope for magic is a deeply rooted one, and so long as there are unscrupulous purveyors who are willing to promise such magic, there will be an ample supply of purchasers! Conceivably, however, the regulating power of governmental and insurance agencies in the decades ahead may serve as a brake on some of the more extreme therapeutic approaches by refusing to honor them for payment.

One of the most significant shifts in psychiatric theory and practice that has been taking place in recent decades has been the increasing recognition of the importance of the milieu in both the production and the amelioration of psychopathology. This has resulted in a shift from the previous, psychoanalytically-influenced, primary preoccupation with intrapsychic factors, to an examination and inclusion in the therapeutic program of other factors in the life system of the individual. Thus we have witnessed not only a movement toward the inclusion of "significant others" in the psychotherapeutic process in the form of conjoint marital therapy and family therapy, but also the entire trend toward community psychiatry with its emphasis on modification of environmental factors wherever possible. In recent years it has become fashionable in some circles to deprecate the community psychiatry movement as promising more than it can deliver, and as tending to minimize intrapsychic considerations in mental disorders. Both points are legitimate criticisms. Intrapsychic mechanisms cannot and must not be ignored in any approach to psychopathology, and there have indeed been foolish excesses in some community psychiatry programs. But the basic premise of the community mental health center concept—to make mental health delivery systems visible and geographically and economically accessible to all people—is a sound one and should not lightly be discarded; neither should its corollary premise, which rests on systems theory, and recognizes the important interrelationships between man's inner and outer worlds, and the need to make changes in both, if preventive psychiatry is ever to become a reality.

This brings me finally to still another major aspect of the current and future psychotherapeutic picture. Even prior to World War II, the development of mental hygiene centers resulted in the beginning use of allied mental health professionals, particularly social workers and psychologists, in the mental health delivery system. After the war, the indication for psychiatric care gradually expanded from its previous emphasis on the care of psychotics and severely disabled neurotics to a concern with the mental health needs of the entire population. Under the emerging concept of the "right to treatment," programs have been established for the treatment of school problems, alcoholism, drug abuse, mental retardation, geriatric problems, and criminal behavior; and nonpsychiatric physicians, psychologists, social workers and nurses, to say nothing of occupational and recreational therapists, special educators, probation officers, vocational, pastoral and marital counselors, have become part of the mental health "team" and are making positive contributions to it. More recently, as part of the community mental health program, new groups of so-called "paraprofessionals," and "indigenous mental health workers" have also been enlisted and trained to function within the mental health delivery system.

To further complicate the problem, increasing numbers of these nonmedical professionals have elected in recent years to leave the clinical and institutional settings, and have moved out into practice to do various forms of psychotherapy.

It is greatly to the credit of the members of the psychiatric profession that after an initial period of resistance to this incursion upon their "territorial rights," they are gradually coming around to a recognition of the fact that the realities of this nation's mental health needs are such that the involvement of nonmedical professionals is both essential and inevitable. Increasing numbers of psychiatrists have begun to participate in the training of these allied groups, as well as to work on various programs involving cooperation and collaboration with them. Within the past year the Assembly of District Branches of the American Psychiatric Association has endorsed payment under medical insurance plans to nonmedical health professionals provided "their services are rendered as part of a plan of treatment that is supervised and/or prescribed by a physician."

One can only guess at what the long-term consequences of these developments for the future practice of psychotherapy by psychiatrists will be. There is, of course, a possibility that economic factors such as lowered third-party payments may function to gradually exclude psychiatrists as the primary providers of psychotherapy, utilizing them only as diagnosticians, consultants, and supervisors of such care. This would mean that people who wanted psychiatrists as their primary psychotherapists would have to pay for such care outside of any governmental or private insurance programs. I consider such a development to be unlikely, however. I cannot conceive of state or federal governments, or of the rest of the medical profession for that matter, condoning the deliberate exclusion of a medical specialty from a major segment of its medical function. Moreover, I do not believe the public would accept such a denial of their right to receive psychotherapeutic help from whomever they considered best qualified to give it to them. One could argue that those who wished to see psychiatrists could supplement their insurance payments to meet the higher fees of the more highly trained professional. Another possibility, however, is that insurance payments for psychotherapy may be graded on the basis of the professional qualifications of the psychotherapist. It is a fact that the psychiatrist is the only one among mental health professionals presently qualified *not only* to do psychotherapy, but also to make a differential diagnosis, to prescribe medication or somatic therapy, and, if need be, to hospitalize a patient for treatment.

There has been an interesting development in just the last few years that may be pertinent to all this. After almost a decade in which applicants for psychoanalytic training had been steadily decreasing, there has been a gradual resurgence in their number. I do not believe this is because an increasing number of young psychiatrists have decided to devote themselves to formal psychoanalytic practice. All of the evidence is that these young men and women are as interested as the rest of their contemporaries in all of the new technical developments in psychotherapy as well as in community psychiatry. I believe rather that this trend is due not only to the fact that they are recognizing the importance of understanding one's self as the basic instrument in all our psychotherapeutic techniques, but also that, when all is said and done, they are realizing that the mere proliferation of techniques in psychotherapy is not enough. In the final analysis, psychotherapy without any rational underpinning and understanding of underlying psychodynamics tends to become a kind of shot in the dark, planless and ultimately unsatisfying. A sound psychodynamic training provides this basic understanding and it is this that I believe these young people are seeking. Thus their search represents a corrective swing of the pendulum away from the blind rejection of cognitive understanding that has characterized so many of the newer psychotherapies.

As I have said elsewhere (16), "the psychotherapeutic challenge of the future is to so improve our theoretical and diagnostic approaches to psychopathology as to be able to most knowledgeably and flexibly apply to each patient the particular treatment technique and the particular kind of therapist that together will most effectively achieve the desired therapeutic goal." To achieve such a goal we need more than just empathy and intuition; we also need to broaden and extend our psychodynamic knowledge and understanding. And so we come full circle, albeit in a somewhat different context, to Freud's perceptive statement: "The voice of the intellect is a soft one, but it does not rest until it has gained a hearing"!

REFERENCES

1. Quoted by Lewis, N. D. C. in "Historical Roots of Psychotherapy," in Masserman, J. and Moreno, J. (ed): *Progress in Psychotherapy*, Vol. III, New York: Grune & Stratton, 1958, p. 25.
2. FREUD, S. *The Future of an Illusion*. London: The Hogarth Press, 1934, p. 93.
3. _____. *Ibid.* p. 77.
4. _____. *New Introductory Lectures*, New York: W. W. Norton, 1933, p. 112.
5. MARMOR, J. "Psychoanalysis and Psychiatric Practice," in Masserman, J. (ed): *Current Psychiatric Therapies*, New York: Grune & Stratton, 1961, pp. 131–138. (Chapter 14, this volume.)
6. _____. "Psychoanalytic Therapy as an Educational Process," in Masserman, J. (ed): *Science and Psychoanalysis*, Vol. V, New York: Grune & Stratton, 1962, pp. 286–299. (Chapter 15, this volume.)
7. _____. "Psychoanalytic Therapy and Theories of Learning," in Masserman,

J. (ed): *Science and Psychoanalysis*, Vol. VII, New York: Grune & Stratton, 1964, pp. 265–279. (Chapter 16, this volume.)

8. _____. "The Nature of the Psychotherapeutic Process," in Usdin, G. L. (ed): *Psychoneurosis and Schizophrenia*, Philadelphia: Lippincott, 1966, pp. 66–75. (Chapter 23, this volume.)

9. Wolpe, J. *Psychotherapy by Reciprocal Inhibition*. Stanford: Stanford University Press, 1958.

10. Rogers, C. *Client Centered Therapy*. Boston: Houghton Mifflin, 1951.

11. Roszak, T. *The Making of the Counter Culture*. New York: Doubleday, 1969.

12. Lazarus, A. A. *Behavior Therapy and Beyond*. New York: McGraw-Hill, 1971.

13. Brady, J. P. "Psychotherapy by a Combined Behavioral and Dynamic Approach," *Comprehensive Psychiatry*, 9:536–543, 1968.

14. Marks, I. M. and Gelder, M. G. "Common Ground Between Behavior Therapy and Psychodynamic Methods," *Brit. J. Med. Psychol.*, 39:11–23, 1966.

15. Feather, B. W. and Rhoads, J. M. "Psychodynamic Behavior Therapy," *Arch. Gen. Psych.*, 26:503–511, 1972.

16. Marmor, J. "Dynamic Psychotherapy and Behavior Therapy," *Arch. Gen. Psych.*, 24:22–28, 1971. (Chapter 24, this volume.)

Part IV

SOCIAL PSYCHIATRY

27

PSYCHODYNAMICS OF GROUP

OPPOSITION TO HEALTH PROGRAMS

(1959)

Health programs generally derive from scientific progress and scientific recommendations. Despite this fact, it is not unusual for such programs to meet with intense and determined opposition on the part of various groups in our society. It is the purpose of this communication to outline the nature of this group opposition, to attempt to delineate its features, and to identify some of the psychodynamic and sociodynamic factors which are involved in its existence.

There is a not infrequent tendency on the part of the scientifically oriented person to generalize about the people who make up this opposition and to characterize them all as being malevolent, ignorant, or members of the so-called "lunatic fringe." A dispassionate study of the problem, however, reveals that such a generalization is unwarranted and is itself the expression of a prejudice which tends to strengthen the very opposition at which it is aimed. The fact is that most group opposition to scientifically motivated health legislation runs a wide gamut of heterogeneity. There is usually a broad spectrum of opposition, with arguments ranging from highly rational and scientific ones to completely irrational and delusional ones; from genuinely selfless considerations to deliberately power-seeking ones; from unconscious motives to consciously manipulative ones.

Drs. Viola W. Bernard and Perry Ottenberg collaborated in the writing of this essay.

Since health legislation is ordinarily introduced only after having been first recommended or endorsed by responsible scientific authorities, it is not surprising to find that, in the opposition which develops, the part which is based on rational considerations tends to occupy a considerably narrower band on the spectrum than that which is irrational and unconsciously motivated or else deliberately dishonest. Nevertheless, the former group is an extremely important one, not only because it lends prestige and scientific authority to the opposition and so influences large numbers of people whose resistances might otherwise not have been aroused, but also because its arguments often point up realistic flaws or inadequate safeguards in the health programs, which might otherwise go unnoticed.

Thus some of the objections raised to the Alaska Mental Health Bill (a bill designed to provide a mental hospital for the territory of Alaska) in its original form dealt with ambiguities in some of its phraseology, which might conceivably have led to misinterpretation or abuse—for example with respect to a patient's right to a jury trial. Similarly, one of the scientific objections raised to water fluoridation has been that, although it indeed protected the enamel, it could lead to pathological bone changes from disturbances in calcification. This sort of honest disagreement, whether it be right or wrong, stimulates further research and observations, which ultimately serve to clarify the issue further.*

Rational opposition to health legislation often grows out of a scientific conservatism, which looks askance at all innovations until they have been proven beyond all peradventure. Such conservatism is by no means without value and serves to protect the public against premature exposure to untested procedures at the hands of misguided enthusiasts. Thus, the American Dental Association and the U.S. Public Health Service both refused to endorse water fluoridation when it was originally proposed. The British Royal Society rejected Jenner's findings concerning cowpox and vaccination when they

---

*An example of this kind of clarifying research, with regard to the above objection, was the ten-year controlled epidemiological study of two population groups which checked, among other things, on possible significant bone changes due to ingestion of fluorides in drinking water and found none. This research was published by Nicholas C. Leone, Michael B. Shimkin, et al., under the title *Medical Aspects of Excessive Fluoride in a Water Supply*, Publ. Hlth. Rep., 69:925–936, 1954 (Reprint 3242).

first appeared. As a rule this kind of scientific resistance tends to melt away when the proof of the adequacy of the new procedures has been fully established. Unfortunately, the original withholding of endorsement by reputable groups or individuals is often used and quoted by less rational opponents of a measure long after the scientific dissidents have withdrawn their opposition.

As one examines this problem more deeply, it becomes apparent that one important aspect of it impinges on the broad problem of social reactions to change in general. Mores and beliefs of people of any given community are not accidental or unrelated phenomena. They are integrated elements in a cultural system that has gradually evolved in time, and a basic change in any one of these elements can have important reverberations affecting the entire network of habits and beliefs.

Not all cultural patterns, however, are of equal importance to the system. Some are more central, others more peripheral. Hence some habits or beliefs are easily altered, while others arouse great resistance. In general, whenever an attempted change challenges established beliefs or practices which are fundamental to the stability of the particular social or cultural or psychological system involved, one may anticipate serious group resistance to change. An example of this is the reaction of a large segment of our Southern white population to desegregation—a social change which threatens cultural patterns, balances of power, and psychological needs which are at the very core of a long-established way of life in that area. On the other hand, the attitude of our population toward the Japanese people has undergone a considerable reversal in the past 15 years without comparable upset to basic cultural integrations.

Among the Zulus, conceptions about tuberculosis are extremely difficult to change, because the symptoms of this disease have long been assumed to be due to witchcraft, and the entire topic is surcharged with powerful feeling.

Similarly, as John and Elaine Cumming (1) recently demonstrated, ideas about mental illness in some groups within our own culture can be just as deeply irrational as those of the Zulus about tuberculosis, and just as resistant to alteration.

The nature and sources of these unconscious and irrational anxieties are of particular interest to us as psychiatrists, and we shall examine them in detail a little later in this communication. For the moment, however, let us continue to survey briefly some of the more conscious and *external* sources of group opposition to health legislation, which often interact with the unconscious and internal sources of opposition.

Sometimes a proposed change threatens or seems to threaten the power, prestige or economic security of certain special segments within a society. This is generally the basis for variations in response to changes that occur on an ecologic or demographic basis—such as differences in response between Northern and Southern areas of our country, or between rural and urban groups. We can expect that specially threatened groups or individuals will do all in their power to mobilize public opinion against the change. Thus, the introduction of vaccination completely displaced the practitioners who favored inoculation by variolation, or the direct transference of smallpox infection. In the antivaccination campaign which followed Jenner's discovery, the opposition of these groups was particularly virulent and all kinds of fantastic charges and slanders were spread by them.

Some of the most powerful opposition to polio vaccination and water fluoridation has come from groups whose vested interests bring them into direct conflict with the theories of organized medicine and dentistry. Prominent among these are naturopaths, chiropractors, cancer quacks, some Christian Science groups, and small but impressive-sounding organizations like the "American Association of Medico-Physical Research," founded by Albert Abrams, who achieved notoriety by the claim that he could diagnose any disease from one drop of the patient's blood, and could, with his "electronic reaction" machine, cure any illness.

Similarly, efforts of governmental experts to introduce a model health, education and welfare project in a Mexican rural community (2) in 1943 met with intense opposition from local officials and wealthy farmers, because they feared the project as an ultimate threat to their power. Such power groups or leaders, whatever their nature, do not hesitate to play deliberately upon the irrational fears, anxieties and prejudices in the population at large to achieve their ends.

Some opponents of the Alaska Mental Health Bill raised the cry that it was an effort to set up a Siberia* for the U.S.A., and darkly hinted that it concealed a nefarious plot by Communists to hospitalize and brainwash their opponents. Others were certain it was part of an international Jewish conspiracy, and one retired general was equally sure that the Bill had been engineered by the Roman Catholic hierarchy in this country as part of its campaign to "destroy our freedoms under the Bill of Rights." In the controversy over fluoridation also, certain groups tied their opposition to the "Communist conspiracy" theme, claiming it was a Communist plan to "rape" the people, weaken their minds and make them "moronic, atheistic slaves."

Sometimes the general public is misled when opponents to health legislation carry the insignia of esteemed authorities. Thus, an M.D. or a Ph.D. degree is not always a reliable indicator of scientific objectivity when borne by individuals whose personal bias outweighs their rationality. Similarly, the position of the *Brooklyn Tablet*, a Catholic weekly, against fluoridation and the Alaska Mental Health Bill gave many people the false impression that the Catholic Church was officially opposed to these projects, and that the undertakings themselves were anti-Catholic—a potent accusation in a city like New York with its large Catholic population.

Another "external" element which plays a partial role in group opposition is the factor of coercion. The word "compulsory" is a negatively loaded semantic concept in societies with a democratic tradition. Occasionally some political liberals may see in compulsory health legislation an invasion of individual freedom. This issue was strongly raised by many in the fight against water fluoridation. It is interesting to note that not infrequently such "liberal" opponents find themselves joined in their opposition to such programs by political conservatives, who see in the same legislation an advance

---

*"This legislation . . . will place every resident of the United States at the mercy of the whims and fancies of any person with whom they might have a disagreement, causing a charge of 'mental illness' to be placed against them with immediate deportation to SIBERIA, USA!" From "Siberia, USA," an article by Mrs. Leigh F. Burkeland, as quoted on Page 141 of the Alaska Mental Health Bill Hearings (H.R. 6376), published by the U.S. Government Printing Office, Washington, 1956

toward the socialistic state. Thus certain opponents of water fluoridation and mental health legislation like the California Community Mental Health Services Act (Short-Doyle Bill) saw, or claimed to see, in these measures dangerous trends toward socialized medicine and governmental infringement upon individual liberty.

Although it is true, therefore, that social changes which are allowed to take place spontaneously, so to speak, are less likely to arouse organized resistance, a governmental agency is faced with the necessity of weighing the pros and cons of such an approach in each specific situation. Where the health or welfare of an entire community is jeopardized, as by a threatened smallpox epidemic, for example, circumstances may not permit the luxury of voluntary gradualism as far as vaccination is concerned.

Related to this factor of coercion is the factor of time. Generally speaking, the more rapid and energetic the attempt at social change, the greater the opposition that is apt to be aroused. When more time is allowed for education and preparation of the group for the proposed change, there is less likely to be misunderstanding or resistance. The historic decision of the Supreme Court on desegregation took cognizance of this temporal factor when it called for its implementation not immediately, but with "deliberate speed" depending on the problems of the local communities. On the other hand, occasionally when an agency allows *too much time* to pass before implementing a proposed change, group resistances to it *may* become more solidly organized and congealed. This was clearly demonstrated in the efforts to introduce water fluoridation and desegregation. In many communities, in which they were introduced with relatively little fanfare, they aroused little anxiety or opposition, while in others, where their adoption was delayed and subjected to prolonged debate, their opponents were able to mobilize sufficient public anxiety and doubt to defeat them. Leonard Duhl (3) has suggested that one of the reasons for popular opposition at such a point may be displaced resentment that some people in modern society feel at being cut off from many areas of governmental decision making.

This raises the question of the value of education of the public in preparation for proposed health legislation. Since, as we shall see later, some of the most important sources of opposition to such legislation come from unconscious and nonrational sources, it is not surprising that educational appeals to conscious reason often fail to dissipate the opposition. This is not to imply, however, that educational efforts are without value. By no means. Often more important, however, than such specific educational campaigns is the *basic* educational and economic level of the various groups within a society. A number of studies have shown that group resistance to scientifically oriented social change is most apt to come from the less educated and lower economic groups within any given community. There are several reasons for this. For one thing, "scientific thinking" tends to be limited to the more highly educated minority, especially those who have gone to college.

Equally important, however, is the overall cultural "climate" as regards science and scientists. In the past decade in America we have witnessed an instance of the periodic emergence of a rather widely prevalent anti-scientific and anti-intellectual attitude, epitomized by the opprobrious term "Egghead." This appears to have been part of a broad, defensive reaction to the threat of Communism, a reaction which led to such political extremes as McCarthyism, and which included in it a distrust of scientists in general as tending to be too "liberal" and hence as being actual or potential "subversives." This distrust has been an important factor in causing various organizations, in the name of patriotism, to link certain scientifically based health proposals to the threat of Communist subversion. Situations in which this link was charged include such diverse proposals as the Alaska Mental Health Bill, the California Community Mental Health Services Act, the polio vaccination program, and fluoridation of water (Figure 1).

The insidious pervasiveness of this anti-scientific attitude in our country was illustrated by a recent study of the "Image of the Scientist Among High School Students," by Margaret Mead and Rhoda Métraux (4). Their study of a nationwide sampling revealed the existence of an "overwhelmingly negative" image of the scientist, when students were asked for their reactions to science as a career, or to the scientist as a person.

Another study was conducted by the National Association of Science Writers in conjunction with New York University and the Survey Research Center of the University of Michigan on "The Public's Image of Science and Scientists" (5). This study, based on

EXAMPLE OF OPPOSITION TO HEALTH PROGRAMS
"THE UNHOLY THREE"

At the Sign of THE UNHOLY THREE

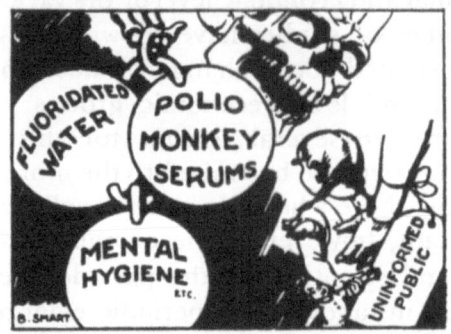

Are you willing to PUT IN PAWN to the UNHOLY THREE all of the
material, mental and spiritual resources of this GREAT REPUBLIC?

FLUORIDATED WATER

1—Water containing Fluorine (rat poison—no antidote) is already
the only water in many of our army camps, making it very easy for
saboteurs to wipe out an entire camp personel. If this happens, every
citizen will be at the mercy of the enemy—already within our gates.

POLIO SERUM

2—Polio Serum, it is reported, has already killed and maimed
children; its future effect on minds and bodies cannot be guaged. This
vaccine drive is the entering wedge for nation-wide socialized medicine, by the U. S. Public Health Service, (heavily infiltrated by Rus-
sian-born doctors, according to Congressman Clare Hoffman.) In
enemy hands it can destroy a whole generation.

MENTAL HYGIENE

3—Mental Hygiene is a subtle and diabolical plan of the enemy
to transform a free and intelligent people into a cringing horde of
zombies.
Rabbi Spitz in the American Hebrew, March 1, 1946: "American
Jews must come to grips with our contemporary anti Semites; we
must fill our insane asylums with anti-Semitic lunatics."

FIGHT COMMUNISTIC WORLD GOVERNMENT by destroying
THE UNHOLY THREE ! ! ! It is later than you think!
———————— KEEP AMERICA COMMITTEE ———————
Box 3094, Los Angeles 54, Calif.   H. W. Courtois, Secy.   May 16, 1955

FIGURE 1

interviews with 1,919 questionnaire respondents in a representative
nationwide sampling, indicated that even though the majority of
the respondents held a positive view of science and the scientist,
there was a significant minority who viewed science with antagonism
and suspicion, and who variously described the scientist as someone
"socially inept, introverted, hard-to-know . . . neurotic, queer, crazy
. . . mildly eccentric, absent-minded, out of touch . . . ideologically
and politically deviant . . . too powerful, able to control lives, with
powerful and dangerous things within his control."

There are some evidences, however, that this anti-scientific cultural climate in the United States has begun to shift recently, mainly as a reaction to the impact of the realization that the Soviet Union has been overtaking and, in some areas, surpassing us scientifically and technologically. Part of this shift, it is true, may merely be the other side of the coin of the image of the scientist as having magical power, power that now is seen as an important ally in the struggle against potential enemies and the frightening mysteries of outer space. Nevertheless, it is possible that with such a change in our society's attitude toward science, there may be some diminution in the distrust encountered by scientifically sponsored health programs.

In any event, this problem of group attitudes tends to highlight the importance of the role of leadership in the fate of such programs. When the leaders of a community are lukewarm or antagonistic to a legislatively ordained change, and consequently make no effort to enforce it legally, it has been found that group resistances become intensified. A dramatic example of contrasting types of leadership and their consequences was afforded in September 1957 in Little Rock, Arkansas, and Nashville, Tennessee. In Little Rock, a plan of gradual desegregation had majority public acceptance and the support of municipal officials. The opposition of the State's governor, however, had the effect of encouraging and legitimizing violence against desegregation. The subsequent chain of events has been such that the desegregation situation in Little Rock is still very tense. Around the same time an elementary school was dynamited in Nashville, where a few Negro children were entering a previously all-white school. Police restrained prosegregationist demonstrators, and arrested a score of them. The State's governor promptly made it clear that the law of the land would be upheld in Tennessee, even though he did not personally like integration. By the end of the month the school scene was peaceful in Nashville and has remained so. Apparently under certain conditions, legally enforced behavioral changes may have to precede attitudinal changes. Such a sequence has been observed following enforced desegregation in the Armed Forces.

The part played by the opposition leaders in the attacks upon health legislation is an extremely important one and impossible to deal fully with here. In general these leaders fall into two main groups, with considerable overlapping: 1) those who are motivated by factors of personal power, prestige or gain; 2) those who are motivated by powerful anxieties or hostilities, the true sources of which are unconscious. They are often individuals of great ability, intelligence, and capacity to arouse intense fervor and passion in others. In extreme forms they assume the role of the godlike crusader, the charismatic leader, who is ready even to endure martyrdom for the sake of the "cause." Their function must be understood not only in terms of their capacity to arouse their followers to what seem to be potential threats; they are also an important factor in trying to hold rigidly to a fundamental conservatism which may provide a sense of security to the group which they lead. Some aspects of the psychology of such leaders and many of their supporters are discussed in what follows.

Granted the existence of all of the external factors which tend to mobilize opposition to certain health programs, the problem still remains to explain the degree of irrational anxiety which these programs often evoke in significant segments of our population. For it is clear that if only external factors were involved, educational campaigns presenting the scientifically proven facts and demonstrating the general benefits involved in the health program ought to have been more successful than they have been. Obviously the appeal to reason fails so often precisely because the popular anxieties which have been aroused have an *irrational* and *unconscious* source.

It is this fact which explains one of the most interesting features of the phenomenon we are considering, namely, the fact that *we find the same groups of people involved over and over again in opposition to widely diverse and disparate health programs.* Thus, many of the same individuals and organizations that are active in the fight against water fluoridation can be found in the ranks of those opposing mental health programs, compulsory vaccination either of animals or humans, and vivisection (Figure 2). As an extreme example, the American Naturopathic Association is on record as opposing not only fluoridation, but also vaccination, immunization, pasteurization, vivisection, drugs, narcotics, alcohol, tobacco, tea, coffee, cocoa, cola drinks and compulsory medication!

What is the common denominator behind the opposition to such

MONTAGE OF EXHIBITS OPPOSING
HEALTH PROGRAMS

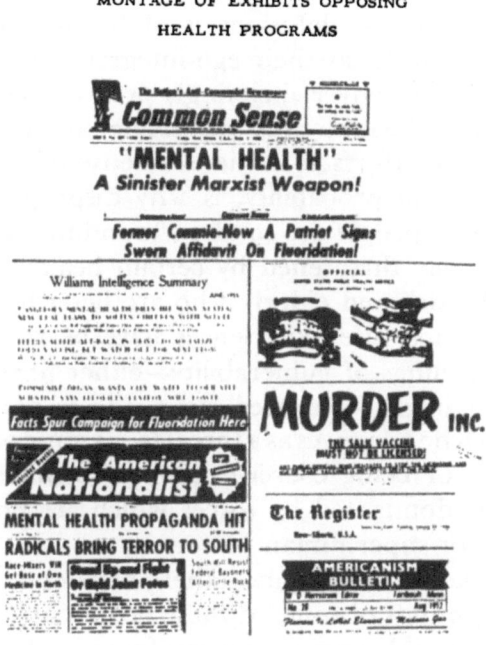

FIGURE 2

varied stimuli? To answer this question we must examine the problem of the psychic significance of health and sickness in the life history of the individual. Good health is linked in the unconscious with basic needs for survival, security and mastery. Ill health is connected with fears of bodily disintegration, dissolution and death. Even more important are the conditioning factors that are experienced in early development, and related to the experience of health or sickness. For all people, for example, what goes into their mouths, and by extension, into any part of their bodies, is very strongly associated with good and evil. "Eat this—it's good for you," and "Don't put that in your mouth—it will make you sick," are among the earliest aspects of enculturation probably in all cultures. "Good" food is "pure," "clean," "wholesome"; "bad" food is "impure," "dirty," "poisonous." To eat well is to be secure, healthy and happy. The converse means insecurity, starvation and death. Little wonder that when psychotics experience a weakening of their ego boundaries, one of their commonest delusions is of being poisoned; or that elderly and sick people, as their ego-integrative capacities become impaired, often become overwhelmingly preoccupied with problems of diet and bodily health, thus regressing to earlier patterns of adaptation in their efforts to achieve a sense of security and ego mastery. (This, in all probability, is why disproportionately large numbers of elderly people are so often found in the ranks of those who feel irrationally threatened by certain health legislation.) But it is not only the sick and elderly who are beset by such anxieties. Any individual whose life experiences have been such as to leave him with deep feelings of vulnerability—either physical or psychological—in the struggle for existence is apt to respond with anxiety to anything which he perceives as a threat to his sense of intactness—or which, by virtue of being coercive, arouses in him fears of being overwhelmed or dominated by forces which are endowed by him with mysterious or superhuman power.

Adorno, Frenkel-Brunswik and others have described the developmental backgrounds of some of these people in *The Authoritarian Personality* (6). Often these people come from homes in which rigid, repressive and authoritarian patterns have dominated their early developmental years, with consequent patterns of deeply repressed hostile, dependent and libidinal strivings. To protect themselves against the emergence of these impulses, such individuals develop patterns of intense characterological rigidity, repression, and an ever-ready tendency to discharge their repressed hostility, or project their repressed sexual strivings, whenever a convenient cultural scapegoat is presented to them.

To such individuals purity is equated with security, and health with wholeness. They are equally concerned with pure food, pure morals, and pure races. They are excessively preoccupied with fears of sexual attack, bodily poisoning, or ideational contamination. Safety lies in what is old and familiar. The new and the unfamiliar are threatening. New habits, new foods, new drugs, or new ideas are all viewed with suspicion and apprehension. Fundamentalism is the cornerstone of their philosophy—a determined and rigid adherence to convention and tradition.

This sense of vulnerability is equivalent to what has been symbolically described in psychoanalytic theory as "castration anxiety" and its developmental precursors. To express this in less technical terms, it is our conviction that the basis for most of the irrational anxiety that some health measures arouse in certain individuals is that the measures are perceived as constituting a threat either to their sense of bodily wholeness, or their sense of psychic wholeness, or else to the wholeness of what we might call their "life-space." These, of course, are often interrelated and interconnected. This is the common denominator which explains our finding the same individuals passionately defending themselves against the forcible entry of any "foreign body"—whether it be a vaccination, a mental health proposal, interracial contact or a wave of immigrants from overseas (Figure 3).

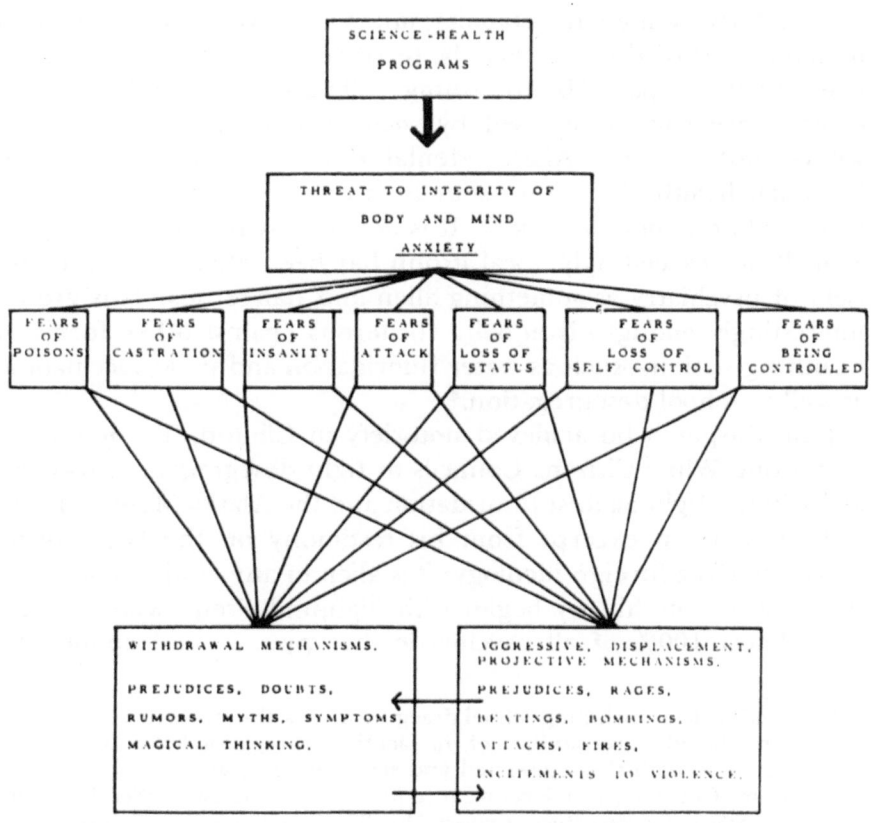

FIGURE 3

Measures which involve introducing something foreign into the human body, such as fluoridation of water, or vaccination, are perceived by such individuals as threatening their bodily integrity. Terms like "rape," "poison," "murder," and "paralysis" figure importantly in their impassioned arguments against these measures. By a simple process of extension or displacement, one generally finds these same people fighting vigorously against similar measures involving animals, such as vivisection, or antirabies inoculation for pets.

On the other hand, the intense fear that mental health proposals arouse in certain people seems to derive from feelings of being threatened psychologically. The reactions of some of these individuals seem to reflect a fear that any psychiatric insights may expose their own underlying mental instability, much as a patient who fears that he has cancer of the lung may be terrified of a chest X-ray. Terms like "mental rape," "brainwashing," "hypnotism," and "thought control" are commonly used by such opponents. As one hostile witness put it in the Alaska Mental Health Bill hearings, "What is mental health? By whose standards can we deduce one person is normal and another is not?" It is noteworthy that in recent years a small but exceedingly vocal group has been attacking the entire field of psychiatry as something alien and dangerous. This group, interestingly enough, is equally vociferous against other forms of health legislation—such as water fluoridation and polio vaccination, as well as school desegregation.*

John Kasper, who achieved notoriety in Clinton, Tennessee, by organizing White Citizens Councils to fight desegregation, was also active in the fight against fluoridation and the Alaska Mental Health Bill. Here is an excerpt from his testimony on the latter issue: "Psychiatry is a foreign ideology; it is alien to any kind of American thinking . . . its history began with Sigmund Freud who is a Jew . . . almost 100% of all psychiatric therapy . . . and about 80%

---

*The rationale of including school desegregation within the context of health legislation is based on recognition of the fact that segregation leads to psychological damage to both the segregated and segregating groups—a fact of which the Supreme Court itself took cognizance in its famous decision. (See *Psychiatric Aspects of School Desegregation,* Report No. 37, Group for the Advancement of Psychiatry, 1957.)

of the psychiatrists are Jewish . . . one particular race is administering this particular thing." The attack on Freud and psychoanalysis is often linked with the implication that psychiatrists, Jews and Communists are somehow involved together in a sinister plot to brainwash loyal Americans. (The hostile association of psychoanalysis and Jews with Communism is particularly ironic when we recall that in the Soviet Union psychoanalysts and Jews have been subjected to the analogous charge that they are tools of Capitalism!) Similar attacks on the mental health movement are being repeatedly made in various extremist publications throughout the country. Regardless of the motives of the publishers of some of these sheets, there is no doubt that many of their readers fall into the group we are describing, and are genuinely frightened by what they are being told.

The concept of the threat to the life-space implies that the individual perceives the threat as going beyond his personal physical and psychic integrity to involve the entire position of himself and his group in the world. It is what he is apt to call a threat to his whole "way of life." The intense panic reactions which many people felt to the news of Russia's Sputnik are an illustration of this kind of response. The reactions of their contemporaries to the discoveries of Galileo, Darwin and Freud are other examples in point.

Up to now, in accordance with our topic, we have concentrated on the psychodynamics of those opposed to health programs. Closely related, however, are the emotional effects of these various kinds of opposition on the programs' supporters. The psychodynamics of the proponents' responses to attack warrant our attention, at least briefly, especially with regard to the deterring effects on scientific progress and the public welfare. Extremist attacks on responsible professional experts and governmental authorities have indeed frequently succeeded, at least temporarily, in blocking various programs such as water fluoridation, desegregation and mental health legislation. Aside from defeating a specific legislative or administrative proposal, however, such attacks can retard or prevent public health programs in ways that are less obvious, harder to assess, and more far-reaching through their psychological effects on initiators, endorsers and advocates of such measures, present and future.

Once a scientific program is rendered socially and politically risky, no matter how irrationally, the extent to which its adherents can withstand the attack and afford, emotionally and practically, to continue its support depends on many variables for each individual. One set of such variables includes personality attributes, values, convictions, motivations, and the person's degree of insight, as well as commitment to the issue. Another set of variables concerns the extent of the threat to his reputation, tenure of office or professional job security. Sometimes people in these situations successfully withstand intimidation and slander from the opposition when they feel that their own leadership and associates are standing firmly together, but become embittered and defeatist if these fail them by capitulating to the power of the anti-scientific opposition. The importance of enlightened and courageous leadership in withstanding the pressures of such opposition can scarcely be overestimated.

Individuals and organizations often face a dilemma in deciding whether or not to continue striving for a particular measure which has aroused intensely heated denunciation. A civic group, for instance, might recognize the merits of the measure, the irrationality of the opposition and the validity of basing its stand solely on the facts and the public welfare. Yet, in deciding on its own course of action, the organization must weigh those considerations which dictate support of the measure against the risk to other valuable parts of its present and future program that may depend on the good will and cooperation of powerful factions or individuals in the community who are currently lined up against the proposal. In such circumstances a realistic and conscious decision is sometimes made to sacrifice a potentially valuable program which has aroused such vehement antagonism in order to safeguard other social objectives of the individual or organization, such as survival and potential for effectiveness. A realistic decision of this type is to be distinguished from the rationalizations that are also a frequent response to a conflict situation of this kind—where actions really based on unacknowledged expediency, and on fears for self which are not ego-acceptable, masquerade under cover of this more respectably altruistic reason. Such rationalizations usually engender guilt feelings and self-contempt that reduce people's overall effectiveness. Contemporary versions of Galileo's famous predicament and recanting of his recanting are still to be found.

Sometimes proponents of scientifically grounded health programs react to unreasonable opposition, not by withdrawal, intimidation, counterattack or unperturbed determination, but by an intensified advocacy. Apparently the experience of being attacked in these ways can stimulate deep personal anxieties and unconscious patterns of defense. As a result, a person's prior scientific basis for supporting a health measure may shift to a blindly emotional espousal of a cause, with all the concomitant drawbacks that this entails. We have already referred to a spectrum of opposition to health legislation which ranges from rational to irrational. The advocacy of these measures can occupy a similar spectrum. The relative proportions of the rational to the irrational bands on this spectrum, however, for the proponents and the opponents are likely to be the reverse of each other.

The general public loses from the inactivation of scientific workers and public officials when, under the pressure of social penalties and demoralization within their own group, they withdraw, emotionally as well as physically, from further endeavors to raise the community health level. Some of those in the health professions retreat into less controversial areas of work. The laboratory may feel safer than the market place. But the public is deprived of the benefits of the laboratory if research findings that are developed and tested there cannot find their way into general application. For each constructive health program that is halted by extremist opposition, it appears likely that an inestimable number of potentially constructive programs fail of inception because officials and scientists fear the real or fantasied power of anti-scientific opposition.

When the social climate renders the risks especially great, as during the height of McCarthyism, not only may the public be deprived of the applications of scientific progress, but that progress itself may be hampered by the extension of the inhibiting forces into certain areas of research. Prejudice, superstition, fear and ignorance have been mobilized against attempted research projects in the fields of preventive mental health and human relations in the same way as against legislative health proposals. Apparently the spur to such opposition is the possibility that the research investigation may produce findings which might lead to broad-scale legislative and administrative applications that threaten these opponents along the lines discussed above. Research in publicly supported institutions is especially vulnerable to this type of attack, and its defenders relatively weak in the face of it. Indirect pressure has also been exerted, however, on nonpublic sources of support, as when private foundations are dissuaded from granting funds to projects because they fear these may foment adverse public opinion and threaten their tax-exempt status.

We are aware that many aspects of this complex topic need further study. How do people who feel compelled to do something actively about their convictions differ from the great majority who may hold similar convictions but never feel the need to commit themselves to action? How does unrealistic *complacency* in the face of realistic danger differ psychodynamically from the unrealistic *anxieties* we have been discussing? We recognize also that today's scientific proposal can end up as tomorrow's fad. Many of us can still remember, for instance, the scientific zeal with which tonsils, teeth and other supposed "foci of infection" were removed in wholesale proportions. How does such "rational" zeal differ from the "irrational" opposition to such measures?

We are aware that not all scientific proposals have been equally validated—witness the differences that exist among reputable scientists as to the degree of harm that is being done by radioactive fallout. Does the degree of validation of a scientific proposal make any difference in the degree of opposition which it arouses? These and many other questions warrant separate communications.

To summarize briefly then: We have tried to demonstrate that opposition to scientifically motivated health legislation covers a wide range of heterogeneity—from groups whose opposition is based on science and reason, to those whose objections appear to be based on self-aggrandizement or political considerations, and finally to those whose opposition stems from irrational anxieties or ignorance. We have indicated that the problem is part of the broader problem of reactions to social change in general. Opposition to social change derives from factors which are external to the individual as well as internal within his psyche. Some of the external factors involved include threats to the power, prestige or economic security of certain groups, the factor of coercion, problems of timing, the attitudes of leadership, and various educational, socioeconomic and cultural factors. The internal factors involved appear to be centered on feelings of vulnerability in relation to the sense of bodily wholeness, psychic wholeness, or wholeness of the individual's "life-space." An awareness of both external and internal factors, and of the way in which they interact in any given "field" situation, is essential for a fuller understanding of this complex group reaction. Although many questions still remain unanswered, it is hoped that this discussion will stimulate further interest in a problem which has, we believe, significant psychiatric as well as social ramifications.

REFERENCES

1. CUMMING, JOHN and ELAINE. "Mental Health Education in a Canadian Community," in *Health, Culture and Community* (B. D. Paul, Ed.), pp. 43–69. New York: Russell Sage Foundation, 1955.
2. LEWIS, OSCAR. "Medicine and Politics in a Mexican Village," in *Health, Culture and Community,* op. cit., pp. 403–434.
3. DUHL, LEONARD. *City Responsibilities in Problems of Mental Health.* Presented at 34th Annual Congress of the American Municipal Assoc., San Francisco, Dec. 3, 1957.
4. MEAD, MARGARET, and RHODA MÉTRAUX. *Image of the Scientist among High School Students.* Science, 126: 384–90, 1957.
5. KREIGHBAUM, HILLIER. "The Public's Image of Science and Scientists," in *Science, the News and the Public,* pp. 35–42. New York, New York Univ. Press, 1958.
6. ADORNO, T. W., et al. *The Authoritarian Personality.* New York: Harper, 1950.

28

THE PSYCHOLOGY OF MAN IN A
WARLESS WORLD
(1962)

Is the personality of man capable of functioning without the outlet of war? Is war so deeply and inexorably a part of man's basic nature that all talk of a world without war must be relegated, reluctantly but hardheadedly, to the wastebasket of utopian, wishful thinking? It is to this question that I wish to address myself first.

The assumption that war is an intrinsic manifestation of human nature grows out of the theory that it is an inevitable social expression of a fundamental instinct toward destructive aggression in man. I shall not attempt here to review the pro and con arguments with regard to this theory, other than to indicate that its validity has been seriously questioned by numerous social and biological scientists. As Fairfield Osborn has pointed out: "Warfare as practiced by man has no parallel in nature. . . . Within the more highly developed animal populations of the earth there is not now nor has there ever been similar destruction within a species itself. In fact one has to go to the lowliest forms of animals, such as certain kinds of ants, to find anything comparable to human warfare" (1).

Most modern behavioral scientists believe that human violence is not spontaneously instinctive, but rather a reactive response either to a sense of frustration or to perceived threats involving some aspect of man's psychological or physical security. This latter view does not deny that the capacity for violence is innate in man but asserts that whether or not this capacity is *expressed* generally depends on external factors.

The crucial point for our discussion, however, is that even if

374

one were to concede, for the sake of argument, that aggression *is* an innate human instinct, it still would not follow logically that wars are inevitable. It is meaningless to talk of modern war as though it were merely the sum total of countless individual human aggressions. Modern war is a complicated social institution—the resultant of the intermeshing of many intricate factors: social, economic, political, and psychological. It involves large and complex social organizations which we call nations. It requires armies, weapons, supplies, scientific research, advanced technology, recruitment and propaganda. Like any other social institution, it is capable of evolution and change. It is precisely its evolution from the techniques of primitive hand-to-hand combat to those of modern nuclear annihilation which confronts the world with its current awesome danger. As a social institution, however, it is also potentially eradicable. Other widespread social institutions of man's past, like slavery, dueling, ritual human sacrifice and cannibalism, which in their times and milieus seemed equally rooted in human nature and destiny, have been, in the course of history, almost totally eliminated. It is also a fact that various societies have existed without recourse to war for many generations.

Although it seems incontrovertible, therefore, that war is not an inevitable expression of human nature, there are, nevertheless, certain aspects of human psychology which strongly predispose man to violence, and which require consideration, since they would be operative even in a warless world.

Perhaps the most fundamental, although not necessarily the most important of these, is *fear*. Abundant clinical experience has shown that panic is a highly potent trigger for hostile behavior, and extreme fear of an adversary is as likely to provoke a violent act as is hatred of him. Yet fear is a basic biological reaction without which an individual might fail to take the proper actions needed for his protection and survival in the face of danger. Unfortunately, however, there is only a thin line between the amount of fear necessary to stimulate corrective behavior and the amount that leads to maladaptive responses. Psychologists have long been aware of what has been called the *primitivizing effect of fear*. The reactions of humans, no less than those of animals, tend to become more archaic and less rational under conditions of extreme fear or panic. The capacity for adaptive discrimination is lost and habitual responses which are no longer appropriate are fallen back upon. When fire breaks out in a movie house, for example, most people will rush for the main exits even though they are jammed, and will ignore the more passable but less customary exitways. In the same way, when fears of an adversary are fanned to great heights by communication media, an unbearable tension is created in many people—tension which seeks relief at nearly any cost. Under such stress, almost any course may seem better than none at all. Hence the cry, so often heard, for "action" and "getting it over with," even though such action might be self-defeating or self-destructive. The certainties of war at such times may appear more endurable than the ambiguities of peace. Fear also shortens time perspective. A fearful person becomes preoccupied with warding off the imminent danger, often to the neglect of the ultimate consequences of his behavior. Similarly, nations may counter what they perceive as an immediate threat by the adversary with action involving long-term consequences which may be much more serious than the initial hazard.

Other common psychological responses to danger that lend themselves to making violence feasible are the mechanisms of *denial* and *isolation*. *Denial* involves the failure to perceive or recognize certain aspects of reality in order to avoid becoming aware of something which might be unduly painful or threatening. It is the psychological equivalent of "burying one's head in the sand." In *isolation* these aspects of reality are perceived, but the painful or disturbing emotions associated with them are blocked out of consciousness. We recognize that mechanisms such as these make it possible for many people to cope with anxieties that might otherwise be incapacitating for them. Nevertheless, it seems incontrovertible that a failure to react with at least some alarm to the possibility of nuclear annihilation must be considered maladaptive.

Denial and isolation are abetted by a number of factors. For one, most human beings cling to an *illusion of personal immortality and invulnerability.* The possibility of war is made tolerable by the thought, "It can't really happen to me; somehow or other *I'll* manage to survive." Another contributing element is the *deep sense of personal helplessness* that most people feel regarding their ability to influence the crucial decisions of war and peace.

Still another element is the *inability of people to conceptualize the magnitude* of a danger with which they have had no prior experience, and which therefore has no reality for them. This is particularly true of nuclear war, the consequences of which are beyond ordinary imagination. Moreover, the inadequacy of language in characterizing such new phenomena is an additional barrier to the accurate perception of such dangers. New words like "megaton" lack emotional impact, since they have no reference to actual experience. The use of old terms, on the other hand, may engender a false sense of security because they fail to convey the impact of the new realities involved. Terms such as "civilian defense" and "national security" are examples of words that arouse reassuring images even though their traditional meanings have been drastically altered by the development of modern weapons.

It follows, then, that even in a warless world anything which aroused intense or prolonged fear in people or abetted the mechanisms of denial and isolation would favor the outbreak of group violence. The elimination of weapons of mass destruction would, of course, remove one of the main potential sources of such reactions. Other factors, however, would still remain.

Perhaps the most serious of these are the mutual distortions of perception which tend to occur between the populations of nations in conflict. These distortions can be subsumed under the general concept of *ethnocentric perception*. This refers to the tendency of members of a group to perceive and evaluate events from the standpoint of their own group's interest and bias. The virtues of one's own side are magnified and its faults are not seen, while the evils of the adversary are exaggerated and his virtues ignored. Thus the identical behavior which is perceived as "standing firm," when exhibited by a member of one's own group, is interpreted as "being pigheaded and obstinate" when manifested by a member of the opposing group.

This often leads to *stereotyped* conceptions, both of one's self and of the adversary, with the development of a self-righteous view of the ingroup and a "bogey-man" view of the opponent. The motives of one's own group are always assumed to be morally honorable, fair, and decent; those of the opposing group are always suspect.

Ethnocentric perception also favors the development of *polarized attitudes,* in which everything is regarded as black or white, never as gray. All truth and morality is regarded as being on one side, all deceit and evil on the other. All who are not 100 percent on one's own side are regarded as being on the opponent's side and neutrality is viewed with suspicion and hostility. Differences with the adversary tend to be exaggerated and similarities to be minimized.

It should not be assumed that ethnocentric perception is necessarily a matter of faulty access to information or of faulty intelligence. Although its extreme manifestations are more apt to be observed among people with lesser educational backgrounds, it occurs in greater or lesser degree among almost all people, in high stations as well as low ones, and even among those who have access to the widest sources of information. The reason for this is rooted in the homeostatic need of all human beings to organize their perceptions to fit into their preexistent conscious and unconscious expectations, needs and wishes, and to reject, minimize, or "fail to see" things that would upset their basic views about the nature of reality. This is an effort to keep the environment as constant and as meaningful as possible, and to avoid whatever might make it appear disturbing or unclear. This "intolerance of ambiguity" or "need for certainty" increases whenever individuals feel threatened, and tends to lessen with feelings of emotional security.

Another basic aspect of human psychology which is involved in ethnocentric distortions is the *tendency to modify one's perceptions and reactions in response to group pressures.* The effect of mob hysteria on individual behavior is a well-known phenomenon, but the ways in which more subtle group pressures affect people often are not as well recognized. This phenomenon was strikingly illustrated by an ingenious experiment performed some years ago by Asch in which a subject is placed in a group of six to eight others, all of whom are asked to make certain perceptual or evaluative judgments (2). What the subject does not know is that the experiment is rigged, that the others have all been instructed to give *false* responses on a predetermined schedule. At first the subject finds himself in agreement with the others, but then finds his responses differing from *all* the others more and more often. He is at first puzzled, but then gets more and more upset, begins to doubt his own judgment, and finally, in about one-third of the cases, begins actually to "see" things the way others presumably do! There is little doubt that this kind of unconsciously influenced perception takes place very widely in all countries, particularly when a conflict with an outside group increases the nationalistic pressures toward conformity.

All of these distortions inevitably lead to a *biased perception of what is fair and reasonable,* and thus not only render meaningful negotiations between adversaries difficult and sometimes impossible, but also fan the winds of fear and hate in their respective populations. The *mutual distrust* that inevitably develops under such circumstances becomes itself one of the most serious of the obstacles to nonviolent resolution of the conflicts between nations. The expectation that no agreement can be reached because "the other side doesn't really want peace" and "can't be trusted" inevitably leads to the anticipated failure and thus becomes a "self-fulfilling prophecy" (Merton).

Finally, no discussion of the psychological obstacles to nonviolence in international conflict can ignore the significant *interactions that exist between heads of governments and their peoples.* Many of the perceptual distortions of an adversary's actions and purposes are often deliberately created and manipulated by political leaders through the withholding of significant information or the dissemination of false information for the purpose of achieving certain strategic objectives in the power struggle with the adversary. Also things may be said by them which are intended only for domestic consumption and domestic power politics but which lend themselves to misinterpretation by the adversary. Once this has been done, however, the tensions, fears, and hostilities created in the minds of their populations become potent forces which control the subsequent freedom of the leaders to act. Thus a constant dialectical interplay exists between national leaders and their followers which often makes them both captives of a vicious cycle of increasing tensions. This is particularly true in open societies like our own, but the significance of such interactions should not be minimized even in Communist societies. Consequently, even when leaders may wish to make realistic compromises with the adversary, they may be unable to do so because of nationalistic pressures, the dictates of political expediency, the influence of power blocs within their own country, and the fears and suspicions that have already been aroused among their own peoples.

We see then that the psychological obstacles to the elimination of organized violence are formidable indeed. Is it possible to modify these barriers or else to find other outlets for them in a world without war? What kinds of psychological changes will be necessary for man to live in such a world without propelling himself once more in the direction of violent internecine conflict with his fellow man?

The first word of caution that needs to be introduced is the reminder that a warless world does not mean a world without conflict. Conflict between individuals, groups, and nations will always be part of the human scene as long as there are diversities of human interests and values. Peace is not a static end-point; it is a dynamic, ongoing process of continuous conflict resolution. Moreover, conflict per se is not necessarily evil. It may have, and often does have, constructive value. The mobilization of energy toward conflict-resolution can have integrative and creative value for a nation as well as for an individual. One of the challenges of a warless world is to enable people and nations to learn to engage in conflict without violence—to find, in William James' apt phrase, the "moral equivalents of war."

That this is psychologically possible for man there can be little doubt. Man has shown himself capable of finding adequate discharge for his aggressive and competitive impulses in all kinds of peacetime activities short of violence. However, many unhealthy current social mores may have to be altered if man's present tendency to erupt into violence is to be significantly modified.

Much has been written, for example, in recent years, about the social and psychological effects of population increases, industrialization, specialization, urbanization, and automation on people. The effect with which I am specifically concerned here is the deindividualization and alienation of man—an alienation which brings with it a sense of non-involvement and indifference to the actual or potential distress of other human beings and thus has a bearing on the capacity of people psychologically to tolerate the implications of mass-destruction and mass-violence. As a result of this process man becomes regarded as a cost factor, an item, or a tool to serve the organization or the mass-machine. He becomes a means to an end, rather than an end in itself. In the semantics of modern military strategy, patterns of thinking are often observable which reflect this "dehumanization" of man. Concepts such as "first-strike," "over-kill," "counter-force deterrence," etc., represent a move-countermove, game-theory type of thinking which treats the millions of potential human victims as mere statistics or pawns in a global chess-game, and psychologically screens out the awesome consequences of the contemplated actions upon individual people—a full appreciation of which would make such actions emotionally intolerable.

One must recognize, however, that the effects of modern technology, automation, and even bureaucracy have not by any means been merely negative. They have also had enormously constructive effects in promoting efficiency, in relieving human drudgery and strain, and in making possible a richer life and increased leisure time for more people. Moreover, intertwined with the trends toward conformity and anonymity in modern society, there are also present persistent impulses toward individuation—in art, in literature, and in the tenacious strivings of men everywhere toward goals of freedom, peace, and human dignity.

Nevertheless, the pressures of modern technology are likely to continue the trend toward the deindividuation of man, and there will be urgent need, in a warless world, to develop psychic antidotes of "rehumanization" to counteract the heightened callousness and the lessened sense of personal responsibility toward the needs or suffering of other human beings which such a trend brings with it.

Still another problem with which a warless world would have to deal would be that of the conceptual stereotypes concerning war which are deeply rooted in our language and traditions, and which foster attitudes conducive to group violence. The history books of every nation justify its wars as brave, righteous, and honorable. This glorification is charged with overtones of patriotism and love of country. Virtues such as heroism and courage are regarded as being "manly" and are traditionally associated with waging war. Conversely, the avoidance of war or the pursuit of peace are generally regarded as "effeminate," passive, cowardly, weak, dishonorable, or subversive. The brutal realities of war are glamorized and obscured in countless tales of heroism and glory, and the warnings of an occasional General Sherman that "War is hell (and) its glory is all moonshine" receive little or no mention.

One of the fundamental points at which a warless society might begin to deal with these stereotypes is in the kinds of influences to which its children are exposed. We often hear it said, for example, that war games and military toys are good for children—that they serve as outlets for their aggressive feelings. It may well be true that they serve as such outlets, but they also prepare the soil for a psychological acceptance of war and violence. One could justify them only if no other kind of toy or game were available which could serve equally well as an outlet for aggressive impulses—an assumption which is patently untrue. The same argument holds, in my opinion, with regard to the show of violence in TV, movies, and comic strips. The oft-heard defense that such violence is merely a mirror of "what goes on in the child's unconscious anyway," and that "healthy, well-adjusted children" are not adversely affected by it, fails to pose the problem in proper perspective. Even if it were true—and it is by no means a proven fact—that aggressive impulses are endogenous and spontaneous in young children, the *forms* and the *outlets* such impulses take are modifiable. There is nothing in the human unconscious which instinctively endows it with the knowledge of "civilized" techniques of torture or killing. To teach children such techniques via our mass communication media is not only to indoctrinate them in methods of brutality but also to progressively desensitize them to the spectacle of human death and violence. This, it seems to me, is a much more serious problem, from the standpoint of society, than whether or not such forms of "entertainment" do or do not cause emotional disturbances in some children. If the organized killing of men is to be rendered obsolete, it is not enough to pay lip-service to nonviolence in terms of our religious mores, when so many other aspects of our social fabric condone or even glorify such killing. To be consistent, every element in the acculturation process which shapes our perceptions and our goals should reinforce the value systems of nonviolence, beginning in early childhood and continuing throughout life. Not only the toys and games of childhood, but our textbooks, our history books, our encyclopedias, and our mass-communications media need to be oriented toward the ennoblement of man's peaceful accomplishments rather than the glamorization of his battles. Our scientists, our educators, and our creative artists, not our generals, need to be the heroes of history.

It may be argued that what I am advocating is a kind of massive indoctrination of people that is incompatible with the ideals of a free society. Such an argument fails to take into account the fact that no society is without a set of mores which it imposes on its members, either implicitly or explicitly. The glorification of military action has been precisely such a value-system. It developed out of the historical necessities of international relationships at a time in which the instrument of armed force appeared to be the only way of achieving urgent national goals. The fact is that we have now entered upon an era in which the resort to war can no longer serve this purpose. In the face of this development it becomes imperative for man, if he is to survive, to consciously alter the outmoded value systems which serve to make war psychologically palatable and to replace them with others which have greater adaptive usefulness. To endeavor to plan our educational, child-training, and mass-communication systems along principles which enhance the dignity and worth of human life is not merely a social necessity in our nuclear age, but also compatible with the most cherished values of a free society.

A world without war may well find it necessary to reexamine others of its values in the light of these criteria. One would expect, for example, that traditional attitudes of punitiveness and vindictiveness toward juvenile delinquents, drug addicts and criminals would give way increasingly to patterns emphasizing their treatment and rehabilitation; and that that ultimate expression of society's violence toward the individual—capital punishment—would become progressively rarer.

However, even if the predisposition to acts of individual violence could be reduced—as I believe it can be—by such modifications in our acculturation processes, what can be done to eliminate the ethnocentric biases which tend to foster *group* attitudes of violence and hatred between nations who are at odds with one another?

Here we have to deal with another significant set of stereotypes which will require changing—those associated with nationalism.* As Stagner reminds us, "Three hundred years ago suggestions of religious tolerance were denounced as evidences of moral weakness. Today we consider religious *intolerance* a sign of moral decay. . . . We may reach a point at which the delusions of national pride and national persecution will be looked upon in the same way" (3).

It is not only psychologically possible, but essential if man is to survive, for the inhabitants of all nations ultimately to demonstrate adherence to an international law which will transcend their own national laws whenever the welfare of the world is involved, just as the people in the 50 states of our Union generally accept the fact that Federal law supersedes their own whenever the national welfare is involved. Signs of such a trend are already apparent in the slowly increasing tendency of many sovereign states to delegate certain powers to the United Nations, or to other international trade or monetary organizations.

But if conflict between nations persists, as it is likely to do over one issue or another, is it psychologically feasible that it can be pursued without violence? There is an accumulating body of evidence to indicate that the nonviolent pursuit of conflict between groups is not only feasible but can actually be very effective. Where traditional approaches of diplomacy, negotiation, or mediation have failed, other techniques such as sanctions or boycotts are still available short of war. The active but nonviolent techniques of carrying on conflict as practiced under the leadership of such men as Gandhi and Martin Luther King are illustrative of the tremendous moral power inherent in such ways of dealing with an adversary; and although not directly applicable to the current East-West conflict, might become more relevant in a world in which the use of lethal mass weapons has been outlawed. Such methods of struggle not only tend to contribute to the restoration of the humanistic values upon which Western civilization prides itself, but also serve to correct the distorted psychological stereotypes which exist concerning violence. For the nonviolent fighter, resort to violence is a sign of weakness, while

---

*See Chapter 29, "Nationalism, Internationalism, and Emotional Maturity."

adherence to nonviolence is a demonstration of inner strength and courage. Psychologically this has considerable validity. Psychiatrists have long known that the resort to violence stems more often from feelings of fear and inner weakness than from strength, and that the customary "common sense" equation of violence with strength and nonviolence with weakness is often a false one in terms of unconscious psychodynamics.

Psychiatrists have also learned that efforts to control an angry patient with force almost always makes him violent in return, while the avoidance of violence tends to inhibit such reactions in him. It has been demonstrated repeatedly that it is possible to set up group standards on a hospital ward which, even under great provocation, will preclude the use of violence by both patients and staff.

At the level of international conflict, some fundamentally different approaches are also worth considering. The great dilemma of our time is that we seem to be faced with an irreconcilable conflict between two powerful ideological, political and economic systems, yet any effort to seek a military solution can result only in mutual annihilation. History has taught us that often the only way out of a dilemma of this kind lies in a critical reexamination of the customary modes of thought out of which it grew. Some of the fundamental paradoxes in the field of natural science, for example, were resolved only when habitual common sense ways of thinking about time and space were transcended by the new modes of thought in Einstein's theory of relativity. Similarly, many paradoxes of human behavior remained obscure until Freud's insight into the existence of unconscious processes was able to clarify what common sense approaches had not been able to. The traditional mode of thinking about international conflicts is in terms of a struggle for power with the only possible ultimate outcome being victory of one side over the other, and finds expression in the "Red or dead" formula which has such wide currency. The leap in our thinking which is necessary to resolve this dilemma is to recognize that it is possible for adversaries to compete with one another *without necessarily encompassing the destruction of either one. Indeed in the process of the competition both sides may even grow stronger.* This implies an acceptance of coexistence which many people find extremely unpalatable. Yet the hard fact is that in our nuclear era there is no alternative but to face and accept this. Actually such coexistence between great ideological adversaries is not alien to human experience. After centuries of futile and bloody violence, Christianity and Mohammedanism settled down to living side by side, and even within Christianity itself, the competitive coexistence of Protestantism and Catholicism is taken for granted. The current Ecumenical Council is an interesting illustration of the fact that given enough time, in the absence of violence, dialectical forces are often set into motion which eventually tend to bring adversaries closer together. Even in the current ideological struggle there is evidence in recent years that there is a trend toward democratization in the Soviet Union which seems to increase as its sense of security increases but diminishes when it feels threatened.

Cooperation between adversaries represents still another nontraditional approach to conflict resolution which tends to be emotionally rejected by many people. The idea that it is possible to collaborate with an opponent, particularly one whose fundamental ideology is so antithetical to our own, appears at first glance to be utterly naive. Yet, as Schelling has pointed out, even in World Wars I and II, some cooperation between the opposing sides took place when their mutual interests were involved (4).

Cooperative activities yield rewards which reinforce positive attitudes between adversaries and inhibit antagonistic ones. Particularly effective are cooperative endeavors toward mutually desired or needed superordinate goals which neither side can achieve alone, such as the researches during the International Geophysical Year. Such activities also include a competitive component which serves as a healthy channel for national rivalries. Other potentially constructive competitions in a warless world would exist in the race toward the exploration of space, in the arts and sciences, and in the rivalry of the great nations to help the underdeveloped nations of the world.

As I bring my remarks to a close, I realize that I may have disappointed some of you by not attempting to project into the future the utopian potentialities which exist for man psychologically in a world without war. If I have not done so, it is not because

I do not believe that such potentialities exist, but because I think it is more realistic to try to understand some of the more immediate psychological problems with which he may be faced in the transitional period in trying to preserve the precious peace that he will have attained. In attempting this, I have no illusions that in this limited presentation I have been able to touch upon more than a fraction of these problems. There is no doubt that they will be many and complex. However, the remarkable brain of man, which has unleashed the secret of the atom and is solving the mysteries of space, is fully capable of coping with them. Most people on our planet yearn consciously for a world at peace; but man's unconscious irrationality may yet destroy him in spite of his conscious wishes. One of the major goals of behavioral science is to increase man's self-understanding so as to bring his unconscious attitudes and impulses under conscious control. Never was such a goal more imperative than in today's world, lest the very machines which man in his ingenuity has constructed become, through his folly, the monsters which encompass his destruction.

REFERENCES

1. OSBORN, F. *Our Plundered Planet,* Boston, Little Brown & Co., 1948.
2. ASCH, S. E. *Social Psychology,* New York, Prentice-Hall, 1952.
3. STAGNER, R. (ed.). *Dimensions of Human Conflict,* Detroit, Wayne State Univ. Press, 1961.
4. SCHELLING, T. C. *The Stragegy of Conflict,* Cambridge, Harvard Univ. Press, 1960.

29

NATIONALISM, INTERNATIONALISM, AND EMOTIONAL MATURITY

(1964)

In a world over which the mushroom cloud of the hydrogen bomb casts its ominous shadow, it becomes increasingly imperative for man to reexamine even his most cherished concepts when they touch upon the urgent question of peaceful relations between nations. Such a concept is that of nationalism—the love of country—in the name of which some of history's most glorious pages and shameful passages have been recorded. Nationalism tends to be a sacrosanct subject in most countries, closely linked to patriotism and fraught with overtones of righteousness, and to question its validity under certain circumstances may call forth accusations of disloyalty or even subversion.

At the same time, and particularly since the end of World War I, aspirations transcending the bounds of nationalism, and based on the ancient Judeo-Christian concept of the universal brotherhood of man, have been finding steadily increasing expression throughout the civilized world.

It is the purpose of this brief communication to subject the concepts of nationalism and of internationalism to psychodynamic scrutiny in the hope that in so doing we can shed some light on their relationship to personality development.

Love of country, of course, is not an uncommon reaction. On the contrary, it is a normal and universal phenomenon. It is present not only in beautiful and prosperous lands, but even in those whose climates are inhospitable and whose soil is so forbidding that its inhabitants can barely draw a marginal subsistence from it. Just

388

as ties to parents normally always remain special, regardless of the objective physical attractiveness or accomplishments of the parents, so too do the ties of motherland or fatherland retain a primary importance. The explanation for this lies in the fact that human beings everywhere tend to find a greater emotional security in what is familiar than in what is unfamiliar, regardless of the extrinsic merits of the situations. The objects and symbols with which we have grown up, with which our earliest identifications have been formed, and from which our earliest gratifications have been derived, always retain a special significance in our minds. The recent findings concerning the importance of the phenomenon of imprinting in lower animals suggests that possibly something akin to this may take place in human beings also, and that not only persons, but even things and symbols, which are linked with our earliest positive perceptions may become favorably and indelibly inscribed in our unconscious. Such deep-seated symbolic images are particularly susceptible to the appeal of emotional slogans, and anything which threatens them can arouse violent defensive reactions.

We also know, however, that one of the fundamental tasks of human growth, among other things, is the ability, as we move out of childhood, to form object-relationships that go beyond the basic attachments of early life. In psychoanalytic parlance, this is generally described in terms of achieving the resolution of the oedipal complex. Success or failure in achieving this task is *reflected not only in individual interpersonal relationships, but also, I submit, in patterns of social behavior.*

When we are very young we love only our parents and our immediate family. If our experiences with the significant parent- and sibling-figures of our childhood have been favorable ones, productive of feelings of trust and self-confidence, we become able, as we grow older and less dependent, to move out of the tight little circle of original family attachments and to begin loving and relating to people outside of it. Persons who fail to resolve their Oedipus complex have difficulties in doing this. They remain uneasy with strangers, and are able to love only people who are like themselves or who resemble significant members of their families. Social reflections of such failures in development often can be seen in adults who remain prolongedly and excessively involved with extended-family symbols such as their fraternities or sororities, their "alma mater," their "home town" or their "home state." At the international level, such individuals remain tied to a parochial kind of nationalism which tends to distrust all "foreigners," and to perceive all actions of one's own government in self-righteous terms, while distrusting and depreciating the motives and actions of "alien" countries. In making this statement, it is not my intention to minimize the importance of all the institutions in a country—e.g., schools, press, movies, radio and television—which constantly foster and reinforce such feelings in people. It is my thesis, however, that the emotionally immature individual is much more susceptible to these institutionalized pressures towards ethnocentrism than is the mature one.

A particularly virulent expression of this kind of reaction is that of the extreme ultranationalist. If my basic formulation is correct it should not surprise us to find that the individual who becomes a "super-patriot" is often a person with a history of profound disturbances in his relationships with the significant authority-figures in his life—relationships which have interfered with his capacity for trusting and satisfying ties with other people, and have also left him with strong unconscious feelings of emotional insecurity. Adorno, Frenkel-Brunswik and others have described the backgrounds of some of these people in their book, *The Authoritarian Personality* (1). Their family relationships are often characterized by rigid, repressive and authoritarian patterns which have led to deeply repressed hostile, dependent and libidinal strivings. As a consequence such individuals develop patterns of intense characterological rigidity with an ever-ready tendency to discharge their repressed hostility onto any convenient scapegoat. Since behind their hostility also lie deep-seated dependency needs and feelings of insecurity, clinging to what is old and familiar becomes particularly important to them, and thus their super-patriotism is often linked with political ultraconservatism. Whatever is new, unfamiliar, or "foreign" is experienced as threatening and viewed with dark distrust and apprehension. This sense of underlying vulnerability is the common denominator which explains the interesting fact that we often find "the same individuals passionately defending themselves against the forcible entry of [anything which symbolizes a] 'foreign body'" (4)—whether it be a vaccination, a new idea, an interracial contact, or a wave of immigrants from overseas.

Erich Fromm, in his classic book, *Escape from Freedom* (3), points out how these psychodynamic factors often lead such individuals to flock behind some strong, charismatic leader, who represents for them the powerful but understanding and benevolent father whom they unconsciously long for, and who, often under slogans of ultranationalism, promises to reverse the tide of history and to return to the traditional patterns of the past.

In contrast, people who lean towards nonethnocentric patterns of thought generally have had less traumatic family relationships in their early lives (2). Their parents tend to be more consistently loving, less rigidly disciplinary, more tolerant to nonconformity, more equalitarian in their relationships to their children. This enables the maturing child to work out his problems of sex and aggression with less conflict and with less repression. He becomes more flexible and has a better developed, better integrated, and less tyrannical superego than does the ethnocentric person. He is able to disagree with authority-figures more openly and with less anxiety, and thus achieves a much greater degree of emotional independence in relation to parents and authority-figures in general. At the same time, since he has less repressed hostility to them, his positive feelings for them are warmer and unambivalent.

Thus, the more emotionally mature an individual is, the more successfully he has transcended both his oedipal attachments and his own primitive narcissism, the more he is able to form attachments to others on the basis of their actual merits as people and not just because they come from the same home town, belong to the same lodge, attend the same church or have the same color skin that he has. This does not mean an abstract and uncritical "love for everybody," but rather the ability, selectively, to like or dislike, or to support or oppose, other individuals on the basis of objective specific experiences with them rather than on the basis of stereotyped ingroup-outgroup preconceptions. By the same token, at the sociopolitical level, the ability to perceive and evaluate the actions and motives of other nations as well as one's own without ethnocentric distortions can be viewed, in most instances, as a reflection of emotional maturity on the part of the individual.

As Charles Osgood (5) has pointed out, the development of social perception in human beings can be divided into three stages. The most primitive and most narcissistic of these is that in which we project our own frame of reference onto others and evaluate them on that basis. At this stage of perception we see anyone who disagrees with us as either deliberately dishonest or evil. The second stage of development involves the ability to recognize that others might disagree honestly with us as a result of their training or life experiences. At this level we are able to be more tolerant and less punitive to differing points of view but still feel smugly superior about the basic "truth" and "rightness" of our own. The third and most mature stage—hardest to achieve and maintain—is that in which we recognize the equally relativistic nature of our own frame of reference, and recognize that our personal or national values, judgments and policies are just as related to our own background and cultural heritage and interests as the other person's are to his. This is a level which precludes ethnocentrism and renders possible a better understanding between people of different nations.

Internationalism per se, however, cannot be regarded as necessarily *always* meaning emotional maturity. In some groups or individuals it may simply be a reflection of specific social or political determinants. For example, it may represent a defence of minority group members against the prejudices of dominant groups in their country and an effort, therefore, to find security in a world in which national differences are abolished.

It must be recognized also that internationalism can be neurotically motivated. Thus in some instances it may be a reflection of distorted early family relationships and rejection of the mother, father, and/or siblings. In such cases the neurotic substrate can be recognized not only in the exaggerated intensity of the individual's attitudes, but also in the fact that he manifests a vehement anti-nationalism and antagonism to authority-symbols more than he does a genuine love for humanity. An example of this is a certain kind of neurotic radical who, growing up with a sense of having been deserted, neglected or mistreated by his father, transfers his resentments to the symbol of his "fatherland." Such individuals, however, have difficulty in relating positively to any authority-symbols, and often are disruptive figures even in the organizations of their own choice.

It must be emphasized that a mature internationalism, with the elimination of patterns of nationalistic bias, does not mean the elimination of love of one's own country. On the contrary, clinical experience (1) suggests that it is precisely those individuals whose favorable early emotional experiences have enabled them to mature successfully in their relationships with parents and siblings, who are most apt to be capable of unambivalent relationships not only with their ingroup but also with outgroup members. A man does not care for his family less because he has a profound love for his country; neither does he love his country less because he has a deep feeling for the welfare of humanity as a whole. But just as a man's love for his family can be overridden by his loyalty to his nation if the latter's existence should be threatened, so also it is possible and even imperative for a man's love of country to be transcended by his loyalty to the human race if *its* existence is threatened, be it by natural catastrophe, pandemic disease or total war. Indeed, just as love of his family is one of the prime factors which motivates a man to be concerned about the health and security of the nation in which they live, so too a genuine love of one's country can be a major compelling factor in a rational concern about the fate of the world.

In conclusion, it has been the thesis of this brief presentation that the capacity to transcend narrow feelings of nationalism when the welfare of humanity itself is involved is in most instances the reflection, at the sociopolitical level, of emotional maturity at the intrapsychic and interpersonal level. As modern techniques of transportation and communication bring the family of nations ever closer together, and reinforce their interdependency, the achievement of such a world-view becomes increasingly important. This value system receives implicit recognition when great humanitarians such as Albert Schweitzer and Eleanor Roosevelt are labeled as "citizens of the world." It is one which must receive universal and explicit recognition if the ethnocentric biases which foster group attitudes of violence and hatred between nations are ultimately to be eliminated, and if man is to survive in our atomic age.

REFERENCES

1. ADORNO, T. W. *et al.: The Authoritarian Personality,* New York: Harper and Brothers, 1950.

2. FRENKEL-BRUNSWIK, E., in Adorno, T. W. *et al.: op. cit.* pp. 482–483.
3. FROMM, E.: *Escape from Freedom.* New York: Farrar and Rinehart, Inc., 1941.
4. MARMOR, J., BERNARD, V., and OTTENBERG, P.: "Psychodynamics of group opposition to health programs," *Am. J. Orthopsychiat.,* 1960, Vol. 30, pp. 330–345. (Chapter 27, this volume.)
5. OSGOOD, C. E.: *An Alternative to War or Surrender.* Urbana, Ill.: University of Illinois Press, 1962.

30

THE PSYCHODYNAMICS OF POLITICAL
EXTREMISM
(1967)

Three preliminary propositions ought to be borne in mind in any discussion involving the psychodynamics of political attitudes.

1. A clear distinction should be made between the psychologic motivations underlying any particular point of view and the point of view itself. Ad hominem discussions of a person's psychodynamic make-up do not necessarily reflect on the correctness or incorrectness of his political ideas.

2. Unconscious psychologic motivations are not confined to those holding unpopular or extreme points of view. Personality factors are just as relevant to an individual's taking a moderate political position. Whether one regards such middle-position motivations as invidious or praiseworthy usually depends on where one stands on the political spectrum oneself. It is not uncommon for extremists at either end to save some of their choicest epithets for those who choose the relative "safety" of the middle.

3. No single psychodynamic formulation can apply universally to every person who takes an extreme left or right position. Any careful and objective study of such individuals will always uncover a range of varying personalities and motivations. However, the percentage of deviants from the "norm" (itself a relative concept derived from the patterns and values of the large center group) will obviously increase as one moves out from the center to either extreme. The psychodynamic patterns that I shall describe for political extremists, therefore, are applicable to many members of such groups but not necessarily to all of them.

What I am chiefly concerned with in this paper are the unconscious psychodynamic patterns that motivate an individual powerfully, and often blindly, to hew to an extremist political position regardless of the realities involved. I shall not deal with those who for purposes of power or monetary gain consciously and deliberately exploit an extremist position in which they themselves do not really believe. Nor shall I concern myself with the idealistic liberal who may be labeled a "communist" by extremists of the right, or of the rational conservative who may be labeled as "fascist" by extremists of the left. Liberals and conservatives serve equally important functions in an evolving democratic society. The former provide the impetus for the progressive change that such a society must have. The latter provide cautionary brakes on such developing programs and thus protect the social organization from ill-considered or hastily conceived utopian schemes that are foredoomed to failure. In this sense, it should be apparent also that I am not equating political extremism with political dissent in general. A great deal of dissent from prevailing governmental policy may take place within the framework of either a liberal or a conservative orientation; such dissent serves an important constructive function in the dynamics of evolutionary cultural change (1). The extremists referred to in this communication are the revolutionary activists at each end of the political spectrum— the militant communists, neo-Nazis, and radical rightists whose publications and public meetings generally reflect a vitriolic hatred of existing institutions and an espousal of violence as a means toward achieving their goals.

One of the most striking aspects of the problem we are considering is the remarkable degree to which such extremists, whether right or left, share certain psychodynamic patterns. Indeed, recent Western political history has illustrated all too often how extremists of the left can become extremists of the right. Mussolini was once a left-wing radical, and prewar Germany had the largest Communist party in Europe. Although I have no factual data upon which to base this, I have little doubt that in the Soviet Union and other Eastern European countries there must be numerous examples of former right-wing extremists who have since become "redder than the rose." What are these shared psychodynamic patterns that set such individuals distinctively apart from political moderates? They are:

1. A tendency toward *blind faith* in a paternalistic leader or leadership. This faith leads to total acceptance without inner or outer questioning of whatever dicta the leader or leadership hands down.

2. *Extreme distortions in the perception of the "enemy,"* accompanied by enormous *suspiciousness* and *distrust* that at times verge on paranoid patterns of reaction. The opposition tends to be thought of in sinister, monolithic terms. On the left, the complex problems of society are blamed on the malevolent machinations of "Wall Street"; on the right, they are attributed to diabolical "communist, Jewish plots" to take over the world. There is an extreme *polarization of attitude* toward those who disagree with them; anyone who is not one hundred percent on their side is considered to be an enemy. Accordingly, both the enemy and the ingroup are perceived in *stereotyped ways:* "We" are all good, "They" are all bad. To the left-wing extremist, even a Franklin Roosevelt is seen as a "warmonger" and a "tool of Wall Street," and the liberal is regarded as a "social fascist." To the right wing extremist, even Eisenhower and Truman are "communist dupes" if not actual communist "agents" and all liberals are considered "Reds."

3. At both extremes the insulation of thought and the distortions of perception lead toward patterns of *grandiosity and egocentricity:* "We've got all the answers, everyone else is confused or duped."

4. At each extreme there is an absolute conviction that the responsibility for saving the world, either from capitalist or communist exploitation, rests upon them and consequently there is a *feeling of justification in imposing their views on others by whatever force or violence may be necessary.* The end is thus seen as justifying the means.

5. Both extremes manifest an *intolerance of ambiguity* and a *need for certainty.* Faced with a world in which ambiguity and uncertainty are the rule, such individuals cry loudly for *immediate action* to put an end to their tension, without regard for the long term consequences of such action. Thus slogans like: "Drop the bomb," "Man the barricades," "Death to the enemy," and "Let's get it over with" are commonly voiced by them.

6. Patterns of repression, denial, rationalization, projection, and reaction formation are strongly evidenced in the effort to maintain or justify patterns of contradictory or illogical beliefs. For years devout communists utilized such mechanisms to justify the brutalities and tyrannies of the Stalinist regime. Similarly, dedicated followers of an Adolf Hitler or a Gerald L. K. Smith employ such mechanisms to justify the genocide of Jews or Negroes.

These qualities, which are shared by extremists of both groups and which stem from similar deep emotional insecurities, make it possible for them, under certain circumstances, to swing from one polar political position to the other. Since their perceptions of reality are grossly distorted, logic and rationality are essentially irrelevant to their ideological stance; the primary determinants are their unconscious security needs.

[The political moderate, in contrast to the extremist, is never quite so sure of his position. He has (depending on one's point of view) the fortunate or unfortunate capacity of being able to see shadings of right and wrong at both ends of the political spectrum and consequently he often finds himself unable to commit himself to a polarized course of action. From the standpoint of others who share his moderate views, this is an indication of his objectivity and more accurate reality perception; but from the standpoint of those at either extreme, it is a reflection of a fear of jeopardizing his security and of an indecisiveness in which ". . . the native hue of resolution is sicklied o'er by the pale cast of thought."]

Apart from the patterns which extremists at both ends share, however, there are a number of other patterns that tend to differentiate the left from the right.

1. Extremists on the left are oriented *against the status quo and in favor of change.* Patterns of sexual freedom, of unorthodox dress, of non-religion or anti-religion, and of racial and ethnic integration are common among them, and reflect their rejection of conventional mores.

In contrast, radical rightists are concerned with *strengthening of the status quo* and are *opposed to change.* They regard the old order of things as natural, sane, and morally correct. They tend to be strongly conventional, sexually prudish, strongly religious, and intensely nationalistic.

> They are equally concerned with pure food, pure morals, and
> pure races. They are excessively preoccupied with fears of sexual
> attack, bodily poisoning, or ideational contamination. Safety lies
> in what is old and familiar. The new and the unfamiliar are
> threatening. New habits, new foods, new drugs, or new ideas
> are all viewed with suspicion and apprehension. Fundamentalism
> is the cornerstone of their philosophy—a determined and rigid
> adherence to convention and tradition. (2)

2. Passive dependent yearnings for security play an important role
in the motivations of extremists at both ends. However, on the
left, these yearnings are linked to the vision of a *future* utopia;
on the right, to the vision of a *past* one, of "the glory that once
was." On this basis, extremists of both types may be united in their
intense opposition to the *present* order, and in their wish to overthrow
it, by force if necessary.

3. The radical leftist, however, usually views his opposition to
the present order as *part of an inevitable historical change* resting
on massive social and economic forces—class struggle, colonial
revolution, the crumbling of imperialistic empires, etc.

In contrast, the extremist of the right tends to attribute all social
change to the sinister plotting of malevolent people, and *never to
historical forces.* Convinced as he is that the old order, about which
his dreams are oriented, was perfect, it follows that the changes
that he sees inexorably taking place all around him can only be
due to the machinations of imperfect, perverse, or subversive
individuals.

> Instead of conflict between capital and labor, there is a plot
> of labor leaders or capitalists or Jews. Instead of an upsurge
> of Negro masses, there is a plot of Negro leaders. Underlying
> all attempts to find solutions for the intellectual problems of
> our times . . . is a cabal of eggheads and longhairs. And . . .
> all of these separate plots are but aspects of a large plot,
> world-encompassing, eternal, evil . . . [that] bears the name
> of Jew, Catholic, communism, the Devil. (3)

4. As Rokeach (4) has perceptively pointed out, even though the
left-wing communist and the right-wing fascist share a common
ideological *structure*, they differ markedly in their ideological *content*.

Thus, organizationally, they both favor leadership by an elite group, unquestioning, disciplined obedience from their members, and repressive measures to stifle opposition or dissent. The ideological content of communism, however, is humanitarian and antiauthoritarian. Theoretically, its ultimate goals are a classless society, the withering away of the state, and an ultimate and perfect security for the individual—"from each according to his abilities, to each according to his needs."

In contrast, the ideological content of the fascist is essentially antihumanitarian and authoritarian. Thus for the Nazi it involved the belief in an aryan master race that would subjugate and rule over the rest of mankind.

It is evident, therefore, that in fascist ideology structure and content are compatible with one another, while in communist ideology they are not. Accordingly, one might anticipate that communists would be more susceptible to inner conflict and guilt feelings than would fascists. Lindner (5) reflected this idea when he commented that there was a neurotic element to communism and a psychopathic one to fascism.

Because of this inherent conflict between communistic political structure and Marxist ideological content, communists are more likely to become disillusioned and to renounce their affiliations than are fascists. The wholesale defections that followed the Nazi-Soviet Pact of 1939 are illustrative of this. Also in communist states, unlike fascist ones, it is possible to have strivings for political democracy without being opposed to Marxian economic ideas—witness recent events within Czechoslovakia.

Moreover, because in fascist ideology structure and content support each other, individuals with authoritarian personality patterns tend in general to become attached more easily to fascist-like ideologies than to communistic ones—as Rokeach's experimental studies have demonstrated (4).

The factors that predispose an individual toward becoming a political extremist are multiple, and are idiosyncratic as well as social and economic. Political extremists at both poles show evidence of considerable anxiety and emotional insecurity, and their political activities represent their efforts to defend against these anxieties. Rokeach (4), however, found somewhat less evidence of conscious anxiety among leftists than among rightists, and speculated that communistic political activity with its emphasis on "comradeship" and group activities may be a more effective reducer of anxiety than the "rugged individualism" and more paranoid ideology of the right.

In general, it seems to me that social and economic factors are greater determinants among working-class leftists than in those of middle- or upper-class origin. Frustrations born of prolonged poverty, unemployment, feelings of deprivation, and experiences of prejudice and discrimination are common in the backgrounds of lower-class radicals. To such individuals the utopian and protective society pictured in Marxist theory has a powerful appeal, and efforts to "sell" them on the advantages of the free enterprise system, as long as they feel themselves to be its prime victims, are clearly doomed to failure. For this group, jobs and economic and social security constitute a far more powerful antidote to communist indoctrination than all the theoretical arguments in the world.

On the other hand, the left-wing extremist who comes from a middle- or upper-class position usually derives his strong identifications with the underdog from more personal factors in his background. A common pattern is rebellion against an authoritarian father. It is my impression, however, that many psychoanalytically oriented writers have tended to overemphasize this factor as being the source of *all* radicalism, not only to the exclusion of the realistic social and economic factors noted above, but also at the expense of other familial factors. Strong identifications with the underdog can also develop on the basis of being a younger or less favored or less adequate sibling, or of having some physical handicap, or through close association with a mistreated or oppressed mother. In other instances, *positive* identifications with a loved or admired radical parent-figure may be the source of such political leanings.

On the right-wing side there is similarly an interplay of various socioeconomic factors and personal ones. Some of the socioeconomic subgroups that tend to be particularly susceptible to radical-right patterns of thinking are: (1) The new rich who feel excluded from established citadels of power, such as some Texas oil millionaires. (2) Southern elite groups trying to maintain their power against the pressure of rising Negro and working class groups. (3) Military elite groups in whom the authoritarian tradition is very strong and who are strongly indoctrinated with an inherent distrust of democratic process. (4) Small businessmen who feel frustrated, threatened, and particularly vulnerable to the changing socioeconomic currents around them. (5) Working-class and lower-middle-class people who feel alienated, isolated, threatened, and frustrated, and are seeking scapegoats for their aggressive feelings. (6) Elderly people who because of weakened egos feel threatened by change and yearn for the security of "the good old days." (7) Members of certain religious groups whose ideological patterns make them more susceptible to authoritarian ways of thinking. Thus orthodox Catholics and fundamentalist Protestants are more apt to be found in the ranks of radical rightists than are, say, Unitarians, Congregationalists, or Reform Jews.

In terms of more personal backgrounds of right-wing extremists, Adorno and his co-workers (6) have described the rigid, repressive, authoritarian home atmosphere commonly encountered in the life-histories of such individuals. This leads to the repression of both hostile and libidinal impulses, with ensuing characterological rigidity, and a tendency to seek external scapegoats on whom their hostility can be discharged. Deutsch (7), on the other hand, in an interesting study of 41 youths, aged eleven to twenty-five, from predominantly working-class families, who had been arrested for smearing swastikas on synagogues in 1960, reported that over half of them had previous police records, and all but eight came from broken or unstable homes with a high incidence of alcoholism, mental illness, and criminal activity. The most common family factors were a lack of communication between family members, a paucity of friends, and an absence of participation or interest in community problems. The values of the youths were consistent with their home values, strongly anti-Semitic, anti-Negro, and sometimes anti-Catholic. They had been highly exposed to much bigoted literature. They had almost all not done well in school—even those with superior intelligence—and were rootless, suspicious, cynical, bitter, and bored. They revealed strong feelings of insecurity and inadequacy. The swastika represented a symbol of compensatory power to them. One of the youths engaged in swastika smearing on several occasions immediately after failure to perform adequately in sexual relations with his wife.

The sense of vulnerability that all of these individuals share in common is "equivalent to what has been symbolically described in psychoanalytic theory as 'castration anxiety' and its development precursors . . ." (2). Irrational anxiety that they generate in response to various programs stems from the fact that these programs

> are perceived as constituting a threat to either their sense of bodily wholeness, or their sense of psychic wholeness, or else the wholeness of what we might call their life-space. These, of course, are often interrelated and interconnected. This is the common denominator which explains our finding the same individuals passionately defending themselves against the forcible entry of any "foreign body"—whether it be a vaccination, a mental health proposal, interracial contact, or a wave of immigrants from overseas (2).

In conclusion, the question may properly be raised as to why there is still only a relatively small percentage of people in the American population who occupy the radical extremes politically. I believe that the answer to this question lies in the democratic structure of the American family, our essentially nonauthoritarian parent-child relationships, and the deeply rooted democratic values of our culture. There is no reason to assume, however, that this constitutes any permanent guarantee against a major swing to the left or the right. If our established values and our political structure should prove inadequate in providing emotional and economic security to a sufficiently large segment of our population, such a swing might well occur. The lessons that recent history have taught us of the price that is paid in terms of personal freedom and self-expression within totalitarian societies, both on the left and on the right, underline more powerfully than ever the importance of the vigilant maintenance of democratic and nonauthoritarian values both within our families and within our social structure. But our society must also not ignore the demands of our poor for economic relief and an end to racial prejudice and discrimination, if the growing frustration and anger in our urban ghettos is to be prevented from increasingly spilling over into patterns of group violence and political extremism (8).

SUMMARY

Extremists at each end of the political spectrum share certain psychodynamic patterns. They are: (1) blind faith in a paternalistic leader or leadership; (2) gross and stereotyped distortions in the perception of the "enemy," with extreme polarization of attitudes toward those who disagree with them; (3) patterns of grandiosity and egocentricity; (4) a feeling of justification in imposing their views on others by whatever force may be necessary, and a feeling that the end justifies the means; (5) an intolerance of ambiguity and a need for certainty; and (6) patterns of repression, denial, rationalization, projection, and reaction formation.

There are other patterns, however, that differentiate the left from the right. (1) Left extremists are oriented against the status quo and in favor of change; those on the right are concerned with maintaining the status quo. (2) Passive dependent yearnings on the left are linked to the visions of a future utopia; on the right, they are tied to a past one. (3) The radical leftist sees himself as part of an inevitable historical change resting on massive social and economic forces. The radical rightist attributes all social change to the sinister plotting of malevolent people and never to historical forces. (4) There is a greater conflict between structure and content in left-wing ideology than there is in right-wing ideology.

The factors that predispose individuals toward becoming political extremists are multiple and idiosyncratic as well as social and economic. Some of these are listed and discussed. The importance of vigilant maintenance of democratic and nonauthoritarian values both within our families and within our social structure is emphasized.

REFERENCES

1. COSER, L. A. The Functions of Dissent. Presented at a meeting of the American Academy of Psychoanalysis, New York City, December 3, 1967.
2. MARMOR, J., BERNARD, VIOLA W., and OTTENBERG, P. Psychodynamics of Group Opposition to Health Programs. *Am. J. Orthopsychiat.*, 30:330, 1960. (Chapter 27, this volume.)
3. SCHNEIDER, E. V. The Radical Right. *The Nation*, Sept. 30, 1961. p. 200.
4. ROKEACH, M. *The Open and Closed Mind.* Basic Books, New York, 1960.
5. LINDNER, R. M. Political Creed and Character. *Psychoanalysis*, 2:10, 1953.
6. ADORNO, T. W., et al. *The Authoritarian Personality.* Harper & Bros., New York, 1950.

7. DEUTSCH, M. The 1960 Swastika-Smearings. Analysis of the Apprehended Youth. *Merrill-Palmer Quart. of Behavior & Development.* April 1962, p. 1.
8. MARMOR, J. Psychosocial Aspects of Urban Violence. *New Mexico Quart.*, 37:335, 1968. (Chapter 31, this volume.)

31

SOME PSYCHOSOCIAL ASPECTS OF CONTEMPORARY URBAN VIOLENCE
(1970)

Violence is a form of behavior intended to injure or destoy an object that is perceived as an actual or potential source of frustration or danger, or as a symbol thereof. Much controversy has raged for many years over the question of whether violence is rooted in an instinctual aggressive urge that is inherent in the nature of man. Many classical psychoanalysts, following the lead of Sigmund Freud, tend to believe that it is. They hold, moreover, that this urge is of autochthonous, spontaneous origin, requiring some external outlet if it is not to be "turned inward" with resultant psychopathology. According to this theory, all assertive behavior, even that which is creative and adaptive, is a form of aggression, although in such instances the aggression is assumed to be "fused" with positive libidinal drives which enable it to have constructive rather than destructive goals.

Most behavioral scientists, however, are of the opinion that although man, like other mammals, is born with an innate *capacity* for violence or aggressive behavior, whether or not this capacity finds *expression* depends almost always on some external factor rather than on a spontaneous inner urge (1). To put it more succinctly, the fact that the capacity for violence is innate in man does not mean that the expression of violence is inevitable.

A distinction needs also to be made between violence and conflict. Conflict in one form or another will always be part of the human scene. The modes by which conflict is expressed and pursued, however, are highly variable, responsive to pressure for change, and amenable to controls that can limit the degree of destructiveness involved.

The sources of most violence can be found in man's life situation. Indeed, the fact that in all societies rates of violent behavior can be demonstrated to be clearly correlated with certain types of social patterning (e.g., poverty, urbanization, social class, etc.) is an effective argument against the assumption that human violence arises spontaneously on the basis of biological needs or simple idiosyncratic propensities (2). Moreover, the common tendency to assume that violent behavior is always correlated with anger or hostility constitutes a considerable oversimplification. In today's world there is at least as great a danger that violence will result from the effects of fear as from hostility. Clinical experience has demonstrated that panic is a potent trigger for violence; and extreme fear of an adversary is just as likely to provoke an aggressive act against him as is hatred of him.

Actually, a great deal of contemporary violence takes place without either anger or fear in relation to the intended victims. This kind of violence, sometimes called "instrumental aggression," is in the service of "just doing a job," a la Eichmann. Much of modern warfare—the dropping of bombs or napalm on faceless, distant, dehumanized dots, or the firing of shells at invisible enemies beyond the horizon—is of such instrumental nature. Indeed, the ultimate achievement of modern war technology, the mathematically precise triggering of intercontinental missiles with nuclear warheads capable of devastating total continents thousands of miles away, is one in which neither anger nor any other passionate emotion has any functional value at all. Thomas Merton, in an essay ironically entitled "A Devout Meditation in Memory of Adolph Eichmann" (3), has recently pointed out that one of the most terrifying aspects of international warfare and genocide is that so much of it takes place on the basis of cold, planned, precise, and deliberate action. As he puts it: "We rely on the sane people of the world to preserve it from barbarism, madness, destruction. And now it begins to dawn on us that it is precisely the *sane* ones who are the most dangerous . . . who can without qualm and without nausea aim the missiles and press the buttons that will initiate the great festival of destruction that they, the *sane ones*, have prepared."

However, another kind of social violence, quantitatively less massive and less destructive than that of modern warfare, is assuming more distressing and frightening proportions for contemporary Americans, because it is close at hand and because "enemy" and "victim" are both highly visible. I refer to the violence in our urban ghettos, which has reached climactic proportions in recent mass riots and which has been dramatically brought home to millions of Americans via television.

In considering the sources of this phenomenon it is useful to distinguish between its basic *underlying roots*, on the one hand, and the *trigger mechanisms* that set it off, on the other. At first glance it would seem to be an obvious truism that the source of much of the contemporary violence in our urban ghettos is rooted in the poverty, poor housing, inadequate education, and generally degraded living conditions with which the residents of these ghettos are confronted. Although no one would deny the relevance of these factors, the question still remains, however, of why these outbursts are taking place now with greater frequency and intensity than in the past. One might point out, for example, that the lot of the blacks under slavery was certainly worse than it is today; or that the lot of poor immigrants at the turn of the century in our urban ghettos, with their sweatshops, twelve-hour day, child labor, etc., was worse than the lot of the poor today. And yet there was not as much violence then in terms of organized mass riots as there is now.

The significant difference between these earlier situations and those of the present lies in what has been called the "revolution of rising expectations." Only when people have been stimulated to hope that their unhappy lot can be changed does it really begin to feel unendurable. As de Tocqueville, referring to the French Revolution, pointed out: "A people which has supported without complaint, as if they were not felt, the most oppressive laws, violently throws them off as soon as their weight is lightened. The social order destroyed by a revolution is always better than that which immediately preceded it . . . . The evil which was suffered patiently as inevitable, seems unendurable as soon as the idea of escaping from it is conceived" (4).

What has happened in contemporary America to account for this revolution of rising expectations, and for the sense of unendurable frustration that many of the masses in our urban ghettos, particularly the black masses, have begun to feel? It seems to me that there are four major factors that account for this change.

1. The first has been the heightened affirmation of the democratic ideals on which our nation was founded. Two world wars have been fought, presumably to make the world safer for democracy, and a succession of American presidents have emphatically publicized these aims. The eloquent idealism of John Kennedy, upon his accession to the Presidency, had a profound influence on young people, in particular, raising their hopes for the realization of the American dream of equality and security for all. The drive to end discrimination took a new lease on life, and American students who had for a generation been "playing it safe" became politically active again through the medium of the civil rights movement. Despite Kennedy's tragic assassination, these hopes for a "great society" received further impetus during the first year of the Johnson Administration, when new civil rights legislation was pushed through Congress in a way that Kennedy himself had not been able to accomplish. The nation's poverty programs, Project Head Start, new housing laws, and apparent progress in desegregation of schools and other public places all seemed to hold high promise for new and hitherto unattained levels of American democracy.

2. The second has been the migration of hundreds of thousands of black people from Southern rural communities to the "promised land" of the Northern cities, where they hoped that they would be able to live with new dignity, and that their children would have opportunities to participate as equals in all the good things of the American way of life.

3. The stimulation of these hopes and expectations has been enormously heightened by the communications explosion growing out of modern technology. There is hardly a house in America today that does not have a radio, and more than ninety percent of all households are now reported to have a television set. This means that the message of democracy is being carried into every community and home in the United States, and can be comprehended even by the totally illiterate. Madison Avenue's visible demonstration via television, magazines, and other mass media of better ways to

live—with constant, tantalizing offers of beautiful homes, tempting foods, attractive clothes, and luxurious holiday resorts—gives increased tangibility and substance to the great promise, in a manner that had never before been possible.

4. The progressive dissolution of colonial empires (at least in their traditional form) in Africa and Asia after World War II, with the emergence on these continents of many new nations whose representatives are accorded full diplomatic respect in the forums and councils of the United Nations, has lent additional strength and impetus to the expectations of our own black population. It has given them renewed pride in their historic traditions, made them less ashamed of their black skin, and heightened their impatience and resentment at the residual manifestations of discrimination which they continue to encounter in their own country.

Given these four factors and the rising hopes and expectations which they have stimulated, it is inevitable that the steady and inexorable escalation of the war in Vietnam, with its inhibiting effect upon the social welfare programs of our country, has tended to create a sense of mounting frustration in our urban ghettos. Poverty programs have had to be curtailed or eliminated, civil rights advances have ground to a standstill, and the massive financing which is needed to rehabilitate the ghettos is no longer available. It is in this context that much of what is going on in contemporary America can be understood. The growing disaffection on our college campuses, the rise of the hippy movement with its rejection of conventional middle-class values, and the mounting anger and frustration of our black populations are all related to the factors described above. Hopes have been stimulated and are not being fulfilled. Among blacks the intense frustration they have experienced has led to intense anger at the whites who have failed them, particularly white liberals. This apparently irrational focusing of their anger on those who have tried hardest to help them is not quite so illogical when we realize that these whites are considered instrumental in stimulating their hopes and then failing to carry through.

Other factors must also be considered. Violence is rarely something that takes place totally unilaterally. It is almost always a transaction involving two parties. The mounting anger of the deprived black and the growing insistence of his demand for equality now have stimulated much anxiety, particularly among lower-middle-class whites, who have then responded with counteraggression and renewed prejudice—the so-called white backlash. This, in turn, has intensified black nationalism, and the chasm between the two groups has grown deeper and wider, with greater polarization of feelings and a greater predisposition to violence on both sides.

Moreover, although the negative aspects of violence are quite obvious, the constructive aspects of violent behavior are often lost sight of. Violent behavior on the part of masses of people represents a kind of crude signaling device or communication to the body politic that something is wrong. Thus riots or acts of violence serve as a means of opening channels of communication between the ghettos and the power structure, channels that in many instances have never existed previously. Also, as has been thoroughly documented in some of the descriptions of recent riots, they provide a release mechanism which gives a sense of power and status to people or groups who have felt inadequate or humiliated. This explains the sense of elation among riot participants that has so frequently been observed, particularly in the early phase of the rioting, before the suppressive weight of control measures has had a chance to take effect.

With these underlying factors, what are the triggers that have set off mass outbursts of urban violence? Not surprisingly, most of these riots have taken place at the height of summer, when the unbearable heat in the central-city ghettos has lowered the threshold of irritability of its inhabitants to dangerous levels. Given the basic setting of chronic anger and frustration and such a lowered threshold of irritability, any police action which seems unwarranted, inconsiderate, or insulting can become the incendiary fuse, as the recent report of the Lemberg Center for the Study of Violence at Brandeis University has pointed out (5). An unjust arrest, or rumors of a black person being injured or unfairly handled by law-enforcement agencies or by some whites, can suddenly release the pent-up anger in the group, anger which then spreads by mass contagion to explosive proportions.

The "treatment" of mass urban violence needs to be dealt with at two levels. The immediate, short-term need is to reduce and eliminate such triggering mechanisms as much as possible. This calls for better police relations and communications with the members of the urban ghettos, for greater use and employment of black police officers, for a greater degree of local rule wherever possible, and for the elimination of the kinds of patterns of behavior that intensify the sense of degradation which the members of these ghettos feel. Thus, while one can appreciate the tensions under which white police officers operate within a black urban ghetto, certain actions that traditionally are often taken by them seem psychologically indefensible. For example, the common practice of spread-eagling a black suspect over the hood of his car while he is searched is a "castrating" procedure that arouses deep feelings of humiliation and resentment among black men, whose masculine self-image has already been rendered deeply vulnerable by chronic unemployment and racial discrimination.

On a more fundamental basis, of course, the deep sources of frustrations in our central cities have to be dealt with. Although it might logically be argued that if one could eliminate the expectations of our poor, they would be better off, this is no longer possible in today's world. Hopes brought to life are not easily stifled, and the American commitment to a democratic ideology is now too deeply rooted in our traditions to be eradicated. It therefore becomes a matter of urgent necessity to tackle the basic sources of frustration of our poor so that their hopes can again acquire the potentiality of realization. In today's explosive urban situation gradualism or tokenism will no longer suffice. To the underprivileged blacks gradualism, through long and bitter experience, has come to mean "never." Only a crash program of massive proportions that will enable them to see results rapidly will have any effect in lessening their level of frustration. Unfortunately, the tragedy of present-day America is that so long as the war in Vietnam continues, there is no prospect that such a crash program will be or can be undertaken.

The special relevance of the war to these urgent urban needs becomes highlighted when we realize that conservative estimates place the cost of the war at $30 billion a year. It is hard for any average person to fully comprehend the meaning of this magnitude of expenditure. Recently, in a somewhat different context, Warren Weaver of the Rockefeller Institute undertook to explore what $30 billion could buy for science and education. Writing in *Medical World*

News on January 5, 1968, he stated: "We could give a ten percent raise in salary, over a ten-year period, to every teacher in the United States, from kindergarten through universities, in both public and private institutions (about $9.8 billion); give $10 million each to 200 of the best smaller colleges ($2 billion); finance seven-year fellowships at $4,000 per person per year for 50,000 new scientists and engineers ($1.4 billion); contribute $200 million each toward the creation of ten new medical schools ($2 billion); build and largely endow complete universities, with medical, engineering, and agricultural faculties for all 53 of the nations which have been added to the United Nations since its original founding ($13.2 billion); create three more permanent Rockefeller Foundations ($1.5 billion); and still have $100 million left over to popularize science."

Perhaps a more relevant example was an estimate that I encountered in 1969 after seeing a heartrending film on the filth, despair, and degradation that characterized a typical urban ghetto area, the Ludlow section of Philadelphia, a section in which even the local residents dared not move around after dusk for fear of being raped, mugged, or otherwise violently assaulted. It was an area characterized by rotting slum tenements, accumulating garbage, and rats that roamed at will. A local civic leader estimated that $20 million was needed to rehabilitate that area and make it a livable place for its inhabitants. Twenty million dollars to clean up one typical urban ghetto: this is an amount approximating six hours' worth of the cost of the Vietnam war! That means that the cost of one year of the Vietnam war could pay for the rehabilitation of fifteen hundred such urban ghettos.

This is not to imply, however, that simply pouring money into the ghettos for improved housing and schools will suffice to solve the problems of the poor in our central cities. Of even higher priority to all our poor—white, black, brown, yellow, and red—is the diginity of full employment at a living wage. Perhaps nothing short of a massive federal work program, and work-training program, along the lines of the Works Progress Administration of the Roosevelt era, will provide that solution, since it seems unlikely that private capital can ever make more than token inroads into this problem.

Finally, there are certain other long-term considerations that are relevant to the prevention of violence in American society. Perhaps the most important of these is the need to alter some of the social institutions and basic values of our present-day culture which subtly tend to glorify violence and, not so subtly, to desensitize people to its manifestations (6). Our history books glorify wars and generals; the millions of victims of war are treated merely as ciphers, and, as Arthur Koestler has so aptly put it, "statistics don't bleed." Our movies, our television stories, our comic books, and our newspapers all "sell" violence in huge doses to our children, our adolescents, and our grownups. War games and toys grow ever more realistic.

The issue here is not whether such marketing of violence "creates" aggression in people. The roots of aggression, as we have seen, are of a deeper sort. Moreover, to argue—as many psychologists and psychiatrists have—that war games and toys, and violence in communications media provide "an outlet for hostility" is completely to miss the essential point. Granting that they are indeed such an outlet, the question is whether this is the kind of outlet that is healthy either for the individual or for society. The insidious fact about such marketing of violence is that it *desensitizes* people to the spectacle of human brutality and killing, and *teaches* them techniques for encompassing such ends. Our society needs institutions that will strengthen the dignity and sanctity of human life, not degrade it. Outlets for hostility do not have to be directed at goals of death and brutality. There are "moral equivalents" of violence, to adapt William James's well-known phrase, that serve such psychological purposes equally well. Cheering for one's side in an athletic contest, or participating in one, is also an outlet for hostility, and a much healthier one socially and individually. There is a crying need in our society to identify the various acculturation processes, subtle and not-so-subtle, that abet patterns of human violence, and try to modify them. Not only can war no longer be considered a rational political instrument in an age of nuclear weapons; the patterns of socially sanctioned violence and brutality in any form need to be eliminated if man is to survive the challenges that face him in the decades ahead.

REFERENCES

1. JUDD MARMOR, "War, Violence and Human Nature," *The Bulletin of the Atomic Scientists*, March, 1964, pp. 19–22.

2. Lewis A. Coser, "Violence and the Social Structure," *Science and Psychoanalysis,* Vol. VI, New York, Grune and Straton, Inc., 1963, pp. 30–42.
3. Thomas Merton, "A Devout Meditation in Memory of Adolph Eichmann," *Raids on the Unspeakable,* New York, New Directions Publishing Company, 1966.
4. Alexis de Tocqueville, *L'Ancien Regime,* trans. by M. W. Patterson. Oxford, England, Basil Blackwell, 1949, p. 186.
5. *Six-City Study. A Survey of Racial Attitudes in Six Northern Cities: Preliminary Findings,* a report of the Lemberg Center for the Study of Violence, Brandeis University, Waltham, Massachusetts, June, 1967 (mimeographed).
6. Judd Marmor, "Psychology of Man in a Warless World" (Chapter 28, this volume).

32

PSYCHIATRY AND THE FUTURE OF MAN
(1972)

Much has been written in the psychiatric literature in recent years about the problems that man will face in the Brave New World of the future—problems of increased leisure, of identity, of creativity, of self-actualization, of spiritual belief, and of altered relationships to his children, to his fellow men, and between the sexes. Now, however, quite another concern has begun to preoccupy us. Does man *have* a future? Our troubled planet has always had its problems, but never before in the history of man has his very existence hung so precariously in the balance. The air we breathe, the water we drink, and the food we eat are all becoming increasingly polluted by by-products of our technology; our forests and wild life are being steadily eroded by the relentless growth of cities and population; our limited mineral wealth is being depleted at an alarming rate; and above all, the shadow of nuclear annihilation looms ominously in the wings of our terrestrial theater. The concerned words of President John F. Kennedy to the United Nations in 1961 are unfortunately no less valid today than they were then. "Every man, woman, and child [on this planet]," he said, "lives under a nuclear sword of Damocles, hanging by the slenderest of threads, capable of being cut at any moment by accident or miscalculation or by madness."

Why have we reached this threatening impasse? How is it possible that the miraculous advances in scientific knowledge that have spanned everything from the mysteries of creation and the origins of life to landing on the distant moon have not been able to help us solve the rather mundane problems of living together in peace and security? Most thoughtful people will agree that the problem

416

is not in the nature of our technology but in the nature of man. "The fault, dear Brutus, is not in our stars but in ourselves." But the consensus stops here. Views still differ sharply concerning man's nature. There are those who would blame our difficulties primarily on the biological nature of man. The essential tenet of these theories is that man is possessed of an instinct for aggression which spontaneously and persistently seeks an outlet—whether it be in self-aggrandizement or in covert, if not overt, acts of cruelty, or at the very least, in competitive efforts to best his fellow-man in one way or another. As Freud said, "*Homo homini lupus.* Who has the courage to dispute this in the face of all the evidence in his own life and history?" (1)

Not surprisingly, in view of the contemporary state of the world, this view of man's nature has received renewed impetus in recent years, particularly in the writings of Robert Ardrey, Desmond Morris, and Konrad Lorenz. In a world in which hostility and destructiveness seem to be so ubiquitous, it is reassuring to be told that this is an inevitable aspect of our biological inheritance, because this provides absolution for the burden of guilt that most people carry with them for their own aggressive fantasies and impulses.

I shall not attempt at this time to analyze the pros and cons of these or other biological explanations for man's violence to his fellow men. I would like instead to present an alternative explanation—one that I believe is not only scientifically more inclusive and valid, but also one that offers a potential solution to the critical dilemma in which we find ourselves.

Within this conceptual framework one does not assume that man's nature is either innately bad, a la Hobbes, or innately good, a la Rousseau, but rather that the behavioral patterns man displays are a consequence of adaptation to the environment in which he finds himself. This does not imply, however, that man at birth is a tabula rasa. Quite the contrary—he comes on the scene with an extraordinarily complex set of inherited structures that have evolved over a million years and that carry with them unique adaptive capacities. Among these are certain neurophysiological structures and mechanisms which, when activated, result in aggressive behavior. Although, as indicated, theorists like Freud and Lorenz argue that these mechanisms operate spontaneously and autonomously, presumably from some internal feedback mechanism, the fact is that no one has ever been able to demonstrate any predictable periodicity or accumulating biochemical or hormonal factor on which such spontaneous activation might be posited. A more acceptable hypothesis—and one that is testable—is that, except in rare instances of specific cerebral pathology, these mechanisms are usually stimulated into action by certain predictable external conditions.

This difference in theory is not a trivial one. As Leon Eisenberg has pointed out in a brilliant essay in *Science* (2), what we choose to believe about the nature of man has social consequences. If one subscribes to the concept of a spontaneous aggressive instinct, one tends to end up with the pessimistic conviction that war and violence are inevitable accompaniments of the human condition, that social and racial inequities are inexorable natural consequences of a Darwinian struggle for survival, and that the only adaptive solutions left to us are those of greater social controls via stronger and bigger police or military forces, or chemical or pharmacological controls (a la Dr. Kenneth Clark) or of some Big-Brotherly techniques of operantly-conditioning the have-nots to passive acceptance of their inferior lot.

If, on the other hand, one takes the position that these mechanisms for aggressive behavior are *not* autonomous, then our attention must be directed to the nature of the environmental factors that call them into play, and the adaptive challenge becomes one of trying to devise psychosocial models that will eliminate these factors.

For most of this century, we psychoanalysts, leaning on the monumental contributions of Sigmund Freud, have sought the reasons for man's wide behavioral variations primarily in the idiosyncratic life histories of individuals. Based on these views, our hopes were raised that if only we could teach mothers and fathers how to properly raise their children, a world of better men would inevitably emerge. Our aspirations went still further. If we could but disseminate our psychotherapeutic techniques and insights widely enough, we might even be able to repair existing behavioral disturbances sufficiently so that psychiatry, by its direct efforts, could contribute significantly to the creation of a better world. I still recall my old teacher, William Alanson White, fervently expressing the conviction that international conflict could be resolved if it were possible to psychoanalyze the national leaders of all the Great Powers!

Unhappily, the current state of our own American society raises serious doubts about the assumptions on which these hopes were based. In spite of two decades of unprecedented expansion of the mental health movement in this country, of the burgeoning of child guidance clinics and family education workshops, and of the extension of psychotherapy to ever wider segments of our population, the degree of violence, cruelty, and unconcern for others has never been greater on our national scene.

In making this point it is not my intention to deprecate the value of the mental health movement or to deny the validity of the important insights which psychodynamic thinking has brought to bear on the understanding of man. I make it only to underline the inescapable conclusion that our explanations have been incomplete, that there must be other factors involved in man's inhumanity to man besides the psychodynamic ones which we have so meticulously explored for the greater part of this century. When we see millions of young people, raised by intelligent and concerned parents, nevertheless becoming alienated from our society and its value-systems; when we see decent, law abiding, average citizens failing even to make a telephone call to save the life of a Kitty Genovese, or when we see clergymen of all faiths and in all countries invoking the name of their deity in defense of their particular brand of patriotism, prejudice, or national war, we are drawn inevitably to the conclusion that significant factors outside of the family, outside of individual psychodynamics, and outside of our biological "nature" must be contributing to these phenomena.

In recent years psychiatric theory has been moving in a direction that sheds some light on this problem. We have begun to recognize that mothers and fathers are not isolated reactors but are themselves part of a larger system whose values and imperatives they consciously or unconsciously purvey to their children. Individual personality development takes place at the core of a series of concentric, interacting spheres of influence beginning with the nuclear family, and extending outward to include the community, the nation, and the world. The generic name for this concept, of course, is systems theory, and I would like to examine a few of its specific implications for man's behavior in today's world and its relevance for his future. Leaving aside, but not underestimating, the profoundly important areas of molecular physics and biochemistry, we begin with the genetic capacities and predispositions which the human infant brings into the world after millions of years of evolutionary development. From the moment of conception on, however, the growing embryo is subjected to vitally important external influences—influences that are nutritional, biochemical, endocrinological, and physical. In our contemporary world the latter may (unhappily) even include the effects of nuclear radiation! The effects of poverty, disease, physical trauma, and environmental pollution continue to be operative when the infant completes the gestational period and emerges into the outer world. For many children in the earliest months of their existence the impact of the larger system outside the family is often profoundly fateful. The effects of protein deficiency, of disease, of cultural deprivation, and of the kinds of child neglect that ensue from lives warped by despair and frustration may leave ego defects from which the developing child may never fully recover.

But it is particularly when we examine the complex acculturation process during which children are exposed to the values and expectations of what we euphemistically continue to call our "civilization" that the answer to our current dilemma begins to emerge.

It has often been argued that man's institutions are an outgrowth of various aspects of man's biological nature. Indeed, such arguments have been used—as Ardrey has done—not only to "justify" various contemporary institutions, but also to raise doubts about whether they can ever be significantly changed. Now clearly, man's genetic constitution *is* a significant factor in shaping his institutions. This seems to me to be incontrovertible.* But to attempt to explain the development of social institutions *primarily* on the basis of man's biological nature is simplistic and reductionistic. One has only to note the enormous diversity of human cultural patterns to recognize

---

*There is strong evidence from comparative ethology, that in pre-agricultural times, in what John Bowlby has called "the environment of evolutionary adaptedness," men, like other higher primates, exhibited strong affiliative tendencies which led them to band together against predators of other species for the protection of their young and their females, as well as of themselves. This deeply ingrained biologically-rooted tendency to become attached to other human beings, which evolved over millions of years precisely because it had species-survival value, is probably the biogenetic nucleus of all of our social institutions.

the obvious fact that other variables must be involved—variables such as climate, terrain, availability of food and water, safety of the environment, and density of population. It is in the *interaction* of man's biological needs with factors such as these that his institutions have emerged and have been adaptively shaped. However—and this is the nub of my thesis—*once these institutions have been formed they acquire a life of their own, a functional autonomy, so to speak, by virtue of which they thenceforth play a profoundly important role in shaping the personalities of human beings who grow up in their sphere of influence.* This is an extremely significant point that is frequently overlooked. Man shapes his institutions, *but he is also shaped by them,* and unless this transactional relationship is understood, the true nature of the complexities underlying many of our contemporary problems will continue to elude us.

Moreover, social institutions undergo evolutionary change and development no less than do biological structures. Those that have survival value for a social system tend to be perpetuated while those that don't get dropped on the way. Thus in a society that is having difficulty in maintaining its numbers due to high infant mortality or a dangerous environment, motherhood and fertility will become highly valued functions and various institutional structures evolve that are designed to protect and enhance these functions. Contrariwise, in a society that is threatened by a scanty food supply, infanticide may emerge as a major institution. In our own culture we are presently in the midst of the gradual evolution of a changing attitude toward abortion from an act that used to be considered abhorrent and illegal to one that is becoming socially sanctioned, a change which, in part at least, is reflective of an adaptive societal reaction to the dangers of overpopulation.

Ethical systems, too, are outgrowths of the needs, aspirations, and circumstances of the societies in which they have developed. In every instance they reflect what each society requires in order to remain functionally effective and homeostatically stable. A slave society does not have the brotherhood of man as a dominant value, nor does a feudal society promote standards of individual liberty and equality. It is not accidental that the ideals of the American and French Revolutions—freedom, equality, and brotherhood—emerged during the Industrial Revolution and the development of capitalism and free enterprise. For capitalism to flourish, it was essential to have free development of science and technology, increased social mobility and freedom of opportunity. Thus the old feudal values of respect for tradition, authority, and the divine rights of kings had to be replaced by a new set of ethical values that were more adaptive to the needs of the new social system. It is not that human beings became more decent people under capitalism, but that the social system required a different set of rules in order to work effectively.

Some 40 years ago, the eminent cultural anthropologist, Ruth Benedict, made some observations concerning values and behavioral patterns in different cultures which are extremely pertinent to this thesis (3). Benedict pointed out that societies that had social orders in which the individual by the same act and at the same time *served his own advantage and that of the group* were characterized by a low incidence of aggressive behavior. This occurred, she suggested, not because people in such societies were unselfish and put social obligations above personal desires, but because when societal institutions were such that personal desires and social obligations coincided, aggressive behavior was not necessary and therefore was not evoked.

Benedict designated societies in which the social structure provided for acts that were mutually advantageous both to the individual and the group as "high synergy" cultures, and those in which the structure elicited activities that were mutually oppositional as "low synergy" ones. In the former societies, what benefited the individual also benefited the group; as a result mutual cooperation was encouraged, and intrasocial competitiveness did not develop. In the latter societies, the advantage of one individual was generally at the expense of another and thus intrasocial competitiveness was fostered. The absolute amount of wealth in a society, she found—and this is important to note—was not the determining factor in the emotional security it afforded. What counted was whether the economic system tended to concentrate the society's riches within a small "have" group, or to disperse them widely. I call special attention to this last point in view of the assumption of many traditional economists that the existence of concentrated wealth does not matter too much so long as the Gross National Product "pie" keeps getting bigger and the general Standard of Living "portions" continue to grow. However, the rising rate of theft and violent crime in this—the richest country in the world, with the highest standard of living man has ever known—would seem to cast doubt on this assumption and to favor Benedict's conclusion.*

In making this point it is not my intention to imply that intrasocial aggression is derived only from economic factors. That would be a simplistic and unwarranted conclusion. But granting the enormously greater complexities and contradictions that exist in our contemporary society, there is still reason to think that Benedict's principle of high- and low-synergy cultures has applicability in our setting also.

It is at this interface between personality and the institutions of our society that I believe we find the most significant challenge for psychiatry in the future of man. There is nothing more important that psychiatry can contribute to that future than to identify those institutional factors that are so shaping the personalities of most contemporary men and women as to render them resistant—as I believe they are—to the fundamental changes that must take place to insure man's survival on this planet. Unless we can recognize these factors and find ways of modifying them nothing else that we as psychiatrists can contribute—our psychotherapies, our mental health centers, our psychobiological researches—will matter very much, for man will almost certainly be doomed.

To put what I am saying in another framework, it seems to me that too many commentators on the current human scene have tended to attribute our problems to defects in individual superegos. Thus there is much talk concerning strengthening the moral fiber of our youth, restoring the influence of the family, or reinforcing our religious teachings. I believe these approaches miss the mark precisely because the problems which threaten our survival lie in our socially-sanctioned, ego-syntonic *group superegos* rather than in our individual ones. It is not the "defective" ones among us, but we the "normal" ones who constitute the problem—all of us, the

---

*A striking and independent confirmation of this principle was provided by another anthropologist, Ralph Linton, in a study of a pair of uniquely related hill tribes in Western Madagascar (4). (See pp. 40–41, this volume.)

pillars of the community, the state, and the church, with our shared and consensually validated group superego attitudes.

As Thomas Merton has put it, "We rely on the sane people of the world to preserve it from barbarism, madness, destruction. And now it begins to dawn on us that it is precisely the *sane* ones who are the most dangerous . . . who can without qualm and without nausea aim the missiles and press the buttons that will initiate the great festival of destruction that they, the *sane* ones, have prepared" (5).

It is we, the *sane ones*, the *"normal" people*, who continue to fight our wars, cut down our forests, pollute our lakes and rivers, poison our atmosphere, destroy our wildlife, discriminate against our minorities, and pursue our profits—we, the "mentally healthy" people, *not* our neurotics or our psychotics.

Recently, for example, a large metropolitan newspaper carried a headline quoting the president of a large industrial conglomerate as saying: "I don't apologize for making profits" (6). And indeed he shouldn't! He is merely doing what his institution expects him to do, even though the maintenance of his corporate profit-level may mean contributing significantly to the pollution of our communal air and water resources, or supporting the exploitation of some miserable colonial population in South America or Asia.

By the same token, leaders of the AFL-CIO are doing what *they* have been programmed to do when they support a war because it provides jobs for their members, or insist on huge wage increases regardless of the effect on other segments of the society. As James Reston has recently commented (7), none of these—neither industrialists nor labor leaders—are evil or insensitive men. They are merely doing what is best for their special interests—and what our competitive system drives most of us to do—even though these interests may not be—and often are not—in the interests of most of our other fellow human beings.

It is in this context that John Gardner's perceptive comment that one of the main reasons it is so difficult to change our institutions is that we ourselves are part of what needs changing becomes understandable. Another way of saying this is that there is a deep resistance in most of us against changing fundamental institutions in our society because our basic personalities—our needs, our expectations, our very language and perceptions—have been so profoundly shaped by those very institutions.

Where does the answer lie? I submit that unless and until we are willing to take a fresh and hard look at those institutions in our society that foster these low-synergy patterns of behavior we shall not find any fundamental solutions to our dilemma. There are many such contemporary institutions—some subtle, others obvious—but I believe that two of the most basic ones are those of capitalism and nationalism—both sacred cows of Western culture which like those of India are objects of widespread veneration, but which no longer are adaptive and which seriously threaten our ultimate survival.

It is important to note that historically both of these institutions *have* been adaptive in the past. The rise of capitalism in the 18th century constituted a major revolutionary social change, of higher synergy than the preceding feudal system. The free enterprise system that accompanied it, with its ideals of rugged individualism, challenged the individual as no previous system had done, to put his best foot forward in the struggle for existence. Whatever creativity, ingenuity, and aggressive potential he possessed were likely to be stimulated and in general rewarded. This was particularly true in an era of frontiers, when an enterprising man could take his fate in his own hands and go forth to create his own opportunities. By so doing, moreover, he not only benefited himself, but usually contributed to the welfare of society as a whole.

Today, however, the situation has changed significantly. The frontiers have largely disappeared. Those that remain are for the most part accessible mainly to people who already have more than their share of economic, technological, or scientific capability. Although social mobility still exists in principle, in practice it is essentially unavailable to underprivileged millions in our own nation, as well as to the vast majority of the rest of mankind who are trapped, generation after generation, in an inexorable matrix of poverty, prejudice and ignorance. As repeated studies have shown, out of that matrix disproportionate amounts of disease, delinquency, crime, violence, mental disorder, and social unrest continuously emerge to threaten us all. In a society in which gross inequities develop and become fixed, and the security of an individual and his family

depends on his ability to acquire material goods in relentless competition with his fellow men, patterns of intrasocial aggression become
inevitable, no matter what kind of Judeo-Christian ethic or its
equivalent is built into the acculturation of its children. In such
a system success depends on the ability to compete aggressively
and with the fewest compunctions, and this in turn brings further
rewards of prestige and power. Once achieved—whether by inheritance or by personal effort—such gains are clung to and defended
tenaciously against the large numbers of have-nots who continue
to struggle, some by fair means, others by foul, to achieve comparable
states of security and power. These struggles, moreover, often become
identified with ideological positions in the name of which wars and
other brutal inhumanities are carried on and justified, usually with
the invoked and assumed blessings of a supportive deity!

We psychiatrists have long noted that there are glaring contradictions in our mores between our ethical teachings on the one
hand, and the aggressive behavior that our competitive system seems
to require. Indeed, many of the patients we work with suffer precisely
because they have difficulty in reconciling these conflicting forces.
Most so-called normal people, however, do not suffer from such conflicts.
They have adapted successfully to the survival requirements of our
society. The ubiquitous aggression which Freud noted is a reflection
of that adaptive success. People cheat, lie, claw, scramble—politely
or impolitely—to "get ahead," and ethical considerations, if they
exist, are usually relegated to the logic-tight compartments of Sunday
church services.

Nevertheless, a cogent argument can be made for the fact that
despite all of its inequities capitalism, as most sharply epitomized
by life in the United States of America, has brought about the
greatest technological and scientific advances, as well as the highest
per capita production, that the world has ever known. The paradox
with which we are now confronted, however, is that the very qualities
that have made this system so successful in the past now threaten
it with extinction. Further technological and scientific advances will
be of no avail to us unless we can find more equitable processes
of *distribution.* In short, we have now reached a point in history
where *consistent centralized social planning is imperative for our survival,*
but capitalism, with its built-in profit motive, and individualistic

motivational base, simply does not lend itself well to such planning. The technological means for controlling pollution, protecting our natural resources, and substantially improving the health, education, and welfare of our underprivileged millions are all within our means, but to achieve these goals requires a communal rather than an individualistic orientation. Unfortunately most of the beneficiaries of our present system who have been taught from early childhood to equate capitalism with freedom, and rugged individualism with virtue, resist any significant changes in these institutions as a serious threat to our "way of life" as do also, of course, the powerful corporate forces whose survival is linked to our profit system.

Let me make clear, however, that I am not naively assuming that all we have to do is adopt a socialistic form of government and all will be well with the world. For one thing, as a psychiatrist I am all too aware that in a complex society such as our own there will always be many other factors besides socioeconomic ones that contribute to human distress and occasional violence. Second, even if by some extraordinary miracle we could transform our social institutions tomorrow to high-synergy ones, the fact that all of our personalities and those of most of our children have already been shaped by our present institutions would mean a substantial cultural lag before a significant change in basic values could be expected. And, finally, any among us who may have harbored such utopian expectations must surely have had them rudely shattered by the historical developments of the past half-century in those countries which have come under the communist sphere of influence. We have learned that the mere achievement of the trappings of socialism is not enough, if we do not at the same time preserve one of man's most precious social heritages, one that has painfully evolved over many centuries of struggle—and one that makes us truly human—the institution of democratic freedom. To eliminate the individual profit motive is one thing; to eliminate individuality and freedom of thought and expression is quite another. We have seen that the subjugation of men by other men can take place at levels other than economic ones, and so long as such subjugation is built into a social system, optimal human development cannot take place. It should be noted, however, that the institution of democracy is not necessarily inherent in capitalism any more than the institution of dictatorship is inherent in socialism. Some of the most dictatorial nations in the world, witness Greece, Portugal, and many of our Central and South American neighbors, are deeply committed to capitalism and the profit system; while it is possible for democracy to evolve even within the framework of a communist nation, witness the short-lived, albeit unhappy example of Czechoslovakia.

It is worth noting also that contrary to popular assumption certain forms of free enterprise are perfectly compatible with a cooperative social order, and may indeed be of a high order of synergy. I refer to patterns of activity such as the provision of human and technical services, the pursuit of scientific discovery, the development of inventions, the exercise of untrammeled artistic and literary creation and the like. Perhaps—and I offer this *most* tentatively—a high-synergy direction in which our modern technological society can move adaptively is one that would encompass certain broad patterns of cooperative social organization without relinquishing the values inherent in democracy, individual freedom and initiative, while maintaining a continuing degree of free enterprise in areas that do not involve the exploitation of natural resources or control over basic means of production.

The second of our contemporary "sacred cows," the institution of nationalism (see Chapter 29), also unquestionably had adaptive value in the historical past when the maintenance of separate areas of territorial integrity was important to a people's survival. Now, however, it has become a maladaptive phenomenon which seriously threatens that survival. The exponential changes in the speed of communication and travel have so eliminated the space-time barriers on our planet as to make national borders increasingly meaningless. No country can be an island unto itself any more, and the interdependence of all nations on the same finite supply of air, water and material resources has become self-evident. If man is to have a future on this shrinking globe, international planning and cooperation cannot be postponed much longer. A One-World ideology, with a genuine acceptance of the brotherhood of all men, will have to supplant the ethnocentric biases, dissensions and suspicions that now set nation against nation and race against race. This does not and need not mean giving up the richness and diversity of ethnic cultural patterns. But ultimately this *will* require the relinquishing to a superordinate world organization of certain aspects of national sovereignty such as the right to wage war. Although this may well seem unthinkable to most national leaders, one can only hope that they will realize before it is too late "that the risks involved in such relinquishment are outweighed by the increasingly grave hazards of not doing so" (8). For with the advent of the nuclear age, we have reached a point in human history where wars in the traditional sense can no longer be won, and where even small wars can become the sparks for a thermonuclear holocaust that can threaten the survival of the entire human race.

But is it at all possible to construct a world order in which more adaptive psychosocial institutions will be operative—institutions that will make possible the kind of international cooperation and planning that can eradicate human poverty and disease, protect our dwindling ecological resources, and eliminate the need for intrasocial violence, aggression and wars? I believe that it is—at least theoretically—but I do not by any means underestimate the obstacles in the way of such a development. My basic thesis, however, is that the so-called nature of man is not one of the obstacles. On the contrary, it is only the extraordinary adaptive capacity of the human brain, with its capacity to anticipate the future and then creatively construct mental models with which to deal with that future, that gives me any reason at all to hope that it is within the realm of possibility to find our way *rationally* to such a social order without having to undergo the violent and cataclysmic upheavals that otherwise seem inevitable.

The massive obstacle in our way—and massive it is—is not our innate biology but our acquired psychology—the programmed set of needs, values, attitudes and prejudices—indeed our very language and our perceptions—which have been shaped and deeply fixed by our existent social institutions and which have rendered most of us extraordinarily resistant to change (see Chapter 27). But the changing of belief-systems and attitudes is one of the prime functions of psychiatry. If man, as I believe, *must* alter many of his fundamental ways in order to survive, then psychiatry has an urgent responsibility to apply its insights toward facilitating such change. We cannot stand aside from political matters and say they are none of our business. Politics is human behavior applied to social action and social change. We, as serious students of man and his ways, must contribute our understanding toward that change, or by our silence become accessories to man's ultimate destruction. Briand's famous comment that "War is much too serious a matter to be left to generals" may be paraphrased to say, "Man's survival is much too serious a matter to be left to politicians."

We must also take cognizance of the fact that we are all products of the very institutions we are trying to change. Pogo's remark that "We have met the enemy and it is us" is particularly pertinent here. This requires that we, as psychiatrists, bend every effort toward becoming less culture-bound in the process of trying to assess these institutions. We are dealing here with the phenomenon of unconscious resistance, both in ourselves as well as in those we are trying to influence, but after all, this is a matter in which we should have a special expertise. It is our responsibility to bring that expertise to bear on the broad manifestations of this phenomenon as it stands in the way of urgently needed social change.

Psychiatry, throughout its more recent history, has been characterized by its willingness to question established mores when it found that they were interfering with optimum mental health and human self-realization. We have dared to challenge conventional attitudes toward insanity, toward sex, toward abortion, and toward racial and ethnic prejudice, to mention only a few. I believe that the time has come when psychiatry, *in the name of mental health,* must find the courage also to challenge the sacrosanct but maladaptive values implicit in certain of our institutional sacred cows. As Erich Fromm has put it, "Man, not techniques, must become the ultimate source of values; optimal human development, not maximal production, the criterion for all planning" (9).

It would be insufferably arrogant, however, to presume that psychiatrists alone can even begin to deal with the extraordinarily complex problems inherent in trying to evolve new institutional forms. Such a task will require the collaborative efforts of people from many disciplines—behavioral, natural and political scientists, economists, educators, legal scholars, spiritual leaders, and representatives of the public-at-large. Most of all, we will need the kind of political leadership in the major nations of the world who will be sufficiently aware of the urgency of bringing such creative and collaborative planning into existence. Unfortunately, governmental leaders no less than the rest of us are products of the very institutions that need to be changed, and thus reflect the needs, prejudices and values that are part of the problem itself. Leaders capable of transcending these cultural and ethnocentric bonds are rare indeed!

There are some who believe and hope, like Charles Reich (10), that our youth are developing an awareness, "Consciousness III," that is inevitably going to transform our institutions into more adaptive ones. I would like to believe that and wish it were so. I am not convinced, however, that the young people Reich describes represent more than a rather small minority of our total youth. Unfortunately, also, many of our Consciousness III young people have disengaged themselves from the mainstream of the social and political process through which any major *evolutionary* institutional change will have to come.

Perhaps in the final analysis we shall have to look to the broad community of science, which traditionally has tended to transcend national boundaries, to dedicate itself to the task of educating both the public and our political leaders to the transcendent gravity of our contemporary dilemma and to the directions in which we must move. It was Albert Einstein who made the comment that if humanity is to survive in the nuclear age "we shall require a substantially new manner of thinking." The adaptive challenge of the decades that lie immediately ahead of us is to acquire that new manner of thinking for the sake of our children and our children's children—and in the common interest of all mankind! To help provide the scientific guidelines that may facilitate such a change may well be the noblest and most important role that psychiatry can play in the future of man.

REFERENCES

1. FREUD, S. *Civilization and its Discontents,* Internat. Psycho-Anal. Library, London: Hogarth Press, Ltd., 1949, 85.
2. EISENBERG, L. "The Human Nature of Human Nature," *Science,* 176 (April, 1972), 123–128.
3. BENEDICT, R. in Maslow, A. and Honigmann, J. "Synergy: Some Notes of Ruth Benedict," *Am. Anthropologist,* (1970), 320–333.
4. LINTON, R. in Kardiner, A. *The Individual and His Society,* New York: Columbia Univ. Press, 1939, 251–290.

5. MERTON, T. "A Devout Meditation in Memory of Adolph Eichman," in *Raids on the Unspeakable*, New York: New Directions Publishing Co., 1966.
6. *Los Angeles Times*, Sunday, May 7, 1972. Business and Finance Section, 1.
7. RESTON, J. *New York Times*, April 16, 1972.
8. Group for the Advancement of Psychiatry. *Psychiatric Aspects of the Prevention of Nuclear War*, New York, 1964, 310.
9. FROMM, E. *The Revolution of Hope: Toward a Humanistic Technology*, New York: Bantam Books, 1968.
10. REICH, C. *The Greening of America*, New York: Random House, 1970.

33

SHORT-TERM DYNAMIC PSYCHOTHERAPY
(1978)

We are living in the midst of a major psychotherapeutic revolution in this second half of the twentieth century. New therapies of all kinds have emerged in astounding numbers, some scientifically based, others reverting to the magical, mystical, and religious roots that were the precursors of scientific psychotherapy. At the same time the development of third-party payers, together with the imminence of some form of national health insurance, places psychiatrists under pressure to find shorter, more broadly applicable, and more efficient techniques of therapy or risk exclusion from these programs for fiscal reasons. As a consequence, we can anticipate that the briefer techniques of group therapy, behavioral therapy, and family therapy will emerge more strongly in the years ahead. The fact is, however, that the vast majority of American psychiatrists are still heavily committed to a one-to-one model of dynamic psychotherapy (1). Therefore, the greatest need to develop more time-effective approaches is in this area.

HISTORICAL BACKGROUND

Brief dynamic psychotherapy is rooted in the psychoanalytic tradition. Its fundamental insights and its basic theoretical principles would not have been possible were it not for the ground-breaking discoveries of Sigmund Freud. Actually, some of the earliest psychoanalytic treatments conducted by Freud tended to be of quite short duration. Bruno Walter, the conductor, described in his autobiography (2) a successful six-session therapeutic experience he had with Freud in 1906. Jones (3, pp. 79–80) related that in 1908 Freud was

433

able to get at the psychodynamic roots of the composer Gustav Mahler's potency problem with his wife and relieve it in a single four-hour session. Even Freud's early didactic analyses were almost all of relatively short duration, ranging from several months to about one year (3, pp. 31–32, 161–162). As the goals of psychoanalysis became more ambitious, however, and its theoretical superstructure grew more complex, analytic treatments began to increase in length to such an extent that in his later years Freud pessimistically concluded that some of them were becoming interminable (4).

Many of the early analysts were aware of and troubled by this trend, but the first psychoanalytic pioneer to methodically explore modifications in psychoanalytic technique for the purpose of shortening the length of classical analysis was Sandor Ferenczi, who, around 1918, began to experiment with a technique that he called "active therapy." Ferenczi (5) claimed that in so doing he was merely following Freud's lead. He referred to a paper that Freud had presented at the Budapest International Congress in 1918 (6) in which Freud stated that in certain cases of phobia or obsessional neurosis it is sometimes necessary, in order to advance the therapy, to institute active measures to induce the patient to face the phobia or anxiety. Ferenczi also pointed out that activity as a technique was inherent in the psychoanalytic process because every interpretation that is given constitutes an interference with the patient's psychic transactions of that moment and thus facilitates the appearance of thoughts that otherwise might not have become conscious.

Ferenczi experimented with various types of activity in the psychoanalytic situation in an effort to overcome what he called a "stagnation of the analysis." Some of his techniques were restrictive or pressuring (e.g., forbidding masturbation or insisting that patients control certain body movements or other actions Ferenczi deemed to be in the service of "unconscious resistance"). Other interventions were loving or indulgent, based on the theory that the analyst as a parent surrogate was thus making amends for the rejections and traumata that the patient may have suffered from his own parents.

Ferenczi's "reparative" efforts included hugging, kissing, and nonerotic fondling of his patients. When Freud heard of these, he wrote Ferenczi the now famous letter (7) expressing his very dim view of these activities and predicting prophetically that they would .

eventually lead to greater excesses on the part of other therapists. He wrote,

> A number of independent thinkers in matters of technique will say to themselves: Why stop at a kiss? . . . Bolder ones will come along who will go further. . . . The younger of our colleagues will find it hard to stop at the point they originally intended, and God the Father Ferenczi, gazing at the lively scene he has created will perhaps say to himself: Maybe after all I should have halted in my technique of motherly affection *before* the kiss.

Ferenczi subsequently abandoned these particular techniques, but he never gave up his efforts to develop a more active approach to analytic therapy.

Ferenczi's efforts brought him into early collaboration with Otto Rank, who had been pursuing similar approaches independently. Ferenczi and Rank worked together for a number of years on evolving various modifications of technique, culminating in 1925 in their publication of the slender but seminal volume *The Development of Psychoanalysis* (8). In this volume they pointed out that early in the history of psychoanalysis "splendid cures . . . were effected, sometimes in a few days or weeks" (p. 52) but that as analytic theory and knowledge expanded analyses became longer and longer. They attributed this to a need for "discovering afresh in every single case the psychological and theoretical knowledge derived from analysis" (p. 59) and to turning every analysis into a proving ground for analytic theory. Ferenczi and Rank characterized this as "making the disastrous mistake of neglecting the actual [therapeutic] task for the sake of the psychological interest" (pp. 24–25).

They pointed out that the technique of psychoanalytic treatment, although dependent on psychoanalytic theory, need not and indeed should not remain tied to the "investigative" methods out of which the theory evolved. In this context they criticized an undue preoccupation in therapy with the historical past and emphasized the paramount importance of focusing on the present analytic situation and its transference implications. Anticipating Franz Alexander's concept of the "corrective emotional experience," Ferenczi and Rank asserted that the goal of psychoanalysis "is to substitute by means of the technique, affective factors of experience for intellectual pro-

cesses" (p. 62). They expressed the conviction that a greater understanding of these practical principles of technique would ultimately
make it possible to "shorten and simplify psychoanalytic treatment."

In some ways Otto Rank may well be the most important historical forerunner of the brief dynamic psychotherapy movement. His
concept of the trauma of birth (9), although biologically and
psychodynamically dubious, laid the groundwork for the subsequent
recognition of the predominant importance in personality development of the pre-oedipal years, particularly the early mother-child
relationship. When Rank published his views, however, the primary
emphasis in psychoanalytic theory was on the oedipal period and
castration anxieties rather than on the pre-oedipal period and the
more basic separation anxieties. Rank's views were vigorously attacked
by Freud's psychoanalytic contemporaries because they were correctly perceived as threatening the fulcrum of Freud's theories at
that time.

It is unfortunate that the issue of disloyalty to Freud has cast a
heavy shadow over the value of Rank's achievements. Looking back
from the vantage point of our present knowledge of the importance
of pre-oedipal relationships in personality development as well as
the nuclear importance of separation and individuation in emotional
maturation, we can now perceive that Rank was the prime theoretical precursor of these developments, without in any way denigrating
the later creative contributions of people like Rene Spitz (10), Margaret Mahler (11), or John Bowlby (12).

As his ideas evolved, Rank himself began to play down the importance of the birth trauma itself and to recognize that the issue of
separation and individuation was really the core problem. He made
its working through the central focus of his psychotherapeutic
method. It is not surprising, therefore, that Rank was the first analyst
to attribute major importance to the setting of a time limit for the
analytic process to promote an earlier therapeutic focus on the problem of separation. However, Rank was not the first analyst to experiment with setting a termination date in advance. Freud did this in
1912 in his analysis of the "Rat Man," which he published in 1918 as
"From the History of an Infantile Neurosis" (13). Although Freud
recognized the usefulness of this technical device, he never made it
a cardinal point in his analytic technique. Rank, on the other hand,

considered the setting of a time limit central to the therapeutic work and the issue of separation and individuation critical to the process of adaptation and maturation in all of human existence. Thus at a very early point in Rank's therapy the analytic work became centered on the anxieties and conflicts surrounding separation and termination and the entire therapeutic process was foreshortened. In recent years Mann has made this technique the focal point of his approach to time-limited psychotherapy, but, surprisingly, he made only a brief and passing reference to the work of Rank in his book (14).

It is also interesting, in the light of current developments in brief psychotherapy, to take a second look at Rank's concept of "will therapy" (15). Rank emphasized the importance of mobilizing the patient's "will" in the course of therapy and claimed that by so doing the therapeutic process could be facilitated. If we were to substitute for the word "will" the more modern term "motivation," we would find that Rank was saying something that has been emphasized by all modern theorists about short-term dynamic psychotherapy, namely, the overwhelming importance in achieving a favorable therapeutic outcome of a strong motivation to change on the part of the patient. In this connection it is noteworthy that four of the seven criteria for motivation to change used by Sifneos (16) in selecting patients for brief psychotherapy employ the concept of willingness (i.e., willingness to actively participate in the treatment situation, willingness to understand oneself, willingness to change, and willingness to make reasonable sacrifices in terms of time and fees). What is willingness in this context but the ability to mobilize one's "will" toward a particular objective?

When, some twenty years after Ferenczi and Rank's contributions, Alexander and French came out with their important and seminal volume on psychoanalytic therapy (17), they were frank to admit that their work was "a continuation and realization of ideas first proposed by Ferenczi and Rank." The work of Alexander and French stands on its own merits, however. Their volume was the culmination of seven years of research and investigation into the development of shorter approaches to psychotherapy that had been carried out at the Chicago Institute of Psychoanalysis.

Alexander, the prime mover in this research, had for years been puzzled by what he called the "baffling discrepancy" between the length and intensity of psychoanalytic treatment and the degree of therapeutic success. He began his investigations by questioning the validity of the following traditional psychoanalytic dogmas: 1) that the depth of therapy is necessarily proportionate to the length of treatment and frequency of interviews; 2) that therapeutic results achieved by a relatively small number of interviews are necessarily superficial and temporary but results of more prolonged therapy are necessarily more stable and profound; and 3) that prolongation of an analysis is justified on the grounds that the desired therapeutic results are more likely to be achieved than through briefer techniques. None of these traditional assumptions proved to be justified.

In the course of their research, Alexander and his colleagues experimented with the frequency of interviews, the optional use of the chair or couch, long or short interruptions of therapy preparatory to termination, and the combination of psychotherapy with drug or other therapy. They also sought to learn how to control and manipulate the transference relationship to fit the particular psychodynamics of each case. The first and most important principle that evolved from these studies, that of flexibility, seems obvious today, but it was revolutionary in an era dominated by the conviction that the standard psychoanalytic method was the optimum method of therapy for most neurotic patients. Alexander insisted that in psychotherapy as in all medical therapy the physician should adapt his technique to the needs of the patient. "Only the nature of the individual case," he said, "can determine what technique is best suited to bring about the curative processes" (17, p. 26).

Alexander also pointed out that in many instances daily interviews prove to be antitherapeutic because they gratify the patient's dependent needs more than is desirable. He questioned the therapeutic value of promoting regression and argued that it should be "a general principle in all psychotherapy to attempt to check this regressive tendency from the very beginning of the treatment" (17, p.30). This principle was subsequently strongly advocated by Sandor Rado (18).

As one way of heightening the emotional intensity of interviews with patients Alexander recommended consciously manipulating the frequency of visits. He felt this was an effective technique for controlling the transference relationship, limiting regression, preventing the development of overdependency on the therapist, and fostering autonomy. He also advocated interruptions of treatment as another way of increasing the emotional intensity and efficiency of the therapeutic process. Interruptions, by virtue of their ability to test the patient's capacity for self-reliance and for more effectively coping with his life situation, could also be used as preparatory indicators enabling both therapist and patient to arrive at a mutually agreed-on termination point.

Like Ferenczi and Rank, Alexander placed great emphasis on the emotional experiences of the patient in relation to the therapist, specifically on what he called the "corrective emotional experience," in which the patient is reexposed under the more favorable circumstances of the transference relationship to emotional situations that he could not handle in the past.

Alexander asserted that in order to know what new emotional experiences are necessary to achieve therapeutic results, the therapist must understand not only the patient's current psycho-dynamics but also the genetic development of his difficulties. In this respect Alexander's technique differs decisively from that of Rank, who tended to minimize the importance of such genetic understanding. The more precise this understanding, according to Alexander, the more adequately the therapist can provide the proper corrective emotional experience. Therefore, he felt that the therapist's reactions had to be planned on the basis of these dynamic insights.

Although Alexander's views were violently attacked by most of the classical psychoanalysts of his time, by now the principles he elucidated have become part of the daily working equipment of almost every psychiatrist and psychoanalyst. It is fair to say that Alexander more than any other modern psychoanalyst is responsible for leading the way toward the application of psychoanalytic principles to more active and shorter dynamic psychotherapy. As a consequence of his germinal work, an increasing number of psychoanalysts began to practice more flexibly during the years following World War II. Psychoanalysts began to see their patients less frequently than the traditionally mandated four or five times weekly, often working with them face to face and, in general, entering into more active communicative transactions with them than the more passive classical model required.

In more recent years, as the demand for psychotherapy has widened to encompass greater and greater segments of the population, the pressures to clarify our therapies and sharpen our skills in the application of psychodynamic theory to briefer forms of psychotherapy have continued to increase. Beginning with the 1960s, a number of psychoanalysts both in the United States and abroad have responded to this challenge by picking up where Alexander and French left off. Malan (19, 20), Wolberg (21), Bellak and Small (22), Sifneos (16), Balint and associates (23), Mann (14), and Davanloo (24) are but a few of the individuals who have contributed significantly to the theory and technique of short-term psychotherapy. In the pages that follow I shall attempt to present a synthesis of their views that will reflect the present state of the art in short-term dynamic psychotherapy.

SELECTION CRITERIA

Short-term dynamic psychotherapy rests on two basic substructures, selection and technique. Each of these is of equal importance. Not all patients are equally suitable for short-term dynamic psychotherapy, but a substantial proportion of those who are ordinarily considered suitable for longer-term analytic procedures are equally suitable for the shorter-term approach.

At the very outset of the selection process it is important to underline the necessity for a good history and a psychodynamic diagnosis. By a psychodynamic diagnosis I do not mean placing the patient into a formal nosologic category but, rather, carefully evaluating both the inner and outer forces that contribute to the patient's psychopathology. Inasmuch as short-term dynamic psychotherapy involves an uncovering and searching out of reievant unconscious intrapsychic factors, the therapist looks for qualities in the patient that will indicate his capacity to work effectively in this way. The following are the most important of these qualities: 1) evidences of ego strength (e.g., intelligence, level of educational achievement, sexual adjustment, type of work, ability to assume responsibility); 2) at least one meaningful interpersonal relationship in the past, indicating a capacity for basic trust, which is essential in the psychotherapeutic process; 3) the ability to interact with the therapist in the first session (i.e., the capacity to form a positive transference); 4) the ability to think in psychological terms (i.e., the ability to accept interpretation or, as it is sometimes called, the capacity for insight, which is usually tested in the initial interview by making a tentative interpretation and evaluating the patient's response to it); and 5) the ability to experience feelings (i.e., the degree to which the individual seems to be in touch with his own emotions).

The above five qualities are essential factors in the selection of patients for any form of dynamic psychotherapy, long-term as well as short-term. Two additional selection factors are particularly relevant to and essential for a short-term psychotherapeutic approach. The first of these is the existence of a focal conflict. The therapist should be able in the first interview or two, at most, to identify a central conflictual problem around which most of the patient's difficulties revolve. Sifneos (16) has stated that this focal conflict must be oedipal, but this view is not shared by others. For example, the focal conflict can also be a dependence-independence conflict, a sibling rivalry situation, or a difficulty in coping with object loss.

The other selection factor of prime relevance to short-term therapy is the existence of a clear-cut and strong motivation to change. Malan (19, 20) properly emphasized that the issue is not simply one of the patient's wish to get rid of his symptoms but of an acceptance of the fact that in the process some basic change in adaptational patterns may be necessary.

As already noted, with the exception of the last two, all of these selection criteria are not very different from the criteria that are usually applied in deciding whether or not a patient is suitable for classical psychoanalytic therapy. However, these selection criteria are not necessarily indicative of the depth of existing psychopathology. Most contemporary workers in the field agree that short-term dynamic psychotherapy can be used with patients who might be described as relatively "sick" as well as for those with relatively minor problems. Patients with a wide variety of personality disorders and psychoneuroses as well as those with transitional crises may be suitable for short-term dynamic psychotherapy provided they fulfill the selection criteria. The critical issue is not diagnosis so much as the possession of certain personality attributes plus the existence of a focal conflict and a high degree of motivation.

TECHNIQUE

In considering the technique of short-term dynamic psychotherapy it is first necessary to emphasize that there are certain common denominators in all psychodynamic therapies. I have described these in detail elsewhere (25–27) and shall merely summarize them here: 1) a release of tension (catharsis) in a setting of hope and expectation of help; 2) a constructive patient-therapist relationship (therapeutic alliance) based on both unconscious factors (transference factors) as well as the real qualities that both patient and therapist bring to their transactions; 3) cognitive learning based on interpretations (insight); 4) operant conditioning based on overt and/or covert indications of approval or disapproval from the therapist that move the patient in the direction of "mental health" (an additional facet of this operant conditioning is the existence of corrective emotional experiences in which the therapist reacts differently and more constructively to the patient than did significant authority figures in the patient's past); 5) identification with the therapist in which the patient (usually unconsciously) models himself after the therapist, incorporating some of the latter's value systems and/or behavioral patterns; 6) elements of suggestion and persuasion, either covert or overt, which are present in all psychotherapies; 7) some aspects of practice and rehearsal of new adaptive techniques and their generalization, sometimes called "working through" or "reality testing," all in a setting of consistent emotional support from the empathic therapist.

Given these general factors common to all dynamic therapies, how does short-term dynamic psychotherapy differ from other therapies? Four factors that are specific to the short-term technique can be identified. First, the patient is always seen sitting up, facing the therapist. Although this factor is essential to short-term dynamic psychotherapy, it is, of course, present in many longer-term dynamic therapies as well. Therefore, it is not as unique as the other three factors are. It is important, however, for creating a structure in which a more active transactional process can occur than would be possible with the patient on the couch.

Second, brief therapy always involves setting a time limit. This is a unique and important element in all short-term psychotherapies. Setting a time limit is essential for the process, and its importance cannot be overemphasized. Mann (14) has discussed the meaning of time in psychotherapy in eloquent philosophical terms. From a purely clinical standpoint, however, three fundamental consequences can be identified as deriving from this technical maneuver. First, the setting of a time limit places a central emphasis from the very beginning of the therapy on the issues of separation and individuation. This colors the entire therapeutic process from beginning to end and creates an entirely different set of expectations than in long-term therapy, where the patient is told at the outset that the length of therapy is open-ended, unpredictable, or may go on for a year or two or more. Second, not only is the issue of separation and individuation relevant, if not central, to the problem presented by most patients, but putting it in the forefront of the therapeutic technique reflects a basic respect for and encouragement of the patient's capacity to be autonomous. This counters the patient's impulse to see himself as helpless, inadequate, and in need of dependent support. Third, the very process of termination constitutes a therapeutic act that tends to encourage the patient's independence and self-confidence. This is not to deny that the initial response of most patients to approaching termination is one of anxiety and often of regression. Nevertheless, the firm and steady insistence on a termination date and the working through of separation anxieties is critical to the process of short-term dynamic psychotherapy.

The issue of how many sessions should be involved is still unsettled among short-term psychotherapists. Mann sets an arbitrary and fixed limit of twelve sessions, but Sifneos, Malan, Wolberg, and Davanloo are rather more flexible, varying the number of visits from fifteen to forty, depending on the severity of the patient's problem as well as his ego-adaptive capacities. For most patients, somewhere between twenty and thirty visits seems to be quite satisfactory. It has been my own practice after termination to leave the door open for a follow-up visit after three or six months, if the patient desires. This removes the element of finality from the separation process and softens its impact, but the majority of patients given such an opportunity do not find a need for it. Indeed, they tend to feel better as time goes on.

The third specific feature of short-term dynamic psychotherapy is the persistent focus throughout therapy on the core conflict and the refusal to permit defensive digressions from that central focus. This in turn leads to the fourth major factor, the activity of the therapist, an essential feature of short-term therapy. This activity has two major and significant psychodynamic elements. First, it is a reflection of the therapist's interest in and concern for the patient and the therapist's wish to be helpful, which are important therapeutic factors. Second, insisting on adhering to the central focus and actively discouraging digressions maintains a high level of therapeutic tension and interaction throughout the therapy more effectively than the traditional "abstinence" patterns of classical psychoanalysis. Sifneos called this technique "anxiety provoking," and it often is.

It should be emphasized that such activity does not mean that the therapist is being directive. On the contrary, the therapist follows essentially the nondirective line of traditional psychoanalytic therapy. The activity consists of persistent confrontations and interpretations and, by means of these confrontations, of the discouragement of regression. Whenever possible, Menninger's "triangle of insight" (28) is used in offering cognitive interpretations; that is, the therapist tries to link interpretations to the historical past, to the patient's present life situation and interpersonal relationships, and to the transference relationship in the therapeutic situation. Active transference interpretations and the bringing out of negative feelings as well as positive ones constitute an essential part of the technique of short-term dynamic psychotherapy.

The emphasis on transference interpretation and on the acquisition of insight clearly demonstrates the close link between short-term dynamic psychotherapy and classical psychoanalytic theory. As I have indicated elsewhere (26), it is questionable that insight in and of itself has the specific therapeutic effect that most psychoanalysts attribute to it, but it nevertheless serves as a powerful reinforcement to all of the other factors that play a role in the psychotherapeutic process.

COMPARISON WITH CRISIS INTERVENTION

The question is often raised as to how short-term therapy differs from crisis intervention. It may be useful in this regard to distinguish emergency care, crisis intervention, and short-term dynamic psychotherapy, which in a sense represent different points on a continuum of psychiatric intervention. Emergency care is concerned with the provision of immediate relief or help to a person who has decompensated in the face of internal or external stress and is totally unable to cope with the situation. In crisis intervention one is dealing with an individual who is in danger of decompensating from internal or external stress and is coping poorly. The goal of crisis intervention is to reduce or remove the stress situation and/or to help the patient deal with it more effectively.* In short-term dynamic psychotherapy we are dealing with individuals in conflict, not necessarily in crisis, although a crisis situation may be involved. The goal in short-term dynamic psychotherapy is primarily on modifying the patient's coping abilities and only secondarily on relieving stress.

It is evident from these definitions that there are no sharp lines of demarcation among these modes of approach. Each can merge into the other. Emergency treatment may proceed from the provision of immediate relief to an effort to reduce the precipitating stress situation, and in crisis intervention it is often necessary to help the patient develop more effective coping mechanisms to deal with the presenting stress situation as well as future ones. To the extent that crisis intervention emphasizes the modification of coping mechanisms it moves closer to short-term dynamic psychotherapy.

The differences are primarily in terms of emphasis. Crisis intervention is usually of shorter duration and limited to five or six sessions, and dynamic psychotherapy is usually of longer duration. The primary goal of crisis intervention is the restoration of homeostasis. A secondary goal is to improve the patient's adaptive capacity when necessary. The basic goal of short-term dynamic psychotherapy is to improve the patient's coping abilities. The termination point of crisis intervention is when the crisis is resolved. The termination point of short-term dynamic therapy is not dictated by the resolution of the crisis. Crisis intervention involves a more supportive approach than does short-term dynamic psychotherapy. It can also be more

*Some crisis theorists divide crisis therapy into two categories: crisis support, which focuses on the patient's current problems and/or relief of symptoms, and crisis intervention, which deals with the patient's adaptive and maladaptive coping mechanisms in the crisis situation. The latter technique clearly merges into short-term dynamic psychotherapy and differs from it primarily in being of shorter duration and crisis oriented.

directive. In short-term dynamic therapy, the approach is active but nondirective. Crisis intervention deals only with the here and now; short-term dynamic psychotherapy includes the exploration of the past to illuminate the present. Finally, crisis intervention may involve a variety of other techniques (e.g., family therapy, group therapy, and dealing with the social network), but short-term dynamic psychotherapy is essentially a one-to-one approach. However, it may well be that the lessons learned from short-term dynamic psychotherapy will find increasing application in conjoint marital, family, and group therapies as time goes on.

INDICATIONS FOR LONGER-TERM PSYCHOTHERAPY

The foregoing does not imply that longer-term dynamic psychotherapy will no longer be necessary or indicated. Given the present state of our knowledge, the substantial number of people now seen in dynamic psychotherapy who do not meet the selection criteria for the short-term approach will continue to require longer-term therapeutic relationships. These patients include individuals with more seriously impaired egointegrative capacities, particularly the more severe character disorders, and borderline syndromes. As every psychiatrist knows, some patients may need a tenuous symbiotic relationship with a psychotherapist for most of their lives in order to be able to continue functioning.

THEORETICAL OBJECTIONS

The opposition of traditional psychoanalysis to the short-term therapeutic model has been based on the preconception that in order to be deep, therapy has to be long. Indeed, when in the course of psychoanalytic therapy patients improved quickly their improvement was usually derogated as a transference cure or a flight into health. The assumption was that the therapy was inevitably incomplete and that sooner or later the patient would be back. However, this often did not occur. The reason for the faulty assumption was another misconception of the traditional psychoanalytic model, namely, that it was a closed-system model in contrast to the open-system model of contemporary psychiatric thought. The closed model posited that unless all aspects of the patient's libidinal fixations and unconscious conflicts were worked through they would sooner or later lead to a recurrence of symptomatology. Open-system thinking recognizes that enabling a patient to function more effectively in a particular area leads not only to heightened self-esteem but also to positive feedback from the environment. These changes, both from within and from without, can modify the internal psychodynamic system without having to work everything through.

The classical method of psychoanalysis arose as a brilliantly innovative research technique created by Freud to explore the furthermost corners of the unconscious. For this purpose it has no equal. A good research technique, however, is not ipso facto a good therapeutic method, and Freud's own later pessimism about the results of psychoanalysis reflected this awareness. Short-term psychodynamic techniques are not in any sense a degradation of the "pure gold" of psychoanalysis. On the contrary, they constitute innovative techniques and approaches that open the way to new objectives and potentials for psychoanalytic psychotherapy. They constitute a historical trend of the first magnitude and point to the direction in which the rational psychotherapies of the future will be moving.

References

1. MARMOR, J.: Psychiatrists and Their Patients. Washington, DC, Joint Information Service of the American Psychiatric Association and the National Association for Mental Health, 1975, p 20.
2. WALTER, B.: Theme and Variation. New York, Alfred A Knopf, 1940.
3. JONES, E.: The Life and Work of Sigmund Freud, vol 2. New York, Basic Books, 1957.
4. FREUD, S.: Analysis, terminable and interminable (1937), in Complete Psychological Works, standard ed, vol 23. Translated and edited by Strachey J. London, Hogarth Press, 1962.
5. FERENCZI, S.: The further development of an active therapy in psychoanalysis (1920), in Further Contributions to the Theory and Technique of Psychoanalysis. By Ferenczi S. London, Hogarth Press, 1950.
6. FREUD, S.: Lines of advance in psychoanalytic therapy (1919), in Complete Psychological Works, standard ed, vol 17. Translated and edited by Strachey J. London, Hogarth Press, 1962.
7. JONES, E.: The Life and Work of Sigmund Freud, vol 3. New York, Basic Books, 1957, pp 163–164.
8. FERENCZI, S., RANK O: The Development of Psychoanalysis. Translated by Newton C. New York, Nervous and Mental Disease Publishing Co, 1925.
9. RANK, O.: The Trauma of Birth (1924). New York, Robert Brunner, 1952.

10. Spitz, R.: Anxiety in infancy.Int J Psychoanal 31:138–143, 1950.
11. Mahler, M.: On Human Symbiosis and the Vicissitudes of Individuation. New York, International Universities Press, 1969.
12. Bowlby, J.: Attachment and Loss, vols 1, 2. New York, Basic Books, 1969, 1973.
13. Freud, S.: From the history of an infantile neurosis (1918). in Complete Psychological Works, standard ed, vol 17. Translated and edited by Strachey J. London, Hogarth Press, 1955.
14. Mann, J.: Time-Limited Psychotherapy. Cambridge, Harvard University Press, 1973.
15. Rank, O.: Will Therapy. New York, Alfred A Knopf, 1947.
16. Sifneos, P.: Short-Term Psychotherapy and Emotional Crisis. Cambridge, Harvard University Press, 1972.
17. Alexander, F., French, T., et al.: Psychoanalytic Therapy. New York, Ronald Press, 1946.
18. Rado, S.: Recent Advances in Psychoanalytic Therapy in Psychoanalysis of Behavior. New York, Grune & Stratton, 1956. pp 251–267.
19. Malan, D.H.: A Study of Brief Psychotherapy. New York, Plenum Press, 1963.
20. Malan, D.H.: The Frontier of Brief Psychotherapy. New York, Plenum Press, 1976.
21. Wolberg, L.R. (ed): Short-Term Psychotherapy. New York, Grune & Stratton, 1965.
22. Bellak, L., Small, L.: Emergency Therapy and Brief Psychotherapy. New York, Grune & Stratton, 1965.
23. Balint, M., Ornstein, P.H., Balint, E.: Focal Psychotherapy. Philadelphia, JB Lippincott Co, 1972.
24. Davanloo, H.: Basic Principles and Techniques in Short-Term Dynamic Psychotherapy. New York, Spectrum Books, 1978.
25. Marmor, J.: Psychoanalytic therapy as an educational process (1962), in Psychiatry in Transition. By Marmor J. New York, Brunner/Mazel, 1974.
26. Marmor, J.: Psychoanalytic therapy and theories of learning (1964). Ibid.
27. Marmor, J.: The nature of the psychotherapeutic process (1964). Ibid.
28. Menninger, K.A., Holzman, P.S.: Theory of Psychoanalytic Technique, 2nd ed. New York, Basic Books, 1973, p 152.

ACKNOWLEDGMENTS

CHAPTER 1. **The Role of Instinct in Human Behavior.** Presented at the Annual Meeting of the Association for the Advancement of Psychoanalysis, Boston, May 19, 1942. Published in *Psychiatry: Journal of the Biology and Pathology of Interpersonal Relations*, Vol. V, No. 4, pp. 509–516, November 1942. Copyright © The William Alanson White Psychiatric Foundation, Inc. Copyright renewed.

CHAPTER 2. **Toward an Integrative Conception of Mental Disorder.** Published in *The Journal of Nervous and Mental Disease*, 3:19–29, 1950.

CHAPTER 3. **Some Observations on Superstition in Contemporary Life.** Presented at the 110th Annual Meeting of the American Psychiatric Association, St. Louis, May 6, 1954. Published in *The American Journal of Orthopsychiatry*, Vol. XXVI, No. 1, January 1956. Copyright © the American Orthopsychiatric Association, Inc.

CHAPTER 4. **The Individual, The Family and The Community.** Published in *Emotional Forces in the Family*, Samuel Liebman, M.D. (Ed.), J. B. Lippincott Co., Philadelphis, 1959. (Pp. 103–118)

CHAPTER 5. **The Cancer Patient and His Family.** Published in *The Psychological Basis of Medical Practice*, H. I. Lief, V. F. Lief, and Nina R. Lief (Eds.), Harper & Row, New York, 1963. (Pp. 309–317)

CHAPTER 6. **The Crisis of Middle Age.** Presented at the 44th Annual Meeting of The American Orthopsychiatric Association, program on "Crises in Adult Life," Washington, D.C., March 22–25, 1967. Published in *Psychiatry Digest*, Vol. 29, No. 5, pp. 17–21, May 1968.

CHAPTER 7. **"Normal" and "Deviant" Sexual Behavior.** Published in *The Journal of the American Medical Association*, Vol. 217, No. 2, pp. 165–170, July 12, 1971.

CHAPTER 8. **The Theory and Practice of Psychoanalysis.** Published in *Science & Society*, Vol. X, No. 1, pp. 54–79, 1946.

CHAPTER 9. **Psychoanalysis and Dialectical Materialism.** Published in *Philosophy for the Future*, Roy Wood Sellars, V. J. McGill, and Marvin Farber (Eds.), The Macmillan Company, New York, 1949. (Pp. 317–339)

CHAPTER 10. **Some Considerations Concerning Orgasm in the Female.** Presented to the Society for Psychoanalytic Medicine of Southern California, November 6, 1952. Published in *Psychosomatic Medicine*, Vol. 16, No. 3, pp. 240–245, May–June 1954.

CHAPTER 11. **Orality in the Hysterical Personality.** Presented at the Annual Meeting of the American Psychoanalytic Association, Los Angeles, May 2, 1953. Published in *Journal of the American Psychoanalytic Association*, Vol. 1, No. 4, October 1953.

CHAPTER 12. **The Psychodynamics of Realistic Worry.** Presented at the Midwinter Meeting of the American Psychoanalytic Association, New York, December 1, 1955. Published in *Psychoanalysis and the Social Sciences*, International Universities Press, New York, 1958. (Pp. 155–163)

CHAPTER 13. **Some Comments on Ego Psychology.** Presented at a panel discussion on "Ego Psychology" at the 113th Annual Meeting of the American Psychiatric Association, Chicago, May 16, 1957. Published in *Journal of the Hillside Hospital*, Vol. 7, No. 1, pp. 26–31, January 1958.

CHAPTER 14. **Psychoanalysis and Psychiatric Practice.** Published in *Current Psychiatric Therapies*, Grune & Stratton, New York, 1961. (Pp. 131–138)

CHAPTER 15. **Psychoanalytic Therapy as an Educational Process.** Published in *Science and Psychoanalysis*, Jules Masserman (Ed.), Vol. V, Grune & Stratton, New York, 1962. (Pp. 286–299)

CHAPTER 16. **Psychoanalytic Therapy and Theories of Learning.** Published in *Science and Psychoanalysis*, Jules Masserman (Ed.), Vol. VII, Grune & Stratton, New York, 1964. (Pp. 265–279)

CHAPTER 17. **Psychoanalysis at the Crossroads.** Presidential Address to the American Academy of Psychoanalysis, Tenth Annual Meeting, May 1966. Published in *Science and Psychoanalysis*, Jules Masserman (Ed.), Vol. X, Grune & Stratton, New York, 1966. (Pp. 1–9)

CHAPTER 18. **Changing Patterns of Femininity.** Published in *The Marriage Relationship*, Salo Rosenbaum and Ian Alger (Eds.), Basic Books, New York, 1968. Copyright © Society of Medical Psychoanalysts.

CHAPTER 19. **New Directions in Psychoanalytic Theory and Therapy.** Published in *Modern Psychoanalysis: New Directions and Perspectives*, Judd Marmor (Ed.), Basic Books, New York, 1968. (Pp. 3–14)

CHAPTER 20. **Limitations of Free Association.** Published in *Archives of General Psychiatry*, Vol. 22, pp. 160–165, February 1970. Copyright © American Medical Association.

CHAPTER 21. **The Feeling of Superiority.** Presented at the 109th Annual Meeting of the American Psychiatric Association, Los Angeles, May 4–8, 1953. Published in *The American Journal of Psychiatry*, Vol. 110, No. 5, pp. 370–376, November 1953. Copyright © The American Psychiatric Association.

CHAPTER 22. **The Doctor-Patient Relationship in Psychotherapy.** Presented at a symposium of The Association for the Advancement of Psychoanalysis. Reprinted by permission of the Editor of *The American Journal of Psychoanalysis*, Vol. 15, No. 1, pp. 7–9, 1955.

CHAPTER 23. **The Nature of the Psychotherapeutic Process.** Presented at the symposium "Psychiatry in the Mid-Sixties," sponsored by the Touro Infirmary, Department of Neurology and Psychiatry, New Orleans, November 19–20, 1964. Published in *Psychoneurosis and Schizophrenia*, Gene Usdin (Ed.), J. B. Lippincott Co., Philadelphia, 1966. (Pp. 66–75)

CHAPTER 24. **Dynamic Psychotherapy and Behavior Therapy.** An earlier version of this paper was read before the Temple University Conference on Dynamic Psychotherapy and Behavior Therapy, Philadelphia, March 6, 1969. Published in *Archives of General Psychiatry*, Vol. 24, pp. 22–28, January 1971. Copyright © American Medical Association.

CHAPTER 25. **Sexual Acting-Out in Psychotherapy.** Revised version of an earlier essay which appeared in *Psychiatry Digest*, October 1970, under the title "The Seductive Psychotherapist." Reprinted by permission of the Editor of *The American Journal of Psychoanalysis*, Vol. 32, No. 1, pp. 3–8, 1972.

CHAPTER 26. **Changing Trends in Psychotherapy.** Presented at the First Combined Teaching Seminar and Annual Meeting, The American College of Psychiatrists, New Orleans, January 26, 1973.

CHAPTER 27. **Psychodynamics of Group Opposition to Health Programs.** Presented at the 36th Annual Meeting of The American Orthopsychiatric Association, 1959. Published in *The American Journal of Orthopsychiatry*, Vol. XXX, No. 2, pp. 330–345, April 1960. Copyright © The American Orthopsychiatric Association.

CHAPTER 28. **The Psychology of Man in a Warless World.** Presented at a symposium on "A Warless World," sponsored by the Center for the Study of Democratic Institutions, Santa Barbara, December 1, 1962. Published in *A Warless World*, Arthur Larson (Ed.), McGraw-Hill Book Co., New York, 1963. (Chapter 10, pp. 117–130)

CHAPTER 29. **Nationalism, Internationalism, and Emotional Maturity.** Presented at the Joint Meeting of the American Psychiatric Association and the Mexican Society of Neurology and Psychiatry, Mexico City, May 11–14, 1964. Published in *The International Journal of Social Psychiatry,* Vol. XII, No. 3, pp. 217–220, 1966.

CHAPTER 30. **The Psychodynamics of Political Extremism.** Based on a paper presented at the Sixth National Scientific Meeting of the Association for the Advancement of Psychotherapy, Detroit, May 7, 1967. Published in *American Journal of Psychotherapy,* Vol. XXII, No. 4, pp. 561–568, October 1968.

CHAPTER 31. **Some Psychosocial Aspects of Contemporary Urban Violence.** Published in *Violence in America,* Thomas Rose (Ed.), Random House Vintage Books, New York, 1970. (Pp. 338–348)

CHAPTER 32. **Psychiatry and the Future of Man.** A fusion of two addresses—one given at the Future of Man Symposium honoring Leo H. Bartemeier on his 75th birthday, Baltimore, September 1970; the other at the Sesquicentennial Celebration of the Institute of Living, Hartford, May 1972. A condensed version was published in *Saturday Review,* May 22, 1971, under the title "Psychiatry and the Survival of Man."

INDEX OF NAMES

Abraham, K., 155
Abrams, A., 358
Adler, A., 4, 94, 189n, 195, 197, 198, 199, 214, 267, 296, 299, 337
Adorno, T. W., 366, 373, 390, 393, 402, 404
Aichhorn, A., 28
Alexander, F., xiii, 28, 138n, 190, 192, 200, 202n, 208, 217, 224, 228, 234, 270, 272, 275, 298, 303, 308, 312, 321, 322, 325
Anderson, S., 49
Angel, E., 76
Ardrey, R., 417, 420
Asch, S. E., 387

Bandura, A., 208, 220–222, 224, 306
Baron, S., 29
Bartemeier, L., 64
Bartlett, F., 94, 103, 110–116, 117, 118, 130n–131n, 141
Beach, F. A., 85, 89, 145, 153
Beam, L. A., 148, 150, 153
Bender, L., 25, 28
Benedek, T., 148, 152
Benedict, R., 10, 15, 28, 142, 422–423, 431
Bentley, M., 193
Bergler, E., 157, 168
Bernard, V. W., 355–373, 394, 404
Bernfeld, S., 183
Bernheim, H., 336
Bertalanfy, L. von, 190
Bingham, H. C., 9, 15
Birk, L., 317–319
Bleuler, E., 227
Bloch, J., 115n
Bohr, N., 215
Bowlby, J., 420
Brady, J. P., 324, 326, 346, 351

Breger, L., 324, 326
Breuer, J., 121, 298, 308
Brill, A. A., xiv, 4, 130n, 187
Brückner, G. H., 7, 15
Bühler, K., 182, 216, 224, 300, 308
Burkeland, L. F., 359n
Burrow, T., 287, 290

Caldwell, J. M., 23, 28, 168
Campbell, C. M., 28, 44
Cannon, W., 189
Caspari, E. W., 79
Cheskin, L., 53
Clark, K., 418
Conradi, E., 6, 15
Coser, L. A., 404, 415
Craig, W., 6–7, 15
Cumming, E., 357, 373
Cumming, J., 357, 373
Cutler, M., 65, 70

Dahlberg, C. C., 327, 335
Darwin, C., 5, 369
Davis, K., 11, 16, 142
de Tocqueville, A., 408, 415
Deutsch, H., 241, 244, 250
Deutsch, M., 402, 405
Dewey, J., 193, 234
Dichter, E., 51
Dickinson, R. L., 145, 147–148, 150, 152, 153, 244, 250
Dittman, A. T., 326
Dollard, J. C., 224
Dubois, P., 336
Duhl, L. J., 260, 263, 360, 373
Dunbar, F., 190

Edel, L., 260, 263
Eichmann, A., 407
Einstein, A., 385, 431

Eisenberg, L., 418, 431
Eliot, T. S., 282
Ellenberger, H. F., 76
Engel, G. L., 190, 260, 263
Engels, F., 115n
Erickson, M. H., 97, 117, 125, 141, 190, 230
Erikson, E. H., 50, 71, 76, 242, 250
Estes, W. K., 219, 224
Eysenck, H. J., 221, 306, 312–313, 325

Feather, B. W., 346, 351
Feldman, M. P., 317, 325
Fenichel, O., 130–132, 142, 160, 164, 165, 168
Ferenczi, S., 44, 94, 266, 271, 328–329
Fiedler, F. E., 197, 198, 208, 297, 308
Fielding, W. J., 44
Fitts, W. T., 67, 70
Ford, C. S., 85, 89, 145, 153
Forel, A., 5, 15
Frank, J. D., 202, 208, 321, 325
Freedman, B., 141
Freedman, L. Z., 260, 263
French, T. M., 138n, 190, 312, 322, 325
Frenkel-Brunswik, E., 366, 390, 394
Freud, A., 117, 181, 184, 185, 189
Freud, S., 16, 44, 89, 117, 118, 141, 153, 168, 178, 185, 209, 224, 250, 275, 290, 308, 350, 431 (See also Index of Subjects)
Friedan, B., 237, 250
Friesen, S. R., 68, 70
Fromm, E., 16, 36, 44, 50, 109, 118, 138n, 189, 196, 197, 214, 245n, 249, 296, 391, 394, 430, 432
Fromm-Reichmann, F., 25, 28, 102n, 118, 191, 289n, 293

Galanter, E., 179
Galileo, 369, 370
Gandhi, M. K., 384
Gardner, J., 424
Gelder, M. G., 324, 326, 346, 351
Gesell, A., 10, 15
Gill, M., 190
Gitelson, M., 234
Glasser, W., 341

Glover, E., 209
Grant, G. L., 8
Grinker, R. R., 28, 117, 190, 193, 209, 226
Guthrie, E. R., 211

Halliday, J. L., 17–18, 29
Hamilton, G. V., 15
Hampson, J. G., 80, 82, 89, 249, 250
Hampson, J. L., 80, 82, 89, 249, 250
Hand, W., 30–31, 44
Harpole, B. P., 68, 70
Hartmann, H., 181–182, 185, 189, 230
Hawthorne, N., 294–295
Hegel, G., 127
Heine, R. W., 197, 209, 297, 308
Hilgard, E. R., 210, 211, 216, 224
Hobbes, T., 130, 417
Hoch, P., 27, 29
Hollingshead, A. B., 188, 194, 259, 263
Horney, K., xiv, 16, 94, 104, 111, 116–117, 118, 138n, 144, 153, 181, 189, 196, 197, 198, 199, 214, 267, 293, 296, 299
Housman, A. E., 35, 44
Hull, C. L., 211, 216, 310, 339

Ibsen, H., 109, 249

Jackson, D. D., 260, 263
Jacobson, E., 177, 178
James, W., 380, 414
Janet, P., 336
Janis, I. L., 173n
Jekels, L., 130n, 141
Jelliffe, S. E., 187
Jenkins, T. N., 14
Jenner, E., 356, 358
Johnson, V. E., 77, 144n, 152n, 245, 250, 315, 319–321, 325, 327, 334, 335
Jones, E., 120, 138–139, 141, 155, 187, 196, 209, 279, 284, 286, 290, 335
Jung, C. G., 4, 23, 29, 123, 168, 195, 197, 198, 214, 296, 299, 300, 331, 337

Kaplan, W. K., 201, 209, 275, 303, 308
Kardiner, A., xiv, 10, 15, 16, 29, 94, 117, 136n–137n, 138n, 142, 189, 190, 196

Karpman, B., 331
Kasanin, J., 28, 29
Kasper, J., 368
Kaufman, L., 44
Kaufman, M. R., 44
Kelly, G. L., 153
Kelly, W. D., 68, 70
Kempf, E. J., 9, 15
Kennedy, J. F., 56, 409, 416
King, M. L., 384
Kinsey, A. C., 29, 87, 145, 153
Klein, D. B., 206, 209, 306, 308
Klein, M., 337, 340
Klein, M. H., 325, 326
Kluckhohn, F., 257, 263
Knight, R. P., 166, 168, 188, 194, 261, 263
Koestler, A., 414
Kohler, W., 216, 300
Komarovsky, M., 250
Krasner, L., 202, 209, 224, 275, 303, 308, 317, 325
Kreighbaum, H., 373
Kubie, L. S., xiv, 142, 190, 255, 262, 263, 264
Kuo, Z. Y., 8, 15

Landis, C., 145, 148, 153
Laplace, P., 136
Lazarus, A. A., 346, 351
Leblond, C. P., 7, 15
Leone, N. C., 356n
Leopold, R. L., 260, 263
Levine, S., 260, 264
Levy, D., 25, 29, 138n, 190
Lewin, B., xiv
Lewin, K., 190, 211, 217, 218, 219, 224
Lewis, O., 373
Liddell, H. S., 173, 177, 178, 189, 190, 222, 314, 322
Lidz, T., 260, 264
Lindner, R. M., 400, 404
Linton, R., 9, 10, 15, 40–41, 44, 423n, 431
Litin, E. M., 68
Locke, J., 116
Longfellow, H. W., 76
Lorand, S., 144, 153

Lorenz, K., 417
Luria, A. R., 97, 113, 117, 123–125, 140, 141

MacCulloch, M. I., 317, 325
Malinowski, B., 10, 15
Mandell, A. J., 260, 264
Mandler, G., 201, 209, 275, 303, 308
Margolin, S., 190
Marks, I. M., 324, 326, 346, 351
Martin, C. E., 29, 153
Marx, K., 115n
Maslow, A. H., 9, 15, 134–135, 142, 250
Masserman, J., 190, 222, 260, 264, 274, 314, 322
Masters, E. L., 49
Masters, W. H., 77, 144n, 152n, 245, 250, 315, 319–321, 325, 327, 334, 335
May, R., 76, 169–170, 178
McCartney, J., 330–331, 335
McDougall, W., 3
McGaugh, J. L., 324, 327
McGill, V. J., 128n, 141
McLuhan, M., 75n, 76
Mead, M., 10, 15, 142, 361, 373
Merton, T., 379, 407, 415, 424, 432
Mesmer, F., 336
Métraux, R., 361, 373
Miller, G. A., 179
Miller, J., 190
Miller, N. E., 224
Miller, W. L., 169n
Miller, W. R., 23, 29, 168
Minuchin, S., 257, 264
Mirsky, A., 190
Money, J., 81–82, 89
Morgan, C. L., 8, 15
Moriarity, J. D., 188, 194
Morris, D., 417
Mullahy, P., 209
Munroe, R. L., 209
Mussolini, B., 396
Myerson, A., 23, 29, 168

Noble, G. K., 6, 15
Novikoff, A. B., 29
Nunberg, H., xiv

Olds, J., 84, 89
Opler, M. K., 82, 89, 248, 250
Osborn, F., 374, 387
Osborn, R., 130, 141
Osgood, C., 391, 394
Ottenberg, P., 355–373, 394, 404

Packard, V., 51, 60
Parloff, M. B., 326
Pattie, F. A., 7, 15
Pavlov, I., 222, 310, 312, 314, 322, 339
Peale, N. V., 169n
Perloff, W. H., 89, 148, 153
Peterson, E., 250
Piers, G., 182, 185
Pomeroy, W. B., 29, 153
Pribram, K. H., 179
Pumpian–Mindlin, E., 17–29, 168, 173, 178
Putnam, J., 187

Rachlin, H. L., 27, 29
Radford, E., 44
Radford, M. A., 44
Rado, S., xiv, 81, 89, 94, 138n, 170, 171, 178, 189, 196, 214
Rank, O., 195, 197, 198, 214, 296, 299, 300
Rapaport, D., 230
Rapaport, J., 141
Ravdin, I. S., 67, 70
Redlich, F. C., 188, 194, 259, 263
Reich, C., 56n, 431, 432
Reich, W., 94, 117, 138, 142, 154, 155–156, 165, 168, 181, 185, 189, 268, 329–330, 335
Renneker, R., 65, 70
Reston, J., 432
Rhoads, J. M., 346, 351
Ribble, M., 190
Riesman, D., 50, 53, 60
Riggs, A., 171, 178
Rogers, C., 205, 339, 351
Rogow, A. A., 260, 264
Róheim, G., 37–39, 45
Rokeach, M., 399, 400, 404
Romanes, G. J., 5
Romm, M., 250
Roosevelt, E., 393

Rosen, J. N., 190, 300, 309
Roszak, T., 342, 351
Rousseau, J. J., 130n, 417
Rubenstein, B. B., 148, 152
Rubinstein, S. L., 141, 142

Salzinger, K., 209, 275
Sapir, E., 10, 15
Saul, L. J., 45
Sayer, G., 269
Schelling, T. C., 386, 387
Schilder, P., 24, 29, 138n, 190
Schneider, E. V., 404
Schneirla, T. C., 15
Schweitzer, A., 393
Scotch, N. A., 260, 264
Scott, W. E., 6, 15
Selesnick, S., 234
Selsam, H., 142
Shakow, D., 177, 178
Shannon, C. E., 190
Sheard, N. M., 7, 15
Sherfey, M. J., 244, 250
Shimkin, M. B., 356n
Shoben, E. J., 200, 209, 224
Singer, M. T., 260, 264
Skinner, B. F., 211, 216, 219, 224, 310, 312, 314, 339
Smith, E. R., 29
Spectorsky, A. C., 52, 60
Spiegel, J. P., 28, 117, 190, 193, 259, 264
Spitz, R., 190
Stagner, R., 384, 387
Stekel, W., 288, 331
Stoffler, E. H., 57, 60
Strachey, J., 200–201, 209, 270
Strupp, H. H., 200, 209, 257, 264
Sullivan, H. S., 16, 138n, 182, 189, 191, 196, 197, 198, 199, 214, 267, 296, 300

Taylor, G. R., 89
Thomas, D., 75n
Thompson, C., xiv, 117, 209, 243, 250
Thorndike, E. L., 211
Tolman, E. C., 211
Twain, M., 49

Ullman, L. P., 317, 325

van Bark, B., 29
Van Clute, W., 141
Veblen, T., 52
Virchow, R., 17

Warden, C. J., 14
Warner, L. H., 14
Weaver, W., 177n, 190, 412–413
Weinstein, E. A., 260, 264
Welch, L., 128n, 141
Weston, R., 64
White, W. A., 4, 187, 418
Whitehead, A. N., 185
Whitehorn, 294
Whyte, W. F., 60
Whyte, W. H., Jr., 50, 60
Wiener, N., 190

Wiesner, B. P., 7, 15
Wilmer, H., 68
Wittels, F., 155, 158, 159, 168
Wolberg, L. R., 29, 190, 325
Wolfe, W. B., 333
Wolpe, J., 221, 306, 307, 309, 315–317,
    325, 339, 351
Wortis, J., 94, 103, 110, 111, 117, 141
Wundt, W. M., 123
Wylie, E., 51
Wynne, L. C., 260, 264

Yerkes, R. M., 216, 225, 300
Young, J. Z., 178

Zilboorg, A., 215n, 225
Zilboorg, G., xiv, 23, 24, 29, 142, 168
Zuckerman, S., 15

INDEX OF SUBJECTS

Abortion, 78, 421
Abreaction, 103, 199–200, 297–298, 341
Acculturation, 83, 183, 382, 420
Addiction, 158, 159
Affective complexes, 113, 125, 140
Aggression, 9, 134–136, 245–246, 374–375, 382–383, 406, 407, 414, 417, 418, 422, 423, 426
Alaska Mental Health Bill, 356, 359, 361, 368
American Academy of Psychoanalysis, 344
American Dental Association, 356
American Naturopathic Association, 364
American Psychiatric Association, 194, 349
American Psychoanalytic Association, 188, 196, 230, 271–272, 344
Anal erogenicity, 83, 84
"Anatomy is fate" theory, 137, 240, 241–243
Anticathexis, 174, 175, 177, 178
Anti-intellectualism, 342–343
Anti-scientific attitude, 361–363
Anxiety
  crisis of middle age and, 74
  as defense mechanism, 138
  existential, 74
  in hysteric, 164
  increase in occurrence of, 99
  physical manifestations of, 111
  of psychotherapist, 282–283, 286–287
  reformulation of concept of, 180, 189
  worry and, 169–173, 175, 176
Authoritarianism, 366, 390, 401–402
Automation, effects of, 51–60

Aversion therapy, 315, 317–319, 339

Behavior, human, see Human behavior
Behavior, sexual, "normal" vs. "deviant," 77–89
Behavior therapies, 128n, 220–223, 306–307, 310–326, 339, 340, 346
Betsileo culture, 41, 136n–137n
Biofeedback, xiii, 340, 343
Bisexuality, 79, 81
Blacks, urban violence and, 406–415
Black women, family life and, 239
British Royal Society, 356

California Community Mental Health Services Act, 360, 361
Cancer, psychological impact of, on patient and family, 61–70
Capitalism, 425–428
Castration anxiety, 164, 330, 366, 403, 412
Cathexis, 174, 177, 178, 179, 252
Catholic Church, 32, 78, 359
Change, group resistance to, 357–373, 423, 424, 430
Character structure, 108, 127, 138
Clitoral orgasm, 143–153, 241n, 244–245
Cognitive learning, 211, 305, 323
Communications theory, 185, 190, 230
Communism, 400–401
Community, interaction of, with individual and family, 46–60
Community psychiatry, 347–348, 350
Compensation, 98
Compulsion neurosis, 158
Conditioning
  in aversion therapy, 317–319
  in dynamic psychotherapy, 323
Conflict, 97–98, 125, 128, 406–407

457

Conformity, 49–51, 53, 55, 381
Conjoint marital therapy, 258, 270
Constitutional factors in mental disorders, 17, 25–28
Couch, use of, in psychoanalysis, 100–101, 191–192, 257, 271, 338
Counterconditioning techniques, 220–223, 306, 315–316
Countertransference, 194, 204, 291–292, 327, 328, 331–332, 334
Cryptogenic, as designation of mental illness, 24
Cybernetics, 185, 190

Death, fear of, 61–62
Decompensation, 75–76
Defensive mechanisms, 64–65, 138
Denial, 64–65, 173, 376, 377, 398
Dependency attitudes and superstition, 34
Desegregation, opposition to, 357, 360, 363, 368–369
Desensitization, 316, 319–320, 339, 346
Destination sickness, 52
Developmental crises, 71
"Deviant" sexual behavior, 77–89
Dialectical materialism, psychoanalysis and, 119–142
Dianetics, 340–341
Didactic analysis, 261, 266, 273–274
Direct analysis, 300–301
Directive psychotherapy, 206
Disease, etiology of, 17–18
Dreams, 97, 122n–123n, 128, 163–164, 172, 204
Drugs, therapeutic use of, 296, 298, 307–308, 341, 346–347
Dynamic psychotherapy
and behavior therapy, 310–326, 346
origins of, 336–337

Eastern Pennsylvania Psychiatric Institute, 325
Ego, 24, 86, 172–173, 175, 177, 178, 180, 183
Ego psychology, 83, 96, 138, 180–185, 189, 195, 230
Ego-reparative strivings, 54–56

Emotional maturity and internationism, 391–393
Emotions and ideas, 112–117
Encounter groups, 56n
Endogenous, as designation of mental illness, 24
Entelechy, 129–130, 130n–131n, 138
Environment
and "human nature," 14
and individual, 18–28
Envy, and superstition, 34–35, 43–44
Ethnocentric perception, 377–378, 390
Evil eye superstition, 37–39
Existential anxiety, 74
Expectancy, as factor in psychotherapy, 321–322
Extragenital orgasm, 87, 150–151
Extramarital sex, 78–79, 85
Extremism, political, 395–405

Family
cancer patient and, 61–70
cultural transmission through, 52–55
interaction of, with individual and community, 46–60
isolation of, 48–49
matrileneal, 236
move to suburbs by, 52, 54–55
personality development within, 139–140
therapy, 258–270
and trend toward conformity, 49–50, 55
urban lower class, 56–59
Fantasies, hysteric orality and, 163–164
Fascist ideology, 400–401
Fear, 169–170, 176–177, 375–376, 407
Feeling–oriented therapies, 339–340
Femininity, 81–82, 96, 108–109, 137, 235–250
Feral children, 10–12
Fetishism, 87, 222
Field theory, 185, 189, 230, 271
Fixation, 156–158, 165–168
Fluoridation, opposition to, 356, 358, 359, 360, 361, 368
Free association, 97, 120, 121–125, 128, 253, 265–275

Free will, 127
Frequency of psychoanalytic visits, 101, 192, 217, 257–258, 338, 344–345
Freud, S. (*See also* Index of Names)
  aggression theories of, 134–136, 406, 417, 426
  anxiety theories of, 164, 169, 170, 180, 189
  application of individual theory to groups by, 115
  criticism of, 93–117
  contemporary reaction to, 186, 227, 229, 369
  definition of psychoanalysis by, 120
  dream theories of, 122n–123n
  on fear of death, 61
  on feminine psychology, 108–109, 137, 143, 144, 151, 235, 237, 240–241, 243, 246, 247–248
  and Ferenczi, 266, 271, 328–329
  free association developed by, 121–122, 125, 266–267, 268
  genital erogenicity theory of, 144–146
  God concept of, 282
  hysteria studies of, 154–157, 298
  instinct theories of, 4, 5, 10, 12–13, 14, 96, 111, 128–138
  on the intellect, 350
  libido theory of, 83, 166–167, 214, 330, 341
  on mourning, 174–175
  neurosis theory of, 103, 105–106, 336–337
  opposition to, 93, 368–369
  psychoanalytic technique developed by, 102–110, 120, 125–126, 191–193, 198, 212, 217, 222, 230, 231, 254–255, 285, 288, 301, 336–338, 344–345
  psychoanalytic theory of, 95–102, 120–139, 180–181, 186, 195–200, 211, 212, 221, 228, 229, 251–254, 293, 299, 310, 313, 336–337, 341, 418
  rejection of, by Marxists, 93–94
  sexual behavior theories of, 77, 81, 83–84, 133–134
  on the unconscious, 229, 385
Frigidity, 143, 144, 148–149, 315, 319–320
Frustration, 218

Game theory, 310
Gender role, 82, 248–250
General systems theory, see Systems theory
Genetic factors in metal disorder, 17, 25–28
Genital erogenicity, 144–146
Gestalt theory, 211, 215–216, 340
Ghettos, causes of violence in, 408–414
God complex of psychotherapists, 279–290
Gratification, 81
Grief, 174, 176
Group opposition to health programs, 355–373
Group therapy, 259, 270, 271, 340, 345

Health programs, group opposition to, 355–373
Heredity
  factors in mental disorder, 25–28
  and "human nature," 14
Historical materialism, 127
Homosexuality
  aversion therapy for, 315, 317–319
  in different societies, 20, 79, 86, 87
  normal vs. pathological, 20
  studies of, 7, 10, 163–164
Hope, cancer patients and, 65–66
Hostility, and superstition, 33, 34, 37, 43
Human behavior
  importance of symbolic abstraction in, 306–307
  role of instinct in, 3–14
  stimulus-response theory of, 211, 313–314
  unified theory of, xvi, 208, 231, 234
"Human nature"
  as biologically determined, 10–15
  changeability of, 99, 417–418
  dialectical conception of, 132, 134
  and war, 374–375

Hypnosis, xiii, 121, 298, 311
Hypnotherapy, 190, 311
Hysteria
and abreaction, 298
decrease in occurrence of, 99
significance of, in development of psychoanalysis, 154, 156–157
Hysterical personality, orality in, 154–168

Id, 24, 86, 180, 183
Ideas and emotions, 112–117
Identification, 182–183, 201, 304, 305, 323, 401
Impotence, 148–150, 315, 319–320
Incest, 331, 334
Individual
interaction of, with family and community, 46–60
interrelationship of, with total environment, 18–28
Information theory, 310, 311
Inner conflict, 97–98, 125, 128, 406–407
Insight, 103, 104, 110, 198–199, 203–204, 211, 212, 213–216, 269, 298–300, 301, 338
Instinct
confusion regarding meaning of, 3–5
Freudian view of, 4, 5, 10, 12–13, 14, 96, 111, 128–138
role of, in human behavior, 3–14
scientific definitions of, 4
vs. learned behavior, 6–14
Institute for Behavioral Research, 190
Instrumental aggression, 407
International Psychoanalytic Association, 230
Internationalism, 388–394
Isolation, 48–49, 54, 376, 377

Jews, 78, 359, 368–369
Juvenile delinquency, 57, 59

Knocking on wood superstition, 31–32, 34, 38, 39, 43–44
Kraepelinian psychiatry, 27n, 187

Latency period of sexual development, 83, 84–85
Lay analysis, 232–233
Learning process, psychoanalysis as, 200–208
Learning theories, and psychoanalytic therapy, 210–225
Learning theory, 310
Left-wing ideology, 395–405
Lemberg Center for the Study of Violence, 411, 415
Libido theory, 13, 83, 166–167, 181, 211, 214, 228, 230, 330, 341
Life-space, threats to, 367, 369
Life-system, of patient, 258, 259

Magic, superstition and, 39–43
Manic–depressive psychosis, 25, 26–27, 158
Marquesan society, 20, 86
Marxist theory, 93, 115, 400, 401
Masculinity, 81–82
Masochism, 241, 245–247
Masturbation, 10, 84, 144, 330
Matrilineal families, 236
Mechanistic materialism, 129–131, 130n–131n, 138
Medical psychotherapy, as new specialty, 263
Men
crisis of middle age in, 74
orgasm in, 146–147, 150
Menopause, 72, 74, 76, 137, 241
Menstruation, 241, 246–247
Mental disorder
environmental stress and, 18–23
differentiation among types of, 26–28
genetic factors in, 17, 25–28
integrative conception of, 17–29
Mental health
definition of, 21
delivery systems, 347–349
Middle age, crisis of, 71–76
Monogamy, 85
Mourning, 174–176

National Association of Science Writers, 361

Nationalism, 384, 388–394, 428–429

Negative transference, 125–126, 271, 289, 291, 301–302

Negroes, urban violence and, 406–415

Negro women, family life and, 239

Neurosis
basic concepts of, 154–155, 157
as changeable state of behavior, 23, 165–166
conflict and, 97–98, 222–223
Freud's theory of cause of, 103, 105–106, 336–337
vs. psychosis, 22–23

New York Psychoanalytic Institute, xiv

Nondirective therapy, 205–206, 305–306

Nonverbal reactions of therapists, 193, 202, 216–217, 268, 292, 302–303

Nonviolence, 384–385

Nymphomania, 20

Obsessional neurotic, and superstition, 42–43

Obsessive compulsive disorders, increase in occurrence of, 99

Objectives of therapy, 197, 199–200, 296–297, 322

Oedipus complex
current research on, 134
Freud's theory of, 13, 105–107, 129, 247
human growth through resolution of, 389
orality in hysterical personality and, 160, 163, 165, 167
superstition and, 33, 41

Operant conditioning, 220, 305, 306, 323, 339

Open-system theory, see Systems theory

Orality, in hysterical personality, 154–168

Orgasm
extragenital, 150–151
female, 143–153, 238–239, 244–245, 246
impotence in, 148–150
male, 146–147, 150

Overcompensation, 75

Passive dependency, 49, 108–109, 214, 299, 399

Passivity, 9, 241, 245–247

Penis envy, 96, 100, 108–109, 137, 237, 241, 243–245

Personality structure, 18–23, 108

Pharmacotherapy, xiii, 296, 298, 307–308, 341, 346–347

Political extremism, 395–405

Politically radical patient, analysis of, 109–110

Polygamy, 85

Polymorphous-perverse sexual behavior, 83, 84, 88

Positive transference, 125, 291, 301–302, 304, 322, 328, 333

Primal scream therapy, 341

Projection, 98, 398

Protestant Ethic, 51, 60

Psychiatrists, psychoanalytically trained, 187, 231, 259, 261, 344

Psychiatry
alienation of, from psychoanalysis, 186, 232
clinical, 187
community, 347–348, 350
dynamic, 231
and the future of man, 416–432
Kraepelinian, 187
psychoanalysis and, 186–194

Psychoanalysis (See also Psychotherapy)
analyst's active participation in, 102, 192–193, 257
changes in basic doctrine of, 138–141
common denominators among schools of, xiv-xv, 206–208, 213–215, 223
critical crossroad in, 226–234
development of, 121–128
and dialectical materialism, 119–141
differences among schools of, 184–185, 195–199, 287
and financial sacrifice, 218, 258
frequency of visits in, 101, 192, 217, 257, 338, 344–345
Freud's definition of, 120
and "instinct," 13
as an investigative tool, 229, 253–254

and Marxist theory, 93–94, 115
and normal mental processes, 177
progressive, 94, 98–102, 104–110,
    126, 140–141
and psychiatric practice, 186–194
as a technique of therapy, 102–110,
    231–233, 253, 254–257
as a theory of human behavior, 94–
    102, 229–231, 253–254
theory and practice of, 93–117, 120,
    251–264
therapeutic goals of, 272–273
use of couch in, 100–101, 191–192,
    257, 271, 338
Psychoanalytic institutes, 186–187,
    227–228, 261, 273–274
Psychoanalytic journals, 186
Psychoanalytic societies, 186
Psychoanalytic therapy
as an educational process, 195–209
and theories of learning, 210–225
Psychoanalytically trained psychia-
    trists, 187, 231, 259, 261, 344
Psychobiological unity, 111, 132–133
Psychopathic personality, 18, 25, 26–
    27, 158
Psychosexual neutrality, 80
Psychosis
as changeable state of behavior, 23,
    165–166
differentiation among types of,
    27–28
interrelationship of individual to en-
    vironment and, 18
vs. neurosis, 22–23
Psychosomatic disorders
environmental stress and, 26–27
increase in occurrence of, 99
Psychosomatic medicine, 136, 190
Psychotherapeutic approaches, dif-
    ferences among, 188, 207
Psychotherapeutic techniques
aversion therapy, 315, 317–319, 339
behavior therapy, 128n, 220–223,
    306–307, 310–326, 339, 340, 346
conjoint marital therapy, 258, 270
dynamic psychotherapy, 310–326,
    336–337, 346
family therapy, 258, 270

feeling-oriented therapies, 339–340
group therapy, 259, 270, 271, 340,
    345
hypnotherapy, 190, 311
operant conditioning, 220, 305, 306,
    323, 339
reality therapy, 341
reciprocal inhibition, 306, 307, 315–
    317, 339
reward-punishment, 211–212, 217–
    220, 339
technological, 343
Psychotherapy (See also Psychoanalysis)
changing trends in, 336–354
common denominators among dif-
    ferent schools of 297, 298–300
differences among schools of, 296–
    297, 298–300
directive, 206
dynamic, 187, 188, 190, 336–337
feeling of superiority as occupational
    hazard in, 279–290, 294
goals of, 197, 199–200, 296–297, 322
as a learning process, 301–306, 338–
    339
main factors in, 305
medical, as new specialty, 263
nature of, 296–309
nondirective, 205–206
patient–therapist relationship in,
    291–295, 305–306
psychoanalytic, 187
role of patient expectancy in, 321–
    322
sexual acting–out in, 327–335
short–term techniques in, 343–345
Puberty, 83–85
Punishment, learning and, 219–220

Radical patients, analysis of, 109–110
Rapport, between patient and
    therapist, 126, 204–205, 291, 302–
    304
Reaction formation, 98, 398
Reality principle, 211
Reality testing, 105, 305, 323
Reality therapy, 341
Reciprocal inhibition technique, 306,
    307, 315–317, 339

Regression, 157, 190
Religion
  coexistence of opposing theologies,
    386
  and ego-reparative strivings, 55
  and sexual behavior, 78–79
  and superstition, 31–33, 42–43
Repetition–compulsion, 106, 252
Repression, 98, 122, 125, 128, 129,
  190, 265, 337, 398
Resistance, 103, 120, 125, 128, 129,
  190, 212–213, 265
Reward–punishment techniques, 211–
  212, 217–220, 339
Right-wing ideology, 395–405
Rivalry, superstition and, 34–36, 41–42
Rogerian therapy, 205–206
Roman Catholic Church, 32, 78, 359

Schizophrenia, 24–25, 27–28, 158–
  159, 260, 289, 300–301, 307
Science, public attitude toward, 361–
  363
Scientology, 341
Sensitivity training, 340
Separation loss, 73
Sexual acting-out in therapy, 327–335
Sexual behavior
  "normal" vs. "deviant," 77–89
  polymorphous-perverse, 83, 84, 88
Sexual disorders, Masters and Johnson
  technique for treatment of, 319–320
Sexuality
  biological and cultural factors, 79–
    83, 133–134
  developmental factors, 83–85
  female, 143–153
  healthy vs. neurotic, 88–89
Sibling rivalry, 41, 44
Silence, rule of, 102n
Slums, effect of, on individuals, 56–59
Social fragmentation, 48, 54
Society
  and "human nature," 12
  value-systems of, 86–87, 419
Socioeconomic forces
  and aggression, 136
  and character structure, 114–116,
    259–260

Soviet Union, 93, 369, 396
Stimulus-response theories of human
  behavior, 211, 313–314
Stress, 18–23, 63
Success
  as criterion of adequacy, 53
  failure to achieve, 72
  fear of, and superstition, 36
Suggestion, 316, 323
Suicide, cancer patients and, 68
Superego, 24, 86, 180, 241, 247–248,
  423
Superiority feelings of psycho-
  therapists, 279–290, 294
Superstition, role of, in contemporary
  life, 30–45
Synergy, 422, 425, 428
Systems theory, xiv, 185, 190, 230, 252,
  257, 261, 310, 311, 419–423

Tanala culture, 20, 40–41, 86, 136n–
  137n
Technological therapeutic techniques,
  343
Termination of therapy, 255, 305
Toda culture of India, 85
Transference
  as basic assumption of psycho-
    analytic therapy, 98, 104, 105, 120,
    125–126, 128, 204, 255, 256, 268,
    304, 328
  in dyadic vs. group therapy, 259
  and expectancy of patient, 202,
    321–322
  and learning process, 201, 304
  negative, 125–126, 271, 289, 291,
    301–302
  positive, 125, 291, 301–302, 304,
    322, 328, 333
  reality factors involved in, 289, 291,
    301–302
  sexual acting-out of, 327, 330, 331–
    332
  and superiority feelings of therapist,
    280–281, 289
  and termination of analysis, 271
  vs. "rapport," 291, 302, 304
Trieb, 12–13
Trobriand society, 20, 39, 86

Ultranationalism, 390–391
Unconscious, 97, 120, 125, 128, 268,
    272, 275, 387, 395–396
U.S. Public Health Service, 356
Urban lower class, 56–59
Urban violence, 406–415

Vaccination, opposition to, 356, 358,
    361, 368
Vaginal orgasm, 143–153, 241n
Value-system
    of parents, 183
    of patient, 322
    of society, 86–87, 383, 419
    of therapist, 193, 201–202, 249, 283,
        293, 302, 306, 322
Vietnam War, 410, 412, 413
Violence, 374–387, 406–415, 417

War, 374–387, 407, 414, 424
Water fluoridation, opposition to, 356,
    358, 359, 360, 361, 368

Womb envy, 243
Women
    changing status of, 236–240
    crisis of middle age and, 74
    Freud's psychology of, 108–109,
        137, 143, 144, 151, 235, 237, 240–
        241, 243, 246, 247–248
    orgasm in, 143–153, 238–239, 244–
        245, 246
    sexuality of, 143–153
    therapy for, 108–109
Word association test, 123–125
"Working-through" process, 103, 198,
    203, 212, 216, 256, 301
World War I, 99, 176, 386
World War II, 21, 99, 176, 343, 386
Worry, realistic, 169–179

Zen, 256, 340
Zulu society, 358
Zũni society, 39, 134